Statistics for Social and Behavioral Sciences

Advisors:

S.E. Fienberg
W.J. van der Linden

T0189774

For other titles published in this series, go to
http://www.springer.com/series/3463

Haruo Yanai • Kei Takeuchi • Yoshio Takane

Projection Matrices, Generalized Inverse Matrices, and Singular Value Decomposition

Springer

Haruo Yanai
Department of Statistics
St. Luke's College of Nursing
10-1 Akashi-cho Chuo-ku Tokyo
104-0044 Japan
hyanai@slcn.ac.jp

Kei Takeuchi
2-34-4 Terabun Kamakurashi
Kanagawa-ken
247-0064 Japan
kei.takeuchi@wind.ocn.ne.jp

Yoshio Takane
Department of Psychology
McGill University
1205 Dr. Penfield Avenue
Montreal Québec
H3A 1B1 Canada
takane@psych.mcgill.ca

ISBN 978-1-4614-2859-6 ISBN 978-1-4419-9887-3 (eBook)
DOI 10.1007/978-1-4419-9887-3
Springer New York Dordrecht Heidelberg London

Printed on acid-free paper

Springer is part of Springer Science+Business Media (www.springer.com)

Preface

All three authors of the present book have long-standing experience in teaching graduate courses in multivariate analysis (MVA). These experiences have taught us that aside from distribution theory, projections and the singular value decomposition (SVD) are the two most important concepts for understanding the basic mechanism of MVA. The former underlies the least squares (LS) estimation in regression analysis, which is essentially a projection of one subspace onto another, and the latter underlies principal component analysis (PCA), which seeks to find a subspace that captures the largest variability in the original space. Other techniques may be considered some combination of the two.

This book is about projections and SVD. A thorough discussion of generalized inverse (g-inverse) matrices is also given because it is closely related to the former. The book provides systematic and in-depth accounts of these concepts from a unified viewpoint of linear transformations in finite dimensional vector spaces. More specifically, it shows that projection matrices (projectors) and g-inverse matrices can be defined in various ways so that a vector space is decomposed into a direct-sum of (disjoint) subspaces. This book gives analogous decompositions of matrices and discusses their possible applications.

This book consists of six chapters. Chapter 1 overviews the basic linear algebra necessary to read this book. Chapter 2 introduces projection matrices. The projection matrices discussed in this book are general oblique projectors, whereas the more commonly used orthogonal projectors are special cases of these. However, many of the properties that hold for orthogonal projectors also hold for oblique projectors by imposing only modest additional conditions. This is shown in Chapter 3.

Chapter 3 first defines, for an n by m matrix $\boldsymbol{A}$, a linear transformation $\boldsymbol{y} = \boldsymbol{Ax}$ that maps an element $\boldsymbol{x}$ in the m-dimensional Euclidean space E^m onto an element $\boldsymbol{y}$ in the n-dimensional Euclidean space E^n. Let $\mathrm{Sp}(\boldsymbol{A}) = \{\boldsymbol{y}|\boldsymbol{y} = \boldsymbol{Ax}\}$ (the range or column space of $\boldsymbol{A}$) and $\mathrm{Ker}(\boldsymbol{A}) = \{\boldsymbol{x}|\boldsymbol{Ax} = \boldsymbol{0}\}$ (the null space of $\boldsymbol{A}$). Then, there exist an infinite number of the subspaces V and W that satisfy

$$E^n = \mathrm{Sp}(\boldsymbol{A}) \oplus W \text{ and } E^m = V \oplus \mathrm{Ker}(\boldsymbol{A}), \tag{1}$$

where $\oplus$ indicates a direct-sum of two subspaces. Here, the correspondence between V and $\mathrm{Sp}(\boldsymbol{A})$ is one-to-one (the dimensionalities of the two subspaces coincide), and an inverse linear transformation from $\mathrm{Sp}(\boldsymbol{A})$ to V can be uniquely defined. Generalized inverse matrices are simply matrix representations of the inverse transformation with the domain extended to E^n. However, there are infinitely many ways in which the generalization can be made, and thus there are infinitely many corresponding generalized inverses $\boldsymbol{A}^-$ of $\boldsymbol{A}$. Among them, an inverse transformation in which $W = \text{Sp}(\boldsymbol{A})^\perp$ (the ortho-complement subspace of $\text{Sp}(\boldsymbol{A})$) and $V = \text{Ker}(\boldsymbol{A})^\perp = \text{Sp}(\boldsymbol{A}')$ (the ortho-complement subspace of $\text{Ker}(\boldsymbol{A})$), which transforms any vector in W to the zero vector in $\text{Ker}(\boldsymbol{A})$, corresponds to the Moore-Penrose inverse. Chapter 3 also shows a variety of g-inverses that can be formed depending on the choice of V and W, and which portion of $\text{Ker}(\boldsymbol{A})$ vectors in W are mapped into.

Chapter 4 discusses generalized forms of oblique projectors and g-inverse matrices, and gives their explicit representations when V is expressed in terms of matrices.

Chapter 5 decomposes $\text{Sp}(\boldsymbol{A})$ and $\text{Sp}(\boldsymbol{A}') = \text{Ker}(\boldsymbol{A})^\perp$ into sums of mutually orthogonal subspaces, namely

$$\text{Sp}(\boldsymbol{A}) = E_1 \overset{\cdot}{\oplus} E_2 \overset{\cdot}{\oplus} \cdots \overset{\cdot}{\oplus} E_r$$

and

$$\text{Sp}(\boldsymbol{A}') = F_1 \overset{\cdot}{\oplus} F_2 \overset{\cdot}{\oplus} \cdots \overset{\cdot}{\oplus} F_r,$$

where $\overset{\cdot}{\oplus}$ indicates an orthogonal direct-sum. It will be shown that E_j can be mapped into F_j by $\boldsymbol{y} = \boldsymbol{A}\boldsymbol{x}$ and that F_j can be mapped into E_j by $\boldsymbol{x} = \boldsymbol{A}'\boldsymbol{y}$. The singular value decomposition (SVD) is simply the matrix representation of these transformations.

Chapter 6 demonstrates that the concepts given in the preceding chapters play important roles in applied fields such as numerical computation and multivariate analysis.

Some of the topics in this book may already have been treated by existing textbooks in linear algebra, but many others have been developed only recently, and we believe that the book will be useful for many researchers, practitioners, and students in applied mathematics, statistics, engineering, behaviormetrics, and other fields.

This book requires some basic knowledge of linear algebra, a summary of which is provided in Chapter 1. This, together with some determination on the part of the reader, should be sufficient to understand the rest of the book. The book should also serve as a useful reference on projectors, generalized inverses, and SVD.

In writing this book, we have been heavily influenced by Rao and Mitra's (1971) seminal book on generalized inverses. We owe very much to Professor

C. R. Rao for his many outstanding contributions to the theory of g-inverses and projectors. This book is based on the original Japanese version of the book by Yanai and Takeuchi published by Todai-Shuppankai (University of Tokyo Press) in 1983. This new English edition by the three of us expands the original version with new material.

January 2011

Haruo Yanai
Kei Takeuchi
Yoshio Takane

Contents

Chapter 1

Fundamentals of Linear Algebra

In this chapter, we give basic concepts and theorems of linear algebra that are necessary in subsequent chapters.

1.1 Vectors and Matrices

1.1.1 Vectors

Sets of n real numbers $a_1, a_2, \cdots, a_n$ and $b_1, b_2, \cdots, b_n$, arranged in the following way, are called n-component column vectors:

$$\boldsymbol{a} = \begin{pmatrix} a_1 \\ a_2 \\ \vdots \\ a_n \end{pmatrix}, \quad \boldsymbol{b} = \begin{pmatrix} b_1 \\ b_2 \\ \vdots \\ b_n \end{pmatrix}. \tag{1.1}$$

The real numbers $a_1, a_2, \cdots, a_n$ and $b_1, b_2, \cdots, b_n$ are called elements or components of $\boldsymbol{a}$ and $\boldsymbol{b}$, respectively. These elements arranged horizontally,

$$\boldsymbol{a}' = (a_1, a_2, \cdots, a_n), \quad \boldsymbol{b}' = (b_1, b_2, \cdots, b_n),$$

are called n-component row vectors.

We define the length of the n-component vector $\boldsymbol{a}$ to be

$$||\boldsymbol{a}|| = \sqrt{a_1^2 + a_2^2 + \cdots + a_n^2}. \tag{1.2}$$

This is also called a norm of vector $\boldsymbol{a}$. We also define an inner product between two vectors $\boldsymbol{a}$ and $\boldsymbol{b}$ to be

$$(\boldsymbol{a}, \boldsymbol{b}) = a_1 b_1 + a_2 b_2 + \cdots + a_n b_n. \tag{1.3}$$

The inner product has the following properties:

(i) $||\boldsymbol{a}||^2 = (\boldsymbol{a}, \boldsymbol{a})$,

(ii) $||\boldsymbol{a} + \boldsymbol{b}||^2 = ||\boldsymbol{a}||^2 + ||\boldsymbol{b}||^2 + 2(\boldsymbol{a}, \boldsymbol{b})$,

(iii) $(a\boldsymbol{a}, \boldsymbol{b}) = (\boldsymbol{a}, a\boldsymbol{b}) = a(\boldsymbol{a}, \boldsymbol{b})$, where a is a scalar,

(iv) $||\boldsymbol{a}||^2 = 0 \iff \boldsymbol{a} = \boldsymbol{0}$, where $\iff$ indicates an equivalence (or "if and only if") relationship.

We define the distance between two vectors by

$$d(\boldsymbol{a}, \boldsymbol{b}) = ||\boldsymbol{a} - \boldsymbol{b}||. \tag{1.4}$$

Clearly, $d(\boldsymbol{a}, \boldsymbol{b}) \geq 0$ and

(i) $d(\boldsymbol{a}, \boldsymbol{b}) = 0 \iff \boldsymbol{a} = \boldsymbol{b}$,

(ii) $d(\boldsymbol{a}, \boldsymbol{b}) = d(\boldsymbol{b}, \boldsymbol{a})$,

(iii) $d(\boldsymbol{a}, \boldsymbol{b}) + d(\boldsymbol{b}, \boldsymbol{c}) \geq d(\boldsymbol{a}, \boldsymbol{c})$.

The three properties above are called the metric (or distance) axioms.

Theorem 1.1 *The following properties hold:*

$$(\boldsymbol{a}, \boldsymbol{b})^2 \leq ||\boldsymbol{a}||^2 ||\boldsymbol{b}||^2, \tag{1.5}$$

$$||\boldsymbol{a} + \boldsymbol{b}|| \leq ||\boldsymbol{a}|| + ||\boldsymbol{b}||. \tag{1.6}$$

Proof. (1.5): The following inequality holds for any real number t:

$$||\boldsymbol{a} - t\boldsymbol{b}||^2 = ||\boldsymbol{a}||^2 - 2t(\boldsymbol{a}, \boldsymbol{b}) + t^2 ||\boldsymbol{b}||^2 \geq 0.$$

This implies

$$\text{Discriminant} = (\boldsymbol{a}, \boldsymbol{b})^2 - ||\boldsymbol{a}||^2 ||\boldsymbol{b}||^2 \leq 0,$$

which establishes (1.5).

(1.6): $(||\boldsymbol{a}|| + ||\boldsymbol{b}||)^2 - ||\boldsymbol{a} + \boldsymbol{b}||^2 = 2\{||\boldsymbol{a}|| \cdot ||\boldsymbol{b}|| - (\boldsymbol{a}, \boldsymbol{b})\} \geq 0$, which implies (1.6). Q.E.D.

Inequality (1.5) is called the Cauchy-Schwarz inequality, and (1.6) is called the triangular inequality.

For two n-component vectors $\boldsymbol{a}$ ($\neq \boldsymbol{0}$) and $\boldsymbol{b}$ ($\neq \boldsymbol{0}$), the angle between them can be defined by the following definition.

Definition 1.1 *For two vectors* $\boldsymbol{a}$ *and* $\boldsymbol{b}$*,* θ *defined by*

$$\cos\theta = \frac{(\boldsymbol{a}, \boldsymbol{b})}{||\boldsymbol{a}|| \cdot ||\boldsymbol{b}||} \tag{1.7}$$

is called the angle between $\boldsymbol{a}$ *and* $\boldsymbol{b}$*.*

1.1.2 Matrices

We call nm real numbers arranged in the following form a matrix:

$$\boldsymbol{A} = \begin{bmatrix} a_{11} & a_{12} & \cdots & a_{1m} \\ a_{21} & a_{22} & \cdots & a_{2m} \\ \vdots & \vdots & \ddots & \vdots \\ a_{n1} & a_{n2} & \cdots & a_{nm} \end{bmatrix}. \tag{1.8}$$

Numbers arranged horizontally are called rows of numbers, while those arranged vertically are called columns of numbers. The matrix $\boldsymbol{A}$ may be regarded as consisting of n row vectors or m column vectors and is generally referred to as an n by m matrix (an $n \times m$ matrix). When $n = m$, the matrix $\boldsymbol{A}$ is called a square matrix. A square matrix of order n with unit diagonal elements and zero off-diagonal elements, namely

$$\boldsymbol{I}_n = \begin{bmatrix} 1 & 0 & \cdots & 0 \\ 0 & 1 & \cdots & 0 \\ \vdots & \vdots & \ddots & \vdots \\ 0 & 0 & \cdots & 1 \end{bmatrix},$$

is called an identity matrix.

Define m n-component vectors as

$$\boldsymbol{a}_1 = \begin{pmatrix} a_{11} \\ a_{21} \\ \vdots \\ a_{n1} \end{pmatrix}, \boldsymbol{a}_2 = \begin{pmatrix} a_{12} \\ a_{22} \\ \vdots \\ a_{n2} \end{pmatrix}, \cdots, \boldsymbol{a}_m = \begin{pmatrix} a_{1m} \\ a_{2m} \\ \vdots \\ a_{nm} \end{pmatrix}.$$

We may represent the m vectors collectively by

$$\boldsymbol{A} = [\boldsymbol{a}_1, \boldsymbol{a}_2, \cdots, \boldsymbol{a}_m]. \tag{1.9}$$

The element of $\boldsymbol{A}$ in the ith row and jth column, denoted as a_{ij}, is often referred to as the (i, j)th element of $\boldsymbol{A}$. The matrix $\boldsymbol{A}$ is sometimes written as $\boldsymbol{A} = [a_{ij}]$. The matrix obtained by interchanging rows and columns of $\boldsymbol{A}$ is called the transposed matrix of $\boldsymbol{A}$ and denoted as $\boldsymbol{A}'$.

Let $\boldsymbol{A} = [a_{ik}]$ and $\boldsymbol{B} = [b_{kj}]$ be n by m and m by p matrices, respectively. Their product, $\boldsymbol{C} = [c_{ij}]$, denoted as

$$\boldsymbol{C} = \boldsymbol{A}\boldsymbol{B}, \tag{1.10}$$

is defined by $c_{ij} = \sum_{k=1}^{m} a_{ik}b_{kj}$. The matrix $\boldsymbol{C}$ is of order n by p. Note that

$$\boldsymbol{A}'\boldsymbol{A} = \boldsymbol{O} \Longleftrightarrow \boldsymbol{A} = \boldsymbol{O}, \tag{1.11}$$

where $\boldsymbol{O}$ is a zero matrix consisting of all zero elements.

Note An n-component column vector $\boldsymbol{a}$ is an n by 1 matrix. Its transpose $\boldsymbol{a}'$ is a 1 by n matrix. The inner product between $\boldsymbol{a}$ and $\boldsymbol{b}$ and their norms can be expressed as

$$(\boldsymbol{a}, \boldsymbol{b}) = \boldsymbol{a}'\boldsymbol{b}, \ ||\boldsymbol{a}||^2 = (\boldsymbol{a}, \boldsymbol{a}) = \boldsymbol{a}'\boldsymbol{a}, \text{ and } ||\boldsymbol{b}||^2 = (\boldsymbol{b}, \boldsymbol{b}) = \boldsymbol{b}'\boldsymbol{b}.$$

Let $\boldsymbol{A} = [a_{ij}]$ be a square matrix of order n. The trace of $\boldsymbol{A}$ is defined as the sum of its diagonal elements. That is,

$$\text{tr}(\boldsymbol{A}) = a_{11} + a_{22} + \cdots + a_{nn}. \tag{1.12}$$

Let c and d be any real numbers, and let $\boldsymbol{A}$ and $\boldsymbol{B}$ be square matrices of the same order. Then the following properties hold:

$$\text{tr}(c\boldsymbol{A} + d\boldsymbol{B}) = c\text{tr}(\boldsymbol{A}) + d\text{tr}(\boldsymbol{B}) \tag{1.13}$$

and

$$\text{tr}(\boldsymbol{A}\boldsymbol{B}) = \text{tr}(\boldsymbol{B}\boldsymbol{A}). \tag{1.14}$$

Furthermore, for $\boldsymbol{A}$ $(n \times m)$ defined in (1.9),

$$||\boldsymbol{a}_1||^2 + ||\boldsymbol{a}_2||^2 + \cdots + ||\boldsymbol{a}_n||^2 = \text{tr}(\boldsymbol{A}'\boldsymbol{A}). \tag{1.15}$$

Clearly,

$$\text{tr}(\boldsymbol{A}'\boldsymbol{A}) = \sum_{i=1}^{n}\sum_{j=1}^{m} a_{ij}^2. \tag{1.16}$$

Thus,

$$\mathrm{tr}(\boldsymbol{A}'\boldsymbol{A}) = 0 \Longleftrightarrow \boldsymbol{A} = \boldsymbol{O}. \tag{1.17}$$

Also, when $\boldsymbol{A}_1'\boldsymbol{A}_1, \boldsymbol{A}_2'\boldsymbol{A}_2, \cdots, \boldsymbol{A}_m'\boldsymbol{A}_m$ are matrices of the same order, we have

$$\mathrm{tr}(\boldsymbol{A}_1'\boldsymbol{A}_1 + \boldsymbol{A}_2'\boldsymbol{A}_2 + \cdots + \boldsymbol{A}_m'\boldsymbol{A}_m) = 0 \Longleftrightarrow \boldsymbol{A}_j = \boldsymbol{O}\ (j = 1, \cdots, m). \tag{1.18}$$

Let $\boldsymbol{A}$ and $\boldsymbol{B}$ be n by m matrices. Then,

$$\mathrm{tr}(\boldsymbol{A}'\boldsymbol{A}) = \sum_{i=1}^{n}\sum_{j=1}^{m} a_{ij}^2,$$

$$\mathrm{tr}(\boldsymbol{B}'\boldsymbol{B}) = \sum_{i=1}^{n}\sum_{j=1}^{m} b_{ij}^2,$$

and

$$\mathrm{tr}(\boldsymbol{A}'\boldsymbol{B}) = \sum_{i=1}^{n}\sum_{j=1}^{m} a_{ij}b_{ij},$$

and Theorem 1.1 can be extended as follows.

Corollary 1

$$\mathrm{tr}(\boldsymbol{A}'\boldsymbol{B}) \leq \sqrt{\mathrm{tr}(\boldsymbol{A}'\boldsymbol{A})\mathrm{tr}(\boldsymbol{B}'\boldsymbol{B})} \tag{1.19}$$

and

$$\sqrt{\mathrm{tr}(\boldsymbol{A}+\boldsymbol{B})'(\boldsymbol{A}+\boldsymbol{B})} \leq \sqrt{\mathrm{tr}(\boldsymbol{A}'\boldsymbol{A})} + \sqrt{\mathrm{tr}(\boldsymbol{B}'\boldsymbol{B})}. \tag{1.20}$$

Inequality (1.19) is a generalized form of the Cauchy-Schwarz inequality.

The definition of a norm in (1.2) can be generalized as follows. Let $\boldsymbol{M}$ be a nonnegative-definite matrix (refer to the definition of a nonnegative-definite matrix immediately before Theorem 1.12 in Section 1.4) of order n. Then,

$$||\boldsymbol{a}||_M^2 = \boldsymbol{a}'\boldsymbol{M}\boldsymbol{a}. \tag{1.21}$$

Furthermore, if the inner product between $\boldsymbol{a}$ and $\boldsymbol{b}$ is defined by

$$(\boldsymbol{a}, \boldsymbol{b})_M = \boldsymbol{a}'\boldsymbol{M}\boldsymbol{b}, \tag{1.22}$$

the following two corollaries hold.

Corollary 2

$$(\boldsymbol{a}, \boldsymbol{b})_M \leq ||\boldsymbol{a}||_M ||\boldsymbol{b}||_M. \tag{1.23}$$

Corollary 1 can further be generalized as follows.

Corollary 3

$$\mathrm{tr}(\boldsymbol{A}'\boldsymbol{M}\boldsymbol{B}) \leq \sqrt{\mathrm{tr}(\boldsymbol{A}'\boldsymbol{M}\boldsymbol{A})\mathrm{tr}(\boldsymbol{B}'\boldsymbol{M}\boldsymbol{B})} \tag{1.24}$$

and

$$\sqrt{\mathrm{tr}\{(\boldsymbol{A}+\boldsymbol{B})'\boldsymbol{M}(\boldsymbol{A}+\boldsymbol{B})\}} \leq \sqrt{\mathrm{tr}(\boldsymbol{A}'\boldsymbol{M}\boldsymbol{A})} + \sqrt{\mathrm{tr}(\boldsymbol{B}'\boldsymbol{M}\boldsymbol{B})}. \tag{1.25}$$

In addition, (1.15) can be generalized as

$$||\boldsymbol{a}_1||_M^2 + ||\boldsymbol{a}_2||_M^2 + \cdots + ||\boldsymbol{a}_m||_M^2 = \mathrm{tr}(\boldsymbol{A}'\boldsymbol{M}\boldsymbol{A}). \tag{1.26}$$

1.2 Vector Spaces and Subspaces

For m n-component vectors $\boldsymbol{a}_1, \boldsymbol{a}_2, \cdots, \boldsymbol{a}_m$, the sum of these vectors multiplied respectively by constants $\alpha_1, \alpha_2, \cdots, \alpha_m$,

$$\boldsymbol{f} = \alpha_1\boldsymbol{a}_1 + \alpha_2\boldsymbol{a}_2 + \cdots + \alpha_m\boldsymbol{a}_m,$$

is called a linear combination of these vectors. The equation above can be expressed as $\boldsymbol{f} = \boldsymbol{A}\boldsymbol{a}$, where $\boldsymbol{A}$ is as defined in (1.9), and $\boldsymbol{a}' = (\alpha_1, \alpha_2, \cdots, \alpha_m)$. Hence, the norm of the linear combination $\boldsymbol{f}$ is expressed as

$$||\boldsymbol{f}||^2 = (\boldsymbol{f}, \boldsymbol{f}) = \boldsymbol{f}'\boldsymbol{f} = (\boldsymbol{A}\boldsymbol{a})'(\boldsymbol{A}\boldsymbol{a}) = \boldsymbol{a}'\boldsymbol{A}'\boldsymbol{A}\boldsymbol{a}.$$

The m n-component vectors $\boldsymbol{a}_1, \boldsymbol{a}_2, \cdots, \boldsymbol{a}_m$ are said to be linearly dependent if

$$\alpha_1\boldsymbol{a}_1 + \alpha_2\boldsymbol{a}_2 + \cdots + \alpha_m\boldsymbol{a}_m = \boldsymbol{0} \tag{1.27}$$

holds for some $\alpha_1, \alpha_2, \cdots, \alpha_m$ not all of which are equal to zero. A set of vectors are said to be linearly independent when they are not linearly dependent; that is, when (1.27) holds, it must also hold that $\alpha_1 = \alpha_2 = \cdots = \alpha_m = 0$.

When $\boldsymbol{a}_1, \boldsymbol{a}_2, \cdots, \boldsymbol{a}_m$ are linearly dependent, $\alpha_j \neq 0$ for some j. Let $\alpha_i \neq 0$. From (1.27),

$$\boldsymbol{a}_i = \beta_1\boldsymbol{a}_1 + \cdots + \beta_{i-1}\boldsymbol{a}_{i-1} + \beta_{i+1}\boldsymbol{a}_{i+1} + \beta_m\boldsymbol{a}_m,$$

where $\beta_k = -\alpha_k/\alpha_i$ $(k = 1, \cdots, m; k \neq i)$. Conversely, if the equation above holds, clearly $\boldsymbol{a}_1, \boldsymbol{a}_2, \cdots, \boldsymbol{a}_m$ are linearly dependent. That is, a set of vectors are linearly dependent if any one of them can be expressed as a linear combination of the other vectors.

Let $\boldsymbol{a}_1, \boldsymbol{a}_2, \cdots, \boldsymbol{a}_m$ be linearly independent, and let

$$W = \left\{ \boldsymbol{d} | \boldsymbol{d} = \sum_{i=1}^{m} \alpha_i \boldsymbol{a}_i \right\},$$

where the α_i's are scalars, denote the set of linear combinations of these vectors. Then W is called a linear subspace of dimensionality m.

Definition 1.2 *Let E^n denote the set of all n-component vectors. Suppose that $W \subset E^n$ (W is a subset of E^n) satisfies the following two conditions:*

(1) *If $\boldsymbol{a} \in W$ and $\boldsymbol{b} \in W$, then $\boldsymbol{a} + \boldsymbol{b} \in W$.*

(2) *If $\boldsymbol{a} \in W$, then $\alpha \boldsymbol{a} \in W$, where α is a scalar.*

Then W is called a linear subspace or simply a subspace of E^n.

When there are r linearly independent vectors in W, while any set of $r + 1$ vectors is linearly dependent, the dimensionality of W is said to be r and is denoted as $\dim(W) = r$.

Let $\dim(W) = r$, and let $\boldsymbol{a}_1, \boldsymbol{a}_2, \cdots, \boldsymbol{a}_r$ denote a set of r linearly independent vectors in W. These vectors are called basis vectors spanning (generating) the (sub)space W. This is written as

$$W = \mathrm{Sp}(\boldsymbol{a}_1, \boldsymbol{a}_2, \cdots, \boldsymbol{a}_r) = \mathrm{Sp}(\boldsymbol{A}), \tag{1.28}$$

where $\boldsymbol{A} = [\boldsymbol{a}_1, \boldsymbol{a}_2, \cdots, \boldsymbol{a}_r]$. The maximum number of linearly independent vectors is called the rank of the matrix $\boldsymbol{A}$ and is denoted as $\mathrm{rank}(\boldsymbol{A})$. The following property holds:

$$\dim(\mathrm{Sp}(\boldsymbol{A})) = \mathrm{rank}(\boldsymbol{A}). \tag{1.29}$$

The following theorem holds.

Theorem 1.2 *Let $\boldsymbol{a}_1, \boldsymbol{a}_2, \cdots, \boldsymbol{a}_r$ denote a set of linearly independent vectors in the r-dimensional subspace W. Then any vector in W can be expressed uniquely as a linear combination of $\boldsymbol{a}_1, \boldsymbol{a}_2, \cdots, \boldsymbol{a}_r$.*

(Proof omitted.)

The theorem above indicates that arbitrary vectors in a linear subspace can be uniquely represented by linear combinations of its basis vectors. In general, a set of basis vectors spanning a subspace are not uniquely determined.

If $\boldsymbol{a}_1, \boldsymbol{a}_2, \cdots, \boldsymbol{a}_r$ are basis vectors and are mutually orthogonal, they constitute an orthogonal basis. Let $\boldsymbol{b}_j = \boldsymbol{a}_j/||\boldsymbol{a}_j||$. Then, $||\boldsymbol{b}_j|| = 1$ $(j = 1, \cdots, r)$. The normalized orthogonal basis vectors $\boldsymbol{b}_j$ are called an orthonormal basis. The orthonormality of $\boldsymbol{b}_1, \boldsymbol{b}_2, \cdots, \boldsymbol{b}_r$ can be expressed as

$$(\boldsymbol{b}_i, \boldsymbol{b}_j) = \delta_{ij},$$

where δ_{ij} is called Kronecker's δ, defined by

$$\delta_{ij} = \begin{cases} 1 & \text{if } i = j \\ 0 & \text{if } i \neq j \end{cases}.$$

Let $\boldsymbol{x}$ be an arbitrary vector in the subspace V spanned by $\boldsymbol{b}_1, \boldsymbol{b}_2, \cdots, \boldsymbol{b}_r$, namely

$$\boldsymbol{x} \in V = \text{Sp}(\boldsymbol{B}) = \text{Sp}(\boldsymbol{b}_1, \boldsymbol{b}_2, \cdots, \boldsymbol{b}_r) \subset E^n.$$

Then $\boldsymbol{x}$ can be expressed as

$$\boldsymbol{x} = (\boldsymbol{x}, \boldsymbol{b}_1)\boldsymbol{b}_1 + (\boldsymbol{x}, \boldsymbol{b}_2)\boldsymbol{b}_2 + \cdots + (\boldsymbol{x}, \boldsymbol{b}_r)\boldsymbol{b}_r. \quad (1.30)$$

Since $\boldsymbol{b}_1, \boldsymbol{b}_2, \cdots, \boldsymbol{b}_r$ are orthonormal, the squared norm of $\boldsymbol{x}$ can be expressed as

$$||\boldsymbol{x}||^2 = (\boldsymbol{x}, \boldsymbol{b}_1)^2 + (\boldsymbol{x}, \boldsymbol{b}_2)^2 + \cdots + (\boldsymbol{x}, \boldsymbol{b}_r)^2. \quad (1.31)$$

The formula above is called Parseval's equality.

Next, we consider relationships between two subspaces. Let $V_A = \text{Sp}(\boldsymbol{A})$ and $V_B = \text{Sp}(\boldsymbol{B})$ denote the subspaces spanned by two sets of vectors collected in the form of matrices, $\boldsymbol{A} = [\boldsymbol{a}_1, \boldsymbol{a}_2, \cdots, \boldsymbol{a}_p]$ and $\boldsymbol{B} = [\boldsymbol{b}_1, \boldsymbol{b}_2, \cdots, \boldsymbol{b}_q]$. The subspace spanned by the set of vectors defined by the sum of vectors in these subspaces is given by

$$V_A + V_B = \{\boldsymbol{a} + \boldsymbol{b} | \boldsymbol{a} \in V_A, \boldsymbol{b} \in V_B\}. \quad (1.32)$$

The resultant subspace is denoted by

$$V_{A+B} = V_A + V_B = \text{Sp}(\boldsymbol{A}, \boldsymbol{B}) \quad (1.33)$$

and is called the sum space of V_A and V_B. The set of vectors common to both V_A and V_B, namely

$$V_{A \cap B} = \{\boldsymbol{x} | \boldsymbol{x} = \boldsymbol{A}\boldsymbol{\alpha} = \boldsymbol{B}\boldsymbol{\beta} \text{ for some } \boldsymbol{\alpha} \text{ and } \boldsymbol{\beta}\}, \quad (1.34)$$

also constitutes a linear subspace. Clearly,

$$V_{A+B} \supset V_A \text{ (or } V_B) \supset V_{A\cap B}. \tag{1.35}$$

The subspace given in (1.34) is called the product space between V_A and V_B and is written as

$$V_{A\cap B} = V_A \cap V_B. \tag{1.36}$$

When $V_A \cap V_B = \{\mathbf{0}\}$ (that is, the product space between V_A and V_B has only a zero vector), V_A and V_B are said to be disjoint. When this is the case, V_{A+B} is written as

$$V_{A+B} = V_A \oplus V_B \tag{1.37}$$

and the sum space V_{A+B} is said to be decomposable into the direct-sum of V_A and V_B.

When the n-dimensional Euclidean space E^n is expressed by the direct-sum of V and W, namely

$$E^n = V \oplus W, \tag{1.38}$$

W is said to be a complementary subspace of V (or V is a complementary subspace of W) and is written as $W = V^c$ (respectively, $V = W^c$). The complementary subspace of $\text{Sp}(A)$ is written as $\text{Sp}(A)^c$. For a given $V = \text{Sp}(A)$, there are infinitely many possible complementary subspaces, $W = \text{Sp}(A)^c$.

Furthermore, when all vectors in V and all vectors in W are orthogonal, $W = V^\perp$ (or $V = W^\perp$) is called the ortho-complement subspace, which is defined by

$$V^\perp = \{\boldsymbol{a} | (\boldsymbol{a}, \boldsymbol{b}) = 0, \forall \boldsymbol{b} \in V\}. \tag{1.39}$$

The n-dimensional Euclidean space E^n expressed as the direct sum of r disjoint subspaces W_j $(j = 1, \cdots, r)$ is written as

$$E^n = W_1 \oplus W_2 \oplus \cdots \oplus W_r. \tag{1.40}$$

In particular, when W_i and W_j $(i \neq j)$ are orthogonal, this is especially written as

$$E^n = W_1 \dot{\oplus} W_2 \dot{\oplus} \cdots \dot{\oplus} W_r, \tag{1.41}$$

where $\dot{\oplus}$ indicates an orthogonal direct-sum.

The following properties hold regarding the dimensionality of subspaces.

Theorem 1.3

$$\dim(V_{A+B}) = \dim(V_A) + \dim(V_B) - \dim(V_{A\cap B}), \tag{1.42}$$

$$\dim(V_A \oplus V_B) = \dim(V_A) + \dim(V_B), \tag{1.43}$$

$$\dim(V^c) = n - \dim(V). \tag{1.44}$$

(Proof omitted.)

Suppose that the n-dimensional Euclidean space E^n can be expressed as the direct-sum of $V = \mathrm{Sp}(\boldsymbol{A})$ and $W = \mathrm{Sp}(\boldsymbol{B})$, and let $\boldsymbol{Ax} + \boldsymbol{By} = \boldsymbol{0}$. Then, $\boldsymbol{Ax} = -\boldsymbol{By} \in \mathrm{Sp}(\boldsymbol{A}) \cap \mathrm{Sp}(\boldsymbol{B}) = \{\boldsymbol{0}\}$, so that $\boldsymbol{Ax} = \boldsymbol{By} = \boldsymbol{0}$. This can be extended as follows.

Theorem 1.4 *The necessary and sufficient condition for the subspaces* $W_1 = \mathrm{Sp}(\boldsymbol{A}_1), W_2 = \mathrm{Sp}(\boldsymbol{A}_2), \cdots, W_r = \mathrm{Sp}(\boldsymbol{A}_r)$ *to be mutually disjoint is*

$$\boldsymbol{A}_1\boldsymbol{a}_1 + \boldsymbol{A}_2\boldsymbol{a}_2 + \cdots + \boldsymbol{A}_r\boldsymbol{a}_r = \boldsymbol{0} \Longrightarrow \boldsymbol{A}_j\boldsymbol{a}_j = \boldsymbol{0} \text{ for all } j = 1, \cdots, r.$$

(Proof omitted.)

Corollary *An arbitrary vector* $\boldsymbol{x} \in W = W_1 \oplus \cdots \oplus W_r$ *can uniquely be expressed as*

$$\boldsymbol{x} = \boldsymbol{x}_1 + \boldsymbol{x}_2 + \cdots + \boldsymbol{x}_r,$$

where $\boldsymbol{x}_j \in W_j$ $(j = 1, \cdots, r)$.

Note Theorem 1.4 and its corollary indicate that the decomposition of a particular subspace into the direct-sum of disjoint subspaces is a natural extension of the notion of linear independence among vectors.

The following theorem holds regarding implication relations between subspaces.

Theorem 1.5 *Let* V_1 *and* V_2 *be subspaces such that* $V_1 \subset V_2$, *and let* W *be any subspace in* E^n. *Then,*

$$V_1 + (V_2 \cap W) = (V_1 + W) \cap V_2. \tag{1.45}$$

Proof. Let $\boldsymbol{y} \in V_1 + (V_2 \cap W)$. Then $\boldsymbol{y}$ can be decomposed into $\boldsymbol{y} = \boldsymbol{y}_1 + \boldsymbol{y}_2$, where $\boldsymbol{y}_1 \in V_1$ and $\boldsymbol{y}_2 \in V_2 \cap W$. Since $V_1 \subset V_2$, $\boldsymbol{y}_1 \in V_2$, and since $\boldsymbol{y}_2 \subset V_2$, $\boldsymbol{y} = \boldsymbol{y}_1 + \boldsymbol{y}_2 \in V_2$. Also, $\boldsymbol{y}_1 \in V_1 \subset V_1 + W$, and $\boldsymbol{y}_2 \in W \subset V_1 + W$, which together imply $\boldsymbol{y} \in V_1 + W$. Hence, $\boldsymbol{y} \in (V_1 + W) \cap V_2$. Thus, $V_1 + (V_2 \cap W) \subset$

$(V_1 + W) \cap V_2$. If $\boldsymbol{x} \in (V_1 + W) \cap V_2$, then $\boldsymbol{x} \in V_1 + W$ and $\boldsymbol{x} \in V_2$. Thus, $\boldsymbol{x}$ can be decomposed as $\boldsymbol{x} = \boldsymbol{x}_1 + \boldsymbol{y}$, where $\boldsymbol{x}_1 \in V_1$ and $\boldsymbol{y} \in W$. Then $\boldsymbol{y} = \boldsymbol{x} - \boldsymbol{x}_1 \in V_2 \cap W \Longrightarrow \boldsymbol{x} \in V_1 + (V_2 \cap W) \Longrightarrow (V_1 + W) \cap V_2 \subset V_1 + (V_2 \cap W)$, establishing (1.45). Q.E.D.

Corollary (a) *For* $V_1 \subset V_2$, *there exists a subspace* $\tilde{W} \subset V_2$ *such that* $V_2 = V_1 \oplus \tilde{W}$.
(b) *For* $V_1 \subset V_2$,

$$V_2 = V_1 \dot{\oplus} (V_2 \cap V_1^{\perp}). \tag{1.46}$$

Proof. (a): Let W be such that $V_1 \oplus W \supset V_2$, and set $\tilde{W} = V_2 \cap W$ in (1.45).
(b): Set $W = V_1^{\perp}$. Q.E.D.

Note Let $V_1 \subset V_2$, where $V_1 = \mathrm{Sp}(\boldsymbol{A})$. Part (a) in the corollary above indicates that we can choose $\boldsymbol{B}$ such that $W = \mathrm{Sp}(\boldsymbol{B})$ and $V_2 = \mathrm{Sp}(\boldsymbol{A}) \oplus \mathrm{Sp}(\boldsymbol{B})$. Part (b) indicates that we can choose $\mathrm{Sp}(\boldsymbol{A})$ and $\mathrm{Sp}(\boldsymbol{B})$ to be orthogonal.

In addition, the following relationships hold among the subspaces V, W, and K in E^n:

$$V \supset W \Longrightarrow W = V \cap W, \tag{1.47}$$

$$V \supset W \Longrightarrow V + K \supset W + K, \text{ (where } K \in E^n), \tag{1.48}$$

$$(V \cap W)^{\perp} = V^{\perp} + W^{\perp}, \;\; V^{\perp} \cap W^{\perp} = (V + W)^{\perp}, \tag{1.49}$$

$$(V + W) \cap K \supseteq (V \cap K) + (W \cap K), \tag{1.50}$$

$$K + (V \cap W) \subseteq (K + V) \cap (K + W). \tag{1.51}$$

Note In (1.50) and (1.51), the distributive law in set theory does not hold. For the conditions for equalities to hold in (1.50) and (1.51), refer to Theorem 2.19.

1.3 Linear Transformations

A function ϕ that relates an m-component vector $\boldsymbol{x}$ to an n-component vector $\boldsymbol{y}$ (that is, $\boldsymbol{y} = \phi(\boldsymbol{x})$) is often called a mapping or transformation. In this book, we mainly use the latter terminology. When ϕ satisfies the following properties for any two n-component vectors $\boldsymbol{x}$ and $\boldsymbol{y}$, and for any constant a, it is called a linear transformation:

$$\text{(i) } \phi(a\boldsymbol{x}) = a\phi(\boldsymbol{x}), \quad \text{(ii) } \phi(\boldsymbol{x} + \boldsymbol{y}) = \phi(\boldsymbol{x}) + \phi(\boldsymbol{y}). \tag{1.52}$$

If we combine the two properties above, we obtain

$$\phi(\alpha_1 \boldsymbol{x}_1 + \alpha_2 \boldsymbol{x}_2 + \cdots + \alpha_m \boldsymbol{x}_m) = \alpha_1 \phi(\boldsymbol{x}_1) + \alpha_2 \phi(\boldsymbol{x}_2) + \cdots + \alpha_m \phi(\boldsymbol{x}_m)$$

for m n-component vectors, $\boldsymbol{x}_1, \boldsymbol{x}_2, \cdots, \boldsymbol{x}_m$, and m scalars, $\alpha_1, \alpha_2, \cdots, \alpha_m$.

Theorem 1.6 *A linear transformation ϕ that transforms an m-component vector $\boldsymbol{x}$ into an n-component vector $\boldsymbol{y}$ can be represented by an n by m matrix $\boldsymbol{A} = [\boldsymbol{a}_1, \boldsymbol{a}_2, \cdots, \boldsymbol{a}_m]$ that consists of m n-component vectors $\boldsymbol{a}_1, \boldsymbol{a}_2, \cdots, \boldsymbol{a}_m$.* (Proof omitted.)

We now consider the dimensionality of the subspace generated by a linear transformation of another subspace. Let $W = \text{Sp}(\boldsymbol{A})$ denote the range of $\boldsymbol{y} = \boldsymbol{A}\boldsymbol{x}$ when $\boldsymbol{x}$ varies over the entire range of the m-dimensional space E^m. Then, if $\boldsymbol{y} \in W$, $\alpha \boldsymbol{y} = \boldsymbol{A}(\alpha \boldsymbol{x}) \in W$, and if $\boldsymbol{y}_1, \boldsymbol{y}_2 \in W$, $\boldsymbol{y}_1 + \boldsymbol{y}_2 \in W$. Thus, W constitutes a linear subspace of dimensionality $\dim(W) = \text{rank}(\boldsymbol{A})$ spanned by m vectors, $\boldsymbol{a}_1, \boldsymbol{a}_2, \cdots, \boldsymbol{a}_m$.

When the domain of $\boldsymbol{x}$ is V, where $V \subset E^m$ and $V \neq E^m$ (that is, $\boldsymbol{x}$ does not vary over the entire range of E^m), the range of $\boldsymbol{y}$ is a subspace of W defined above. Let

$$W_V = \{\boldsymbol{y} | \boldsymbol{y} = \boldsymbol{A}\boldsymbol{x}, \boldsymbol{x} \in V\}. \tag{1.53}$$

Then,

$$\dim(W_V) \leq \min\{\text{rank}(\boldsymbol{A}), \dim(W)\} \leq \dim(\text{Sp}(\boldsymbol{A})). \tag{1.54}$$

Note The W_V above is sometimes written as $W_V = \text{Sp}_V(\boldsymbol{A})$. Let $\boldsymbol{B}$ represent the matrix of basis vectors. Then W_V can also be written as $W_V = \text{Sp}(\boldsymbol{AB})$.

We next consider the set of vectors $\boldsymbol{x}$ that satisfies $\boldsymbol{A}\boldsymbol{x} = \boldsymbol{0}$ for a given linear transformation $\boldsymbol{A}$. We write this subspace as

$$\text{Ker}(\boldsymbol{A}) = \{\boldsymbol{x} | \boldsymbol{A}\boldsymbol{x} = \boldsymbol{0}\}. \tag{1.55}$$

Since $\boldsymbol{A}(\alpha \boldsymbol{x}) = \boldsymbol{0}$, we have $\alpha \boldsymbol{x} \in \text{Ker}(\boldsymbol{A})$. Also, if $\boldsymbol{x}, \boldsymbol{y} \in \text{Ker}(\boldsymbol{A})$, we have $\boldsymbol{x} + \boldsymbol{y} \in \text{Ker}(\boldsymbol{A})$ since $\boldsymbol{A}(\boldsymbol{x} + \boldsymbol{y}) = \boldsymbol{0}$. This implies $\text{Ker}(\boldsymbol{A})$ constitutes a subspace of E^m, which represents a set of m-dimensional vectors that are mapped into the zero vector by the linear transformation $\boldsymbol{A}$. It is called an annihilation space or a kernel. Since $\boldsymbol{BAx} = \boldsymbol{0}$, if $\boldsymbol{A} = \boldsymbol{0}$, it follows that

$$\text{Ker}(\boldsymbol{A}) \subset \text{Ker}(\boldsymbol{BA}).$$

The following three theorems hold concerning the dimensionality of subspaces.

Theorem 1.7 *Let* $\text{Ker}(\boldsymbol{A}') = \{\boldsymbol{y}|\boldsymbol{A}'\boldsymbol{y} = 0\}$ *for* $\boldsymbol{y} \in E^n$. *Then*

$$\text{Ker}(\boldsymbol{A}') = \text{Sp}(\boldsymbol{A})^{\perp}, \tag{1.56}$$

where $\text{Sp}(\boldsymbol{A})^{\perp}$ *indicates the subspace in* E^n *orthogonal to* $\text{Sp}(\boldsymbol{A})$.

Proof. Let $\boldsymbol{y}_1 \in \text{Ker}(\boldsymbol{A}')$ and $\boldsymbol{y}_2 = \boldsymbol{A}\boldsymbol{x}_2 \in \text{Sp}(\boldsymbol{A})$. Then, $\boldsymbol{y}_1'\boldsymbol{y}_2 = \boldsymbol{y}_1'\boldsymbol{A}\boldsymbol{x}_2 = (\boldsymbol{A}'\boldsymbol{y}_1)'\boldsymbol{x}_2 = 0$. Thus, $\boldsymbol{y}_1 \in \text{Sp}(\boldsymbol{A})^{\perp} \Longrightarrow \text{Ker}(\boldsymbol{A}') \subset \text{Sp}(\boldsymbol{A})^{\perp}$. Conversely, let $\boldsymbol{y}_1 \in \text{Sp}(\boldsymbol{A})^{\perp}$. Then, because $\boldsymbol{A}\boldsymbol{x}_2 \in \text{Sp}(\boldsymbol{A})$, $\boldsymbol{y}_1'\boldsymbol{A}\boldsymbol{x}_2 = (\boldsymbol{A}'\boldsymbol{y}_1)'\boldsymbol{x}_2 = 0 \Longrightarrow \boldsymbol{A}'\boldsymbol{y}_1 = \boldsymbol{0} \Longrightarrow \boldsymbol{y}_1 \in \text{Ker}(\boldsymbol{A}') \Longrightarrow \text{Sp}(\boldsymbol{A}')^{\perp} \subset \text{Ker}(\boldsymbol{A}')$, establishing $\text{Ker}(\boldsymbol{A}') = \text{Sp}(\boldsymbol{A})^{\perp}$. Q.E.D.

Corollary

$$\text{Ker}(\boldsymbol{A}) = \text{Sp}(\boldsymbol{A}')^{\perp}, \tag{1.57}$$

$$\{\text{Ker}(\boldsymbol{A})\}^{\perp} = \text{Sp}(\boldsymbol{A}'). \tag{1.58}$$

Theorem 1.8

$$\text{rank}(\boldsymbol{A}) = \text{rank}(\boldsymbol{A}'). \tag{1.59}$$

Proof. We use (1.57) to show $\text{rank}(\boldsymbol{A}') \geq \text{rank}(\boldsymbol{A})$. An arbitrary $\boldsymbol{x} \in E^m$ can be expressed as $\boldsymbol{x} = \boldsymbol{x}_1 + \boldsymbol{x}_2$, where $\boldsymbol{x}_1 \in \text{Sp}(\boldsymbol{A}')$ and $\boldsymbol{x}_2 \in \text{Ker}(\boldsymbol{A})$. Thus, $\boldsymbol{y} = \boldsymbol{A}\boldsymbol{x} = \boldsymbol{A}\boldsymbol{x}_1$, and $\text{Sp}(\boldsymbol{A}) = \text{Sp}_V(\boldsymbol{A})$, where $V = \text{Sp}(\boldsymbol{A}')$. Hence, it holds that $\text{rank}(\boldsymbol{A}) = \dim(\text{Sp}(\boldsymbol{A})) = \dim(\text{Sp}_V(\boldsymbol{A})) \leq \dim(V) = \text{rank}(\boldsymbol{A}')$. Similarly, we can use (1.56) to show $\text{rank}(\boldsymbol{A}) \geq \text{rank}(\boldsymbol{A}')$. (Refer to (1.53) for Sp_V.) Q.E.D.

Theorem 1.9 *Let* $\boldsymbol{A}$ *be an* n *by* m *matrix. Then,*

$$\dim(\text{Ker}(\boldsymbol{A})) = m - \text{rank}(\boldsymbol{A}). \tag{1.60}$$

Proof. Follows directly from (1.57) and (1.59). Q.E.D.

Corollary

$$\text{rank}(\boldsymbol{A}) = \text{rank}(\boldsymbol{A}'\boldsymbol{A}) = \text{rank}(\boldsymbol{A}\boldsymbol{A}'). \tag{1.61}$$

In addition, the following results hold:

(i) Let $\boldsymbol{A}$ and $\boldsymbol{B}$ be p by n and p by q matrices, respectively, and $[\boldsymbol{A}, \boldsymbol{B}]$ denote a row block matrix obtained by putting $\boldsymbol{A}$ and $\boldsymbol{B}$ side by side. Then,

$$\begin{aligned}&\text{rank}(\boldsymbol{A}) + \text{rank}(\boldsymbol{B}) - \text{rank}([\boldsymbol{A}, \boldsymbol{B}])\\ &\quad \leq \text{rank}(\boldsymbol{A}'\boldsymbol{B}) \leq \min(\text{rank}(\boldsymbol{A}), \text{rank}(\boldsymbol{B})),\end{aligned} \tag{1.62}$$

where $\text{rank}(\boldsymbol{A}) + \text{rank}(\boldsymbol{B}) - \text{rank}([\boldsymbol{A}, \boldsymbol{B}]) = \dim(\text{Sp}(\boldsymbol{A}) \cap \text{Sp}(\boldsymbol{B}))$.

(ii) Let $\boldsymbol{U}$ and $\boldsymbol{V}$ be nonsingular matrices (see the next paragraph). Then,

$$\text{rank}(\boldsymbol{UAV}) = \text{rank}(\boldsymbol{A}). \tag{1.63}$$

(iii) Let $\boldsymbol{A}$ and $\boldsymbol{B}$ be matrices of the same order. Then,

$$\text{rank}(\boldsymbol{A} + \boldsymbol{B}) \leq \text{rank}(\boldsymbol{A}) + \text{rank}(\boldsymbol{B}). \tag{1.64}$$

(iv) Let $\boldsymbol{A}$, $\boldsymbol{B}$, and $\boldsymbol{C}$ be n by p, p by q, and q by r matrices. Then,

$$\text{rank}(\boldsymbol{ABC}) \geq \text{rank}(\boldsymbol{AB}) + \text{rank}(\boldsymbol{BC}) - \text{rank}(\boldsymbol{B}). \tag{1.65}$$

(See Marsaglia and Styan (1974) for other important rank formulas.)

Consider a linear transformation matrix $\boldsymbol{A}$ that transforms an n-component vector $\boldsymbol{x}$ into another n-component vector $\boldsymbol{y}$. The matrix $\boldsymbol{A}$ is a square matrix of order n. A square matrix $\boldsymbol{A}$ of order n is said to be nonsingular (regular) when $\text{rank}(\boldsymbol{A}) = n$. It is said to be a singular matrix when $\text{rank}(\boldsymbol{A}) < n$.

Theorem 1.10 *Each of the following three conditions is necessary and sufficient for a square matrix* $\boldsymbol{A}$ *to be nonsingular:*

(i) *There exists an* $\boldsymbol{x}$ *such that* $\boldsymbol{y} = \boldsymbol{Ax}$ *for an arbitrary* n*-dimensional vector* $\boldsymbol{y}$.

(ii) *The dimensionality of the annihilation space of* $\boldsymbol{A}$ (Ker($\boldsymbol{A}$)) *is zero; that is,* $\text{Ker}(\boldsymbol{A}) = \{\boldsymbol{0}\}$.

(iii) *If* $\boldsymbol{Ax}_1 = \boldsymbol{Ax}_2$, *then* $\boldsymbol{x}_1 = \boldsymbol{x}_2$. (Proof omitted.)

As is clear from the theorem above, a linear transformation ϕ is one-to-one if a square matrix $\boldsymbol{A}$ representing ϕ is nonsingular. This means that $\boldsymbol{Ax} = \boldsymbol{0}$ if and only if $\boldsymbol{x} = \boldsymbol{0}$. The same thing can be expressed as $\mathrm{Ker}(\boldsymbol{A}) = \{\boldsymbol{0}\}$.

A square matrix $\boldsymbol{A}$ of order n can be considered as a collection of n n-component vectors placed side by side, i.e., $\boldsymbol{A} = [\boldsymbol{a}_1, \boldsymbol{a}_2, \cdots, \boldsymbol{a}_n]$. We define a function of these vectors by

$$\psi(\boldsymbol{a}_1, \boldsymbol{a}_2, \cdots, \boldsymbol{a}_n) = |\boldsymbol{A}|.$$

When ψ is a scalar function that is linear with respect to each $\boldsymbol{a}_i$ and such that its sign is reversed when $\boldsymbol{a}_i$ and $\boldsymbol{a}_j$ $(i \neq j)$ are interchanged, it is called the determinant of a square matrix $\boldsymbol{A}$ and is denoted by $|\boldsymbol{A}|$ or sometimes by $\det(\boldsymbol{A})$. The following relation holds:

$$\begin{aligned}&\psi(\boldsymbol{a}_1, \cdots, \alpha\boldsymbol{a}_i + \beta\boldsymbol{b}_i, \cdots, \boldsymbol{a}_n)\\&\quad = \alpha\psi(\boldsymbol{a}_1, \cdots, \boldsymbol{a}_i, \cdots, \boldsymbol{a}_n) + \beta\psi(\boldsymbol{a}_1, \cdots, \boldsymbol{b}_i, \cdots, \boldsymbol{a}_n).\end{aligned}$$

If among the n vectors there exist two identical vectors, then

$$\psi(\boldsymbol{a}_1, \cdots, \boldsymbol{a}_n) = 0.$$

More generally, when $\boldsymbol{a}_1, \boldsymbol{a}_2, \cdots, \boldsymbol{a}_n$ are linearly dependent, $|\boldsymbol{A}| = 0$.

Let $\boldsymbol{A}$ and $\boldsymbol{B}$ be square matrices of the same order. Then the determinant of the product of the two matrices can be decomposed into the product of the determinant of each matrix. That is,

$$|\boldsymbol{AB}| = |\boldsymbol{A}| \cdot |\boldsymbol{B}|.$$

According to Theorem 1.10, the $\boldsymbol{x}$ that satisfies $\boldsymbol{y} = \boldsymbol{Ax}$ for a given $\boldsymbol{y}$ and $\boldsymbol{A}$ is determined uniquely if $\mathrm{rank}(\boldsymbol{A}) = n$. Furthermore, if $\boldsymbol{y} = \boldsymbol{Ax}$, then $\alpha\boldsymbol{y} = \boldsymbol{A}(\alpha\boldsymbol{x})$, and if $\boldsymbol{y}_1 = \boldsymbol{Ax}_1$ and $\boldsymbol{y}_2 = \boldsymbol{Ax}_2$, then $\boldsymbol{y}_1 + \boldsymbol{y}_2 = \boldsymbol{A}(\boldsymbol{x}_1 + \boldsymbol{x}_2)$. Hence, if we write the transformation that transforms $\boldsymbol{y}$ into $\boldsymbol{x}$ as $\boldsymbol{x} = \varphi(\boldsymbol{y})$, this is a linear transformation. This transformation is called the inverse transformation of $\boldsymbol{y} = \boldsymbol{Ax}$, and its representation by a matrix is called the inverse matrix of $\boldsymbol{A}$ and is written as $\boldsymbol{A}^{-1}$. Let $\boldsymbol{y} = \phi(\boldsymbol{x})$ be a linear transformation, and let $\boldsymbol{x} = \varphi(\boldsymbol{y})$ be its inverse transformation. Then, $\varphi(\phi(\boldsymbol{x})) = \varphi(\boldsymbol{y}) = \boldsymbol{x}$, and $\phi(\varphi(\boldsymbol{y})) = \phi(\boldsymbol{x}) = \boldsymbol{y}$. The composite transformations, $\varphi(\phi)$ and $\phi(\varphi)$, are both identity transformations. Hence, we have $\boldsymbol{A}\boldsymbol{A}^{-1} = \boldsymbol{A}^{-1}\boldsymbol{A} = \boldsymbol{I}_n$. The inverse matrix can also be defined as the matrix whose product with $\boldsymbol{A}$ is equal to the identity matrix.

If $\boldsymbol{A}$ is regular (nonsingular), the following relation holds:

$$|\boldsymbol{A}^{-1}| = |\boldsymbol{A}|^{-1}.$$

If $\boldsymbol{A}$ and $\boldsymbol{B}$ are nonsingular matrices of the same order, then

$$(\boldsymbol{A}\boldsymbol{B})^{-1} = \boldsymbol{B}^{-1}\boldsymbol{A}^{-1}.$$

Let $\boldsymbol{A}$, $\boldsymbol{B}$, $\boldsymbol{C}$, and $\boldsymbol{D}$ be n by n, n by m, m by n, and m by m matrices, respectively. If $\boldsymbol{A}$ and $\boldsymbol{D}$ are nonsingular, then

$$\begin{vmatrix} \boldsymbol{A} & \boldsymbol{B} \\ \boldsymbol{C} & \boldsymbol{D} \end{vmatrix} = |\boldsymbol{A}||\boldsymbol{D} - \boldsymbol{C}\boldsymbol{A}^{-1}\boldsymbol{B}| = |\boldsymbol{D}||\boldsymbol{A} - \boldsymbol{B}\boldsymbol{D}^{-1}\boldsymbol{C}|. \tag{1.66}$$

Furthermore, the inverse of a symmetric matrix of the form $\begin{bmatrix} \boldsymbol{A} & \boldsymbol{B} \\ \boldsymbol{B}' & \boldsymbol{C} \end{bmatrix}$, if (1.66) is nonzero and $\boldsymbol{A}$ and $\boldsymbol{C}$ are nonsingular, is given by

$$\begin{bmatrix} \boldsymbol{A} & \boldsymbol{B} \\ \boldsymbol{B}' & \boldsymbol{C} \end{bmatrix}^{-1} = \begin{bmatrix} \boldsymbol{A}^{-1} + \boldsymbol{F}\boldsymbol{E}^{-1}\boldsymbol{F}' & -\boldsymbol{F}\boldsymbol{E}^{-1} \\ -\boldsymbol{E}^{-1}\boldsymbol{F}' & \boldsymbol{E}^{-1} \end{bmatrix}, \tag{1.67}$$

where $\boldsymbol{E} = \boldsymbol{C} - \boldsymbol{B}'\boldsymbol{A}^{-1}\boldsymbol{B}$ and $\boldsymbol{F} = \boldsymbol{A}^{-1}\boldsymbol{B}$, or

$$\begin{bmatrix} \boldsymbol{A} & \boldsymbol{B} \\ \boldsymbol{B}' & \boldsymbol{C} \end{bmatrix}^{-1} = \begin{bmatrix} \boldsymbol{H}^{-1} & -\boldsymbol{H}^{-1}\boldsymbol{G}' \\ -\boldsymbol{G}\boldsymbol{H}^{-1} & \boldsymbol{C}^{-1} + \boldsymbol{G}\boldsymbol{H}^{-1}\boldsymbol{G}' \end{bmatrix}, \tag{1.68}$$

where $\boldsymbol{H} = \boldsymbol{A} - \boldsymbol{B}\boldsymbol{C}^{-1}\boldsymbol{B}'$ and $\boldsymbol{G} = \boldsymbol{C}^{-1}\boldsymbol{B}'$.

In Chapter 3, we will discuss a generalized inverse of $\boldsymbol{A}$ representing an inverse transformation $\boldsymbol{x} = \varphi(\boldsymbol{y})$ of the linear transformation $\boldsymbol{y} = \boldsymbol{A}\boldsymbol{x}$ when $\boldsymbol{A}$ is not square or when it is square but singular.

1.4 Eigenvalues and Eigenvectors

Definition 1.3 *Let $\boldsymbol{A}$ be a square matrix of order n. A scalar λ and an n-component vector $\boldsymbol{x}(\neq \boldsymbol{0})$ that satisfy*

$$\boldsymbol{A}\boldsymbol{x} = \lambda\boldsymbol{x} \tag{1.69}$$

are called an eigenvalue (or characteristic value) and an eigenvector (or characteristic vector) of the matrix $\boldsymbol{A}$, respectively. The matrix equation *above determines an n-component vector $\boldsymbol{x}$ whose direction remains unchanged by the linear transformation $\boldsymbol{A}$.*

The vector $\boldsymbol{x}$ that satisfies (1.69) is in the null space of the matrix $\tilde{\boldsymbol{A}} = \boldsymbol{A} - \lambda \boldsymbol{I}_n$ because $(\boldsymbol{A} - \lambda \boldsymbol{I}_n)\boldsymbol{x} = \boldsymbol{0}$. From Theorem 1.10, for the dimensionality of this null space to be at least 1, its determinant has to be 0. That is,

$$|\boldsymbol{A} - \lambda \boldsymbol{I}_n| = 0.$$

Let the determinant on the left-hand side of the equation above be denoted by

$$\psi_A(\lambda) = \begin{vmatrix} a_{11} - \lambda & a_{12} & \cdots & a_{1n} \\ a_{21} & a_{22} - \lambda & \cdots & a_{2n} \\ \vdots & \vdots & \ddots & \vdots \\ a_{n1} & a_{n2} & \cdots & a_{nn} - \lambda \end{vmatrix}. \tag{1.70}$$

The equation above is clearly a polynomial function of λ in which the coefficient on the highest-order term is equal to $(-1)^n$, and it can be written as

$$\psi_A(\lambda) = (-1)^n \lambda^n + \alpha_1 (-1)^{n-1} \lambda^{n-1} + \cdots + \alpha_n, \tag{1.71}$$

which is called the eigenpolynomial of $\boldsymbol{A}$. The equation obtained by setting the eigenpolynomial to zero (that is, $\psi_A(\lambda) = 0$) is called an eigenequation. The eigenvalues of $\boldsymbol{A}$ are solutions (roots) of this eigenequation.

The following properties hold for the coefficients of the eigenpolynomial of $\boldsymbol{A}$. Setting $\lambda = 0$ in (1.71), we obtain

$$\psi_A(0) = \alpha_n = |\boldsymbol{A}|.$$

In the expansion of $|\boldsymbol{A} - \lambda \boldsymbol{I}_n|$, all the terms except the product of the diagonal elements, $(a_{11} - \lambda), \cdots (a_{nn} - \lambda)$, are of order at most $n - 2$. So α_1, the coefficient on λ^{n-1}, is equal to the coefficient on λ^{n-1} in the product of the diagonal elements $(a_{11} - \lambda) \cdots (a_{nn} - \lambda)$; that is, $(-1)^{n-1}(a_{11} + a_{22} + \cdots + a_{nn})$. Hence, the following equality holds:

$$\alpha_1 = \text{tr}(\boldsymbol{A}) = a_{11} + a_{22} + \cdots + a_{nn}. \tag{1.72}$$

Let $\boldsymbol{A}$ be a square matrix of order n not necessarily symmetric. Assume that $\boldsymbol{A}$ has n distinct eigenvalues, λ_i $(i = 1, \cdots, n)$. Then $\boldsymbol{u}_i$ that satisfies

$$\boldsymbol{A}\boldsymbol{u}_i = \lambda_i \boldsymbol{u}_i \quad (i = 1, \cdots, n) \tag{1.73}$$

is called a right eigenvector, and $\boldsymbol{v}_i$ that satisfies

$$\boldsymbol{A}'\boldsymbol{v}_i = \lambda_i \boldsymbol{v}_i \quad (i = 1, \cdots, n) \tag{1.74}$$

is called a left eigenvector. The following relations hold:

$$(\boldsymbol{u}_i, \boldsymbol{v}_j) = 0 \quad (i \neq j), \tag{1.75}$$

$$(\boldsymbol{u}_i, \boldsymbol{v}_i) \neq 0 \quad (i = 1, \cdots, n).$$

We may set $\boldsymbol{u}_i$ and $\boldsymbol{v}_i$ so that

$$\boldsymbol{u}_i'\boldsymbol{v}_i = 1. \tag{1.76}$$

Let $\boldsymbol{U}$ and $\boldsymbol{V}$ be matrices of such $\boldsymbol{u}_i$'s and $\boldsymbol{v}_i$'s, that is,

$$\boldsymbol{U} = [\boldsymbol{u}_1, \boldsymbol{u}_2, \cdots, \boldsymbol{u}_n], \quad \boldsymbol{V} = [\boldsymbol{v}_1, \boldsymbol{v}_2, \cdots, \boldsymbol{v}_n].$$

Then, from (1.75) and (1.76), we have

$$\boldsymbol{V}'\boldsymbol{U} = \boldsymbol{I}_n. \tag{1.77}$$

Furthermore, it follows that $\boldsymbol{v}_j'\boldsymbol{A}\boldsymbol{u}_i = 0$ $(j \neq i)$ and $\boldsymbol{v}_j'\boldsymbol{A}\boldsymbol{u}_j = \lambda_j \boldsymbol{v}_j'\boldsymbol{u}_j = \lambda_j$, and we have

$$\boldsymbol{V}'\boldsymbol{A}\boldsymbol{U} = \begin{bmatrix} \lambda_1 & 0 & \cdots & 0 \\ 0 & \lambda_2 & \cdots & 0 \\ \vdots & \vdots & \ddots & \vdots \\ 0 & 0 & \cdots & \lambda_n \end{bmatrix} = \boldsymbol{\Delta}. \tag{1.78}$$

Pre- and postmultiplying the equation above by $\boldsymbol{U}$ and $\boldsymbol{V}'$, respectively, and noting that $\boldsymbol{V}'\boldsymbol{U} = \boldsymbol{I}_n \Longrightarrow \boldsymbol{U}\boldsymbol{V}' = \boldsymbol{I}_n$ (note that $\boldsymbol{V}' = \boldsymbol{U}^{-1}$), we obtain the following theorem.

Theorem 1.11 *Let $\lambda_1, \lambda_2, \cdots, \lambda_n$ denote the eigenvalues of $\boldsymbol{A}$, which are all assumed distinct, and let $\boldsymbol{U} = [\boldsymbol{u}_1, \boldsymbol{u}_2, \cdots, \boldsymbol{u}_n]$ and $\boldsymbol{V} = [\boldsymbol{v}_1, \boldsymbol{v}_2, \cdots, \boldsymbol{v}_n]$ denote the matrices of the right and left eigenvectors of $\boldsymbol{A}$, respectively. Then the following decompositions hold:*

$$\begin{aligned} \boldsymbol{A} &= \boldsymbol{U}\boldsymbol{\Delta}\boldsymbol{V}' \quad (\text{or } \boldsymbol{A} = \boldsymbol{U}\boldsymbol{\Delta}\boldsymbol{U}^{-1}) \\ &= \lambda_1 \boldsymbol{u}_1\boldsymbol{v}_1' + \lambda_2 \boldsymbol{u}_2\boldsymbol{v}_2' + \cdots, + \lambda_n \boldsymbol{u}_n\boldsymbol{v}_n' \end{aligned} \tag{1.79}$$

and

$$\boldsymbol{I}_n = \boldsymbol{U}\boldsymbol{V}' = \boldsymbol{u}_1\boldsymbol{v}_1' + \boldsymbol{u}_2\boldsymbol{v}_2' + \cdots, + \boldsymbol{u}_n\boldsymbol{v}_n'. \tag{1.80}$$

(Proof omitted.)

If $\boldsymbol{A}$ is symmetric (i.e., $\boldsymbol{A} = \boldsymbol{A}'$), the right eigenvector $\boldsymbol{u}_i$ and the corresponding left eigenvector $\boldsymbol{v}_i$ coincide, and since $(\boldsymbol{u}_i, \boldsymbol{u}_j) = 0$, we obtain the following corollary.

Corollary *When $\boldsymbol{A} = \boldsymbol{A}'$ and λ_i are distinct, the following decompositions hold:*

$$\begin{aligned} \boldsymbol{A} &= \boldsymbol{U\Delta U}' \\ &= \lambda_1 \boldsymbol{u}_1 \boldsymbol{u}_1' + \lambda_2 \boldsymbol{u}_2 \boldsymbol{u}_2' + \cdots + \lambda_n \boldsymbol{u}_n \boldsymbol{u}_n' \end{aligned} \tag{1.81}$$

and

$$\boldsymbol{I}_n = \boldsymbol{u}_1 \boldsymbol{u}_1' + \boldsymbol{u}_2 \boldsymbol{u}_2' + \cdots + \boldsymbol{u}_n \boldsymbol{u}_n'. \tag{1.82}$$

Decomposition (1.81) is called the spectral decomposition of the symmetric matrix $\boldsymbol{A}$.

When all the eigenvalues of a symmetric matrix $\boldsymbol{A}$ are positive, $\boldsymbol{A}$ is regular (nonsingular) and is called a positive-definite (*pd*) matrix. When they are all nonnegative, $\boldsymbol{A}$ is said to be a nonnegative-definite (*nnd*) matrix. The following theorem holds for an *nnd* matrix.

Theorem 1.12 *The necessary and sufficient condition for a square matrix $\boldsymbol{A}$ to be an nnd matrix is that there exists a matrix $\boldsymbol{B}$ such that*

$$\boldsymbol{A} = \boldsymbol{BB}'. \tag{1.83}$$

(Proof omitted.)

1.5 Vector and Matrix Derivatives

In multivariate analysis, we often need to find an extremum (a maximum or minimum) of a scalar function of vectors and matrices. A necessary condition for an extremum of a function is that its derivatives vanish at a point corresponding to the extremum of the function. For this we need derivatives of a function with respect to the vector or matrix argument. Let $f(\boldsymbol{x})$ denote a scalar function of the p-component vector $\boldsymbol{x}$. Then the derivative of $f(\boldsymbol{x})$ with respect to $\boldsymbol{x}$ is defined by

$$f_d(\boldsymbol{x}) \equiv \partial f(\boldsymbol{x})/\partial \boldsymbol{x} = (\partial f(\boldsymbol{x})/\partial x_1, \partial f(\boldsymbol{x})/\partial x_2, \cdots, \partial f(\boldsymbol{x})/\partial x_p)'. \tag{1.84}$$

Similarly, let $f(\boldsymbol{X})$ denote a scalar function of the n by p matrix $\boldsymbol{X}$. Then its derivative with respect to $\boldsymbol{X}$ is defined as

$$f_d(\boldsymbol{X}) \equiv \frac{\partial f(\boldsymbol{X})}{\partial \boldsymbol{X}} = \begin{bmatrix} \frac{\partial f(\boldsymbol{X})}{\partial x_{11}} & \frac{\partial f(\boldsymbol{X})}{\partial x_{12}} & \cdots & \frac{\partial f(\boldsymbol{X})}{\partial x_{1p}} \\ \frac{\partial f(\boldsymbol{X})}{\partial x_{21}} & \frac{\partial f(\boldsymbol{X})}{\partial x_{22}} & \cdots & \frac{\partial f(\boldsymbol{X})}{\partial x_{2p}} \\ \vdots & \vdots & \ddots & \vdots \\ \frac{\partial f(\boldsymbol{X})}{\partial x_{n1}} & \frac{\partial f(\boldsymbol{X})}{\partial x_{n2}} & \cdots & \frac{\partial f(\boldsymbol{X})}{\partial x_{np}} \end{bmatrix}. \tag{1.85}$$

Below we give functions often used in multivariate analysis and their corresponding derivatives.

Theorem 1.13 *Let* $\boldsymbol{a}$ *be a constant vector, and let* $\boldsymbol{A}$ *and* $\boldsymbol{B}$ *be constant matrices. Then,*

(i) $f(\boldsymbol{x}) = \boldsymbol{x}'\boldsymbol{a} = \boldsymbol{a}'\boldsymbol{x}$ $\quad f_d(\boldsymbol{x}) = \boldsymbol{a}$,
(ii) $f(\boldsymbol{x}) = \boldsymbol{x}'\boldsymbol{A}\boldsymbol{x}$ $\quad f_d(\boldsymbol{x}) = (\boldsymbol{A}+\boldsymbol{A}')\boldsymbol{x}$ $(= 2\boldsymbol{A}\boldsymbol{x}$ if $\boldsymbol{A}' = \boldsymbol{A})$,
(iii) $f(\boldsymbol{X}) = \mathrm{tr}(\boldsymbol{X}'\boldsymbol{A})$ $\quad f_d(\boldsymbol{X}) = \boldsymbol{A}$,
(iv) $f(\boldsymbol{X}) = \mathrm{tr}(\boldsymbol{A}\boldsymbol{X})$ $\quad f_d(\boldsymbol{X}) = \boldsymbol{A}'$,
(v) $f(\boldsymbol{X}) = \mathrm{tr}(\boldsymbol{X}'\boldsymbol{A}\boldsymbol{X})$ $\quad f_d(\boldsymbol{X}) = (\boldsymbol{A}+\boldsymbol{A}')\boldsymbol{X}$ $(= 2\boldsymbol{A}\boldsymbol{X}$ if $\boldsymbol{A}' = \boldsymbol{A})$,
(vi) $f(\boldsymbol{X}) = \mathrm{tr}(\boldsymbol{X}'\boldsymbol{A}\boldsymbol{X}\boldsymbol{B})$ $\quad f_d(\boldsymbol{X}) = \boldsymbol{A}\boldsymbol{X}\boldsymbol{B} + \boldsymbol{A}'\boldsymbol{X}\boldsymbol{B}'$,
(vii) $f(\boldsymbol{X}) = \log(|\boldsymbol{X}|)$ $\quad f_d(\boldsymbol{X}) = \boldsymbol{X}^{-1}|\boldsymbol{X}|$.

Let $f(\boldsymbol{x})$ and $g(\boldsymbol{x})$ denote two scalar functions of $\boldsymbol{x}$. Then the following relations hold, as in the case in which $\boldsymbol{x}$ is a scalar:

$$\frac{\partial(f(\boldsymbol{x}) + g(\boldsymbol{x}))}{\partial \boldsymbol{x}} = f_d(\boldsymbol{x}) + g_d(\boldsymbol{x}), \tag{1.86}$$

$$\frac{\partial(f(\boldsymbol{x})g(\boldsymbol{x}))}{\partial \boldsymbol{x}} = f_d(\boldsymbol{x})g(\boldsymbol{x}) + f(\boldsymbol{x})g_d(\boldsymbol{x}), \tag{1.87}$$

and

$$\frac{\partial(f(\boldsymbol{x})/g(\boldsymbol{x}))}{\partial \boldsymbol{x}} = \frac{f_d(\boldsymbol{x})g(\boldsymbol{x}) - f(\boldsymbol{x})g_d(\boldsymbol{x})}{g(\boldsymbol{x})^2}. \tag{1.88}$$

The relations above still hold when the vector $\boldsymbol{x}$ is replaced by a matrix $\boldsymbol{X}$.

Let $\boldsymbol{y} = \boldsymbol{X}\boldsymbol{b} + \boldsymbol{e}$ denote a linear regression model where $\boldsymbol{y}$ is the vector of observations on the criterion variable, $\boldsymbol{X}$ the matrix of predictor variables, and $\boldsymbol{b}$ the vector of regression coefficients. The least squares (LS) estimate of $\boldsymbol{b}$ that minimizes

$$f(\boldsymbol{b}) = ||\boldsymbol{y} - \boldsymbol{X}\boldsymbol{b}||^2 \tag{1.89}$$

is obtained by taking the first derivative of (1.89) with respect to $\boldsymbol{b}$ and setting the result to zero. This derivative is

$$\frac{\partial f(\boldsymbol{b})}{\partial \boldsymbol{b}} = -2\boldsymbol{X}'\boldsymbol{y} + 2\boldsymbol{X}'\boldsymbol{X}\boldsymbol{b} = -2\boldsymbol{X}'(\boldsymbol{y} - \boldsymbol{X}\boldsymbol{b}), \tag{1.90}$$

obtained by expanding $f(\boldsymbol{b})$ and using (1.86). Similarly, let $f(\boldsymbol{B}) = ||\boldsymbol{Y} - \boldsymbol{X}\boldsymbol{B}||^2$. Then,

$$\frac{\partial f(\boldsymbol{B})}{\partial \boldsymbol{B}} = -2\boldsymbol{X}'(\boldsymbol{Y} - \boldsymbol{X}\boldsymbol{B}). \tag{1.91}$$

Let

$$h(\boldsymbol{x}) \equiv \lambda = \frac{\boldsymbol{x}'\boldsymbol{A}\boldsymbol{x}}{\boldsymbol{x}'\boldsymbol{x}}, \tag{1.92}$$

where $\boldsymbol{A}$ is a symmetric matrix. Then,

$$\frac{\partial \lambda}{\partial \boldsymbol{x}} = \frac{2(\boldsymbol{A}\boldsymbol{x} - \lambda\boldsymbol{x})}{\boldsymbol{x}'\boldsymbol{x}} \tag{1.93}$$

using (1.88). Setting this to zero, we obtain $\boldsymbol{A}\boldsymbol{x} = \lambda\boldsymbol{x}$, which is the eigenequation involving $\boldsymbol{A}$ to be solved. Maximizing (1.92) with respect to $\boldsymbol{x}$ is equivalent to maximizing $\boldsymbol{x}'\boldsymbol{A}\boldsymbol{x}$ under the constraint that $\boldsymbol{x}'\boldsymbol{x} = 1$. Using the Lagrange multiplier method to impose this restriction, we maximize

$$g(\boldsymbol{x}) = \boldsymbol{x}'\boldsymbol{A}\boldsymbol{x} - \lambda(\boldsymbol{x}'\boldsymbol{x} - 1), \tag{1.94}$$

where λ is the Lagrange multiplier. By differentiating (1.94) with respect to $\boldsymbol{x}$ and λ, respectively, and setting the results to zero, we obtain

$$\boldsymbol{A}\boldsymbol{x} - \lambda\boldsymbol{x} = \boldsymbol{0} \tag{1.95}$$

and

$$\boldsymbol{x}'\boldsymbol{x} - 1 = 0, \tag{1.96}$$

from which we obtain a normalized eigenvector $\boldsymbol{x}$. From (1.95) and (1.96), we have $\lambda = \boldsymbol{x}'\boldsymbol{A}\boldsymbol{x}$, implying that $\boldsymbol{x}$ is the (normalized) eigenvector corresponding to the largest eigenvalue of $\boldsymbol{A}$.

Let $f(\boldsymbol{b})$ be as defined in (1.89). This $f(\boldsymbol{b})$ can be rewritten as a composite function $f(\boldsymbol{g}(\boldsymbol{b})) = \boldsymbol{g}(\boldsymbol{b})'\boldsymbol{g}(\boldsymbol{b})$, where $\boldsymbol{g}(\boldsymbol{b}) = \boldsymbol{y} - \boldsymbol{X}\boldsymbol{b}$ is a vector function of the vector $\boldsymbol{b}$. The following chain rule holds for the derivative of $f(\boldsymbol{g}(\boldsymbol{b}))$ with respect to $\boldsymbol{b}$:

$$\frac{\partial f(\boldsymbol{g}(\boldsymbol{b}))}{\partial \boldsymbol{b}} = \frac{\partial \boldsymbol{g}(\boldsymbol{b})}{\partial \boldsymbol{b}} \frac{\partial f(\boldsymbol{g}(\boldsymbol{b}))}{\partial \boldsymbol{g}(\boldsymbol{b})}. \tag{1.97}$$

Applying this formula to $f(\boldsymbol{b})$ defined in (1.89), we obtain

$$\frac{\partial f(\boldsymbol{b})}{\partial \boldsymbol{b}} = -\boldsymbol{X}' \cdot 2(\boldsymbol{y} - \boldsymbol{X}\boldsymbol{b}), \tag{1.98}$$

where

$$\frac{\partial g(\boldsymbol{b})}{\partial \boldsymbol{b}} = \frac{\partial(\boldsymbol{y} - \boldsymbol{X}\boldsymbol{b})}{\partial \boldsymbol{b}} = -\boldsymbol{X}'. \tag{1.99}$$

(This is like replacing $\boldsymbol{a}'$ in (i) of Theorem 1.13 with $-\boldsymbol{X}$.) Formula (1.98) is essentially the same as (1.91), as it should be.

See Magnus and Neudecker (1988) for a more comprehensive account of vector and matrix derivatives.

1.6 Exercises for Chapter 1

1. (a) Let $\boldsymbol{A}$ and $\boldsymbol{C}$ be square nonsingular matrices of orders n and m, respectively, and let $\boldsymbol{B}$ be an n by m matrix. Show that

$$(\boldsymbol{A} + \boldsymbol{B}\boldsymbol{C}\boldsymbol{B}')^{-1} = \boldsymbol{A}^{-1} - \boldsymbol{A}^{-1}\boldsymbol{B}(\boldsymbol{B}'\boldsymbol{A}^{-1}\boldsymbol{B} + \boldsymbol{C}^{-1})^{-1}\boldsymbol{B}'\boldsymbol{A}^{-1}. \tag{1.100}$$

(b) Let $\boldsymbol{c}$ be an n-component vector. Using the result above, show the following:

$$(\boldsymbol{A} + \boldsymbol{c}\boldsymbol{c}')^{-1} = \boldsymbol{A}^{-1} - \boldsymbol{A}^{-1}\boldsymbol{c}\boldsymbol{c}'\boldsymbol{A}^{-1}/(1 + \boldsymbol{c}'\boldsymbol{A}^{-1}\boldsymbol{c}).$$

2. Let $\boldsymbol{A} = \begin{bmatrix} 1 & 2 \\ 2 & 1 \\ 3 & 3 \end{bmatrix}$ and $\boldsymbol{B} = \begin{bmatrix} 3 & -2 \\ 1 & 3 \\ 2 & 5 \end{bmatrix}$. Obtain $\mathrm{Sp}(\boldsymbol{A}) \cap \mathrm{Sp}(\boldsymbol{B})$.

3. Let $\boldsymbol{M}$ be a *pd* matrix. Show

$$\{\mathrm{tr}(\boldsymbol{A}'\boldsymbol{B})\}^2 \le \mathrm{tr}(\boldsymbol{A}'\boldsymbol{M}\boldsymbol{A})\mathrm{tr}(\boldsymbol{B}'\boldsymbol{M}^{-1}\boldsymbol{B}).$$

4. Let $E^n = V \oplus W$. Answer true or false to the following statements:
(a) $E^n = V^{\perp} \oplus W^{\perp}$.
(b) $\boldsymbol{x} \notin V \Longrightarrow \boldsymbol{x} \in W$.
(c) Let $\boldsymbol{x} \in V$ and $\boldsymbol{x} = \boldsymbol{x}_1 + \boldsymbol{x}_2$. Then, $\boldsymbol{x}_1 \in V$ and $\boldsymbol{x}_2 \in V$.
(d) Let $V = \mathrm{Sp}(\boldsymbol{A})$. Then $V \cap \mathrm{Ker}(\boldsymbol{A}) = \{\boldsymbol{0}\}$.

5. Let $E^n = V_1 \oplus W_1 = V_2 \oplus W_2$. Show that

$$\dim(V_1 + V_2) + \dim(V_1 \cap V_2) + \dim(W_1 + W_2) + \dim(W_1 \cap W_2) = 2n. \tag{1.101}$$

6. (a) Let $\boldsymbol{A}$ be an n by m matrix, and let $\boldsymbol{B}$ be an m by p matrix. Show the following:

$$\mathrm{Ker}(\boldsymbol{A}\boldsymbol{B}) = \mathrm{Ker}(\boldsymbol{B}) \Longleftrightarrow \mathrm{Sp}(\boldsymbol{B}) \cap \mathrm{Ker}(\boldsymbol{A}) = \{\boldsymbol{0}\}.$$

(b) Let $\boldsymbol{A}$ be a square matrix. Show the following:

$$\text{Ker}(\boldsymbol{A}) \cap \text{Sp}(\boldsymbol{A}) = \{\boldsymbol{0}\} \Longleftrightarrow \text{Ker}(\boldsymbol{A}) = \text{Ker}(\boldsymbol{A}').$$

7. Let $\boldsymbol{A}, \boldsymbol{B}$, and $\boldsymbol{C}$ be m by n, n by m, and r by m matrices, respectively.

(a) Show that $\text{rank}\left(\begin{bmatrix} \boldsymbol{A} & \boldsymbol{AB} \\ \boldsymbol{CA} & \boldsymbol{O} \end{bmatrix}\right) = \text{rank}(\boldsymbol{A}) + \text{rank}(\boldsymbol{CAB})$.

(b) Show that

$$\begin{aligned} \text{rank}(\boldsymbol{A} - \boldsymbol{ABA}) &= \text{rank}(\boldsymbol{A}) + \text{rank}(\boldsymbol{I}_n - \boldsymbol{BA}) - n \\ &= \text{rank}(\boldsymbol{A}) + \text{rank}(\boldsymbol{I}_m - \boldsymbol{AB}) - m, \end{aligned}$$

8. Let $\boldsymbol{A}$ be an n by m matrix, and let $\boldsymbol{B}$ be an m by r matrix. Answer the following questions:
(a) Let $W_1 = \{\boldsymbol{x}|\boldsymbol{Ax} = \boldsymbol{0} \text{ for all } \boldsymbol{x} \in \text{Sp}(\boldsymbol{B})\}$ and $W_2 = \{\boldsymbol{Ax}|\boldsymbol{x} \in \text{Sp}(\boldsymbol{B})\}$. Show that $\dim(W_1) + \dim(W_2) = \text{rank}(\boldsymbol{B})$.
(b) Use (a) to show that $\text{rank}(\boldsymbol{AB}) = \text{rank}(\boldsymbol{A}) - \dim(\text{Sp}(\boldsymbol{A}') \cap \text{Sp}(\boldsymbol{B})^{\perp})$.

9. (a) Assume that the absolute values of the eigenvalues of $\boldsymbol{A}$ are all smaller than unity. Show the following:

$$(\boldsymbol{I}_n - \boldsymbol{A})^{-1} = \boldsymbol{I}_n + \boldsymbol{A} + \boldsymbol{A}^2 + \cdots.$$

(b) Obtain $\boldsymbol{B}^{-1}$, where $\boldsymbol{B} = \begin{bmatrix} 1 & 1 & 1 & 1 & 1 \\ 0 & 1 & 1 & 1 & 1 \\ 0 & 0 & 1 & 1 & 1 \\ 0 & 0 & 0 & 1 & 1 \\ 0 & 0 & 0 & 0 & 1 \end{bmatrix}$.

(Hint: Set $\boldsymbol{A} = \begin{bmatrix} 0 & 1 & 0 & 0 & 0 \\ 0 & 0 & 1 & 0 & 0 \\ 0 & 0 & 0 & 1 & 0 \\ 0 & 0 & 0 & 0 & 1 \\ 0 & 0 & 0 & 0 & 0 \end{bmatrix}$, and use the formula in part (a).)

10. Let $\boldsymbol{A}$ be an m by n matrix. If $\text{rank}(\boldsymbol{A}) = r$, $\boldsymbol{A}$ can be expressed as $\boldsymbol{A} = \boldsymbol{MN}$, where $\boldsymbol{M}$ is an m by r matrix and $\boldsymbol{N}$ is an r by n matrix. (This is called a rank decomposition of $\boldsymbol{A}$.)

11. Let $\boldsymbol{U}$ and $\tilde{\boldsymbol{U}}$ be matrices of basis vectors of E^n, and let $\boldsymbol{V}$ and $\tilde{\boldsymbol{V}}$ be the same for E^m. Then the following relations hold: $\tilde{\boldsymbol{U}} = \boldsymbol{UT}_1$ for some $\boldsymbol{T}_1$, and $\tilde{\boldsymbol{V}} = \boldsymbol{VT}_2$ for some $\boldsymbol{T}_2$. Let $\boldsymbol{A}$ be the representation matrix with respect to $\boldsymbol{U}$ and $\boldsymbol{V}$. Show that the representation matrix with respect to $\tilde{\boldsymbol{U}}$ and $\tilde{\boldsymbol{V}}$ is given by

$$\tilde{\boldsymbol{A}} = \boldsymbol{T}_1^{-1}\boldsymbol{A}(\boldsymbol{T}_2^{-1})'.$$

12. Consider a multiple regression equation $\boldsymbol{y} = \boldsymbol{X\beta} + \boldsymbol{e}$, where $\boldsymbol{y}$ is the vector of observations on the criterion variable, $\boldsymbol{X}$ the matrix of predictor variables, $\boldsymbol{\beta}$ the vector of regression coefficients, and $\boldsymbol{e}$ the vector of disturbance terms. Show that it can be assumed without loss of generality that $\boldsymbol{\beta} \in \text{Sp}(\boldsymbol{X}')$.

Chapter 2

Projection Matrices

2.1 Definition

Definition 2.1 *Let* $\boldsymbol{x} \in E^n = V \oplus W$. *Then* $\boldsymbol{x}$ *can be uniquely decomposed into*

$$\boldsymbol{x} = \boldsymbol{x}_1 + \boldsymbol{x}_2 \text{ (where } \boldsymbol{x}_1 \in V \text{ and } \boldsymbol{x}_2 \in W).$$

The transformation that maps $\boldsymbol{x}$ *into* $\boldsymbol{x}_1$ *is called the projection matrix (or simply projector) onto* V *along* W *and is denoted as* ϕ. *This is a linear transformation; that is,*

$$\phi(a_1\boldsymbol{y}_1 + a_2\boldsymbol{y}_2) = a_1\phi(\boldsymbol{y}_1) + a_2\phi(\boldsymbol{y}_2) \tag{2.1}$$

for any $\boldsymbol{y}_1$, $\boldsymbol{y}_2 \in E^n$. *This implies that it can be represented by a matrix. This matrix is called a projection matrix and is denoted by* $\boldsymbol{P}_{V \cdot W}$. *The vector transformed by* $\boldsymbol{P}_{V \cdot W}$ *(that is,* $\boldsymbol{x}_1 = \boldsymbol{P}_{V \cdot W}\boldsymbol{x}$*) is called the projection (or the projection vector) of* $\boldsymbol{x}$ *onto* V *along* W.

Theorem 2.1 *The necessary and sufficient condition for a square matrix* $\boldsymbol{P}$ *of order* n *to be the projection matrix onto* $V = \mathrm{Sp}(\boldsymbol{P})$ *along* $W = \mathrm{Ker}(\boldsymbol{P})$ *is given by*

$$\boldsymbol{P}^2 = \boldsymbol{P}. \tag{2.2}$$

We need the following lemma to prove the theorem above.

Lemma 2.1 *Let* $\boldsymbol{P}$ *be a square matrix of order* n, *and assume that (2.2) holds. Then*

$$E^n = \mathrm{Sp}(\boldsymbol{P}) \oplus \mathrm{Ker}(\boldsymbol{P}) \tag{2.3}$$

and

$$\mathrm{Ker}(\boldsymbol{P}) = \mathrm{Sp}(\boldsymbol{I}_n - \boldsymbol{P}). \tag{2.4}$$

Proof of Lemma 2.1. (2.3): Let $\boldsymbol{x} \in \mathrm{Sp}(\boldsymbol{P})$ and $\boldsymbol{y} \in \mathrm{Ker}(\boldsymbol{P})$. From $\boldsymbol{x} = \boldsymbol{Pa}$, we have $\boldsymbol{Px} = \boldsymbol{P}^2\boldsymbol{a} = \boldsymbol{Pa} = \boldsymbol{x}$ and $\boldsymbol{Py} = \boldsymbol{0}$. Hence, from $\boldsymbol{x}+\boldsymbol{y} = \boldsymbol{0} \Rightarrow \boldsymbol{Px}+\boldsymbol{Py} = \boldsymbol{0}$, we obtain $\boldsymbol{Px} = \boldsymbol{x} = \boldsymbol{0} \Rightarrow \boldsymbol{y} = \boldsymbol{0}$. Thus, $\mathrm{Sp}(\boldsymbol{P}) \cap \mathrm{Ker}(\boldsymbol{P}) = \{\boldsymbol{0}\}$. On the other hand, from $\dim(\mathrm{Sp}(\boldsymbol{P})) + \dim(\mathrm{Ker}(\boldsymbol{P})) = \mathrm{rank}(\boldsymbol{P}) + (n - \mathrm{rank}(\boldsymbol{P})) = n$, we have $E^n = \mathrm{Sp}(\boldsymbol{P}) \oplus \mathrm{Ker}(\boldsymbol{P})$.

(2.4): We have $\boldsymbol{Px} = \boldsymbol{0} \Rightarrow \boldsymbol{x} = (\boldsymbol{I}_n - \boldsymbol{P})\boldsymbol{x} \Rightarrow \mathrm{Ker}(\boldsymbol{P}) \subset \mathrm{Sp}(\boldsymbol{I}_n - \boldsymbol{P})$ on the one hand and $\boldsymbol{P}(\boldsymbol{I}_n - \boldsymbol{P}) \Rightarrow \mathrm{Sp}(\boldsymbol{I}_n - \boldsymbol{P}) \subset \mathrm{Ker}(\boldsymbol{P})$ on the other. Thus, $\mathrm{Ker}(\boldsymbol{P}) = \mathrm{Sp}(\boldsymbol{I}_n - \boldsymbol{P})$. Q.E.D.

Note When (2.4) holds, $\boldsymbol{P}(\boldsymbol{I}_n - \boldsymbol{P}) = \boldsymbol{O} \Rightarrow \boldsymbol{P}^2 = \boldsymbol{P}$. Thus, (2.2) is the necessary and sufficient condition for (2.4).

Proof of Theorem 2.1. (Necessity) For $\forall \boldsymbol{x} \in E^n$, $\boldsymbol{y} = \boldsymbol{Px} \in V$. Noting that $\boldsymbol{y} = \boldsymbol{y} + \boldsymbol{0}$, we obtain

$$\boldsymbol{P}(\boldsymbol{Px}) = \boldsymbol{Py} = \boldsymbol{y} = \boldsymbol{Px} \Longrightarrow \boldsymbol{P}^2\boldsymbol{x} = \boldsymbol{Px} \Longrightarrow \boldsymbol{P}^2 = \boldsymbol{P}.$$

(Sufficiency) Let $V = \{\boldsymbol{y}|\boldsymbol{y} = \boldsymbol{Px}, \boldsymbol{x} \in E^n\}$ and $W = \{\boldsymbol{y}|\boldsymbol{y} = (\boldsymbol{I}_n - \boldsymbol{P})\boldsymbol{x}, \boldsymbol{x} \in E^n\}$. From Lemma 2.1, V and W are disjoint. Then, an arbitrary $\boldsymbol{x} \in E^n$ can be uniquely decomposed into $\boldsymbol{x} = \boldsymbol{Px} + (\boldsymbol{I}_n - \boldsymbol{P})\boldsymbol{x} = \boldsymbol{x}_1 + \boldsymbol{x}_2$ (where $\boldsymbol{x}_1 \in V$ and $\boldsymbol{x}_2 \in W$). From Definition 2.1, $\boldsymbol{P}$ is the projection matrix onto $V = \mathrm{Sp}(\boldsymbol{P})$ along $W = \mathrm{Ker}(\boldsymbol{P})$. Q.E.D.

Let $E^n = V \oplus W$, and let $\boldsymbol{x} = \boldsymbol{x}_1 + \boldsymbol{x}_2$, where $\boldsymbol{x}_1 \in V$ and $\boldsymbol{x}_2 \in W$. Let $\boldsymbol{P}_{W\cdot V}$ denote the projector that transforms $\boldsymbol{x}$ into $\boldsymbol{x}_2$. Then,

$$\boldsymbol{P}_{V\cdot W}\boldsymbol{x} + \boldsymbol{P}_{W\cdot V}\boldsymbol{x} = (\boldsymbol{P}_{V\cdot W} + \boldsymbol{P}_{W\cdot V})\boldsymbol{x}. \tag{2.5}$$

Because the equation above has to hold for any $\boldsymbol{x} \in E^n$, it must hold that

$$\boldsymbol{I}_n = \boldsymbol{P}_{V\cdot W} + \boldsymbol{P}_{W\cdot V}.$$

Let a square matrix $\boldsymbol{P}$ be the projection matrix onto V along W. Then, $\boldsymbol{Q} = \boldsymbol{I}_n - \boldsymbol{P}$ satisfies $\boldsymbol{Q}^2 = (\boldsymbol{I}_n - \boldsymbol{P})^2 = \boldsymbol{I}_n - 2\boldsymbol{P} + \boldsymbol{P}^2 = \boldsymbol{I}_n - \boldsymbol{P} = \boldsymbol{Q}$, indicating that $\boldsymbol{Q}$ is the projection matrix onto W along V. We also have

$$\boldsymbol{PQ} = \boldsymbol{P}(\boldsymbol{I}_n - \boldsymbol{P}) = \boldsymbol{P} - \boldsymbol{P}^2 = \boldsymbol{O}, \tag{2.6}$$

implying that $\mathrm{Sp}(\boldsymbol{Q})$ constitutes the null space of $\boldsymbol{P}$ (i.e., $\mathrm{Sp}(\boldsymbol{Q}) = \mathrm{Ker}(\boldsymbol{P})$). Similarly, $\boldsymbol{QP} = \boldsymbol{O}$, implying that $\mathrm{Sp}(\boldsymbol{P})$ constitutes the null space of $\boldsymbol{Q}$ (i.e., $\mathrm{Sp}(\boldsymbol{P}) = \mathrm{Ker}(\boldsymbol{Q})$).

Theorem 2.2 *Let $E^n = V \oplus W$. The necessary and sufficient conditions for a square matrix $\boldsymbol{P}$ of order n to be the projection matrix onto V along W are:*

$$\text{(i) } \boldsymbol{Px} = \boldsymbol{x} \text{ for } \forall \boldsymbol{x} \in V, \quad \text{(ii) } \boldsymbol{Px} = \boldsymbol{0} \text{ for } \forall \boldsymbol{x} \in W. \tag{2.7}$$

Proof. (Sufficiency) Let $\boldsymbol{P}_{V \cdot W}$ and $\boldsymbol{P}_{W \cdot V}$ denote the projection matrices onto V along W and onto W along V, respectively. Premultiplying (2.5) by $\boldsymbol{P}$, we obtain $\boldsymbol{P}(\boldsymbol{P}_{V \cdot W}\boldsymbol{x}) = \boldsymbol{P}_{V \cdot W}\boldsymbol{x}$, where $\boldsymbol{PP}_{W \cdot V}\boldsymbol{x} = \boldsymbol{0}$ because of (i) and (ii) above, and $\boldsymbol{P}_{V \cdot W}\boldsymbol{x} \in V$ and $\boldsymbol{P}_{W \cdot V}\boldsymbol{x} \in W$. Since $\boldsymbol{Px} = \boldsymbol{P}_{V \cdot W}\boldsymbol{x}$ holds for any $\boldsymbol{x}$, it must hold that $\boldsymbol{P} = \boldsymbol{P}_{V \cdot W}$.

(Necessity) For any $\boldsymbol{x} \in V$, we have $\boldsymbol{x} = \boldsymbol{x} + \boldsymbol{0}$. Thus, $\boldsymbol{Px} = \boldsymbol{x}$. Similarly, for any $\boldsymbol{y} \in W$, we have $\boldsymbol{y} = \boldsymbol{0} + \boldsymbol{y}$, so that $\boldsymbol{Py} = \boldsymbol{0}$. Q.E.D.

Example 2.1 In Figure 2.1, $\overrightarrow{OA}$ indicates the projection of $\boldsymbol{z}$ onto $\mathrm{Sp}(\boldsymbol{x})$ along $\mathrm{Sp}(\boldsymbol{y})$ (that is, $\overrightarrow{OA} = \boldsymbol{P}_{Sp(\boldsymbol{x}) \cdot Sp(\boldsymbol{y})}\boldsymbol{z}$), where $\boldsymbol{P}_{Sp(\boldsymbol{x}) \cdot Sp(\boldsymbol{y})}$ indicates the projection matrix onto $\mathrm{Sp}(\boldsymbol{x})$ along $\mathrm{Sp}(\boldsymbol{y})$. Clearly, $\overrightarrow{OB} = (\boldsymbol{I}_2 - \boldsymbol{P}_{Sp(\boldsymbol{y}) \cdot Sp(\boldsymbol{x})}) \times \boldsymbol{z}$.

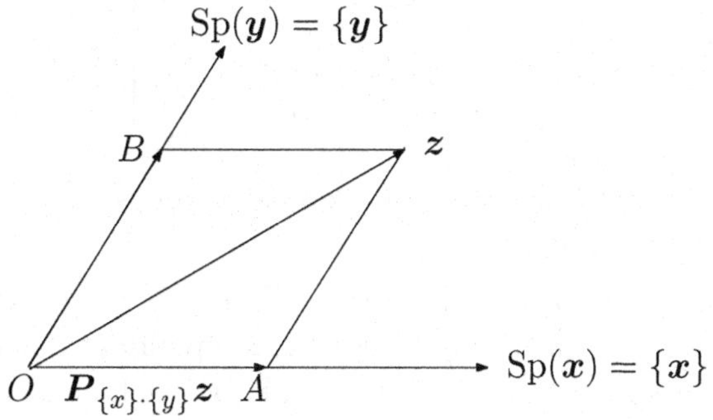

Figure 2.1: Projection onto $\mathrm{Sp}(\boldsymbol{x}) = \{\boldsymbol{x}\}$ along $\mathrm{Sp}(\boldsymbol{y}) = \{\boldsymbol{y}\}$.

Example 2.2 In Figure 2.2, $\overrightarrow{OA}$ indicates the projection of $\boldsymbol{z}$ onto $V = \{\boldsymbol{x} | \boldsymbol{x} = \alpha_1\boldsymbol{x}_1 + \alpha_2\boldsymbol{x}_2\}$ along $\mathrm{Sp}(\boldsymbol{y})$ (that is, $\overrightarrow{OA} = \boldsymbol{P}_{V \cdot Sp(\boldsymbol{y})}\boldsymbol{z}$), where $\boldsymbol{P}_{V \cdot Sp(\boldsymbol{y})}$ indicates the projection matrix onto V along $\mathrm{Sp}(\boldsymbol{y})$.

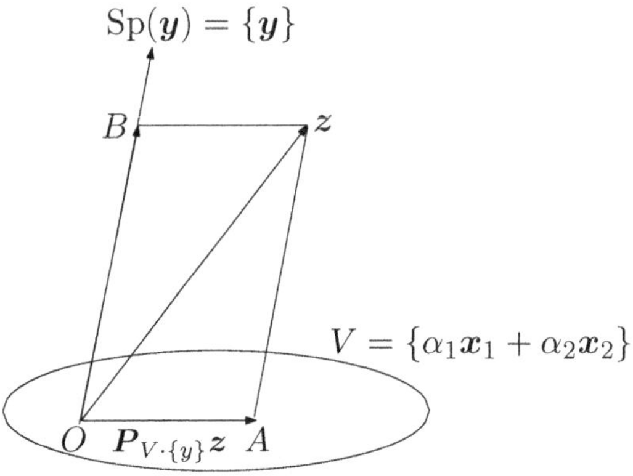

Figure 2.2: Projection onto a two-dimensional space V along $\mathrm{Sp}(\boldsymbol{y}) = \{\boldsymbol{y}\}$.

Theorem 2.3 *The necessary and sufficient condition for a square matrix* $\boldsymbol{P}$ *of order* n *to be a projector onto* V *of dimensionality* r $(\dim(V) = r)$ *is given by*

$$\boldsymbol{P} = \boldsymbol{T}\boldsymbol{\Delta}_r\boldsymbol{T}^{-1}, \tag{2.8}$$

where $\boldsymbol{T}$ *is a square nonsingular matrix of order* n *and*

$$\boldsymbol{\Delta}_r = \begin{bmatrix} 1 & \cdots & 0 & 0 & \cdots & 0 \\ \vdots & \ddots & \vdots & \vdots & \ddots & \vdots \\ 0 & \cdots & 1 & 0 & \cdots & 0 \\ 0 & \cdots & 0 & 0 & \cdots & 0 \\ \vdots & \ddots & \vdots & \vdots & \ddots & \vdots \\ 0 & \cdots & 0 & 0 & \cdots & 0 \end{bmatrix}.$$

(There are r *unities on the leading diagonals,* $1 \le r \le n$*.)*

Proof. (Necessity) Let $E^n = V \oplus W$, and let $\boldsymbol{A} = [\boldsymbol{a}_1, \boldsymbol{a}_2, \cdots, \boldsymbol{a}_r]$ and $\boldsymbol{B} = [\boldsymbol{b}_1, \boldsymbol{b}_2, \cdots \boldsymbol{b}_{n-r}]$ be matrices of linearly independent basis vectors spanning V and W, respectively. Let $\boldsymbol{T} = [\boldsymbol{A}, \boldsymbol{B}]$. Then $\boldsymbol{T}$ is nonsingular, since $\mathrm{rank}(\boldsymbol{A}) + \mathrm{rank}(\boldsymbol{B}) = \mathrm{rank}(\boldsymbol{T})$. Hence, $\forall \boldsymbol{x} \in V$ and $\forall \boldsymbol{y} \in W$ can be expressed as

$$\boldsymbol{x} = \boldsymbol{A}\boldsymbol{\alpha} = [\boldsymbol{A}, \boldsymbol{B}]\begin{pmatrix} \boldsymbol{\alpha} \\ \boldsymbol{0} \end{pmatrix} = \boldsymbol{T}\begin{pmatrix} \boldsymbol{\alpha} \\ \boldsymbol{0} \end{pmatrix},$$

$$\boldsymbol{y} = \boldsymbol{A}\boldsymbol{\alpha} = [\boldsymbol{A}, \boldsymbol{B}]\begin{pmatrix} \boldsymbol{0} \\ \boldsymbol{\beta} \end{pmatrix} = \boldsymbol{T}\begin{pmatrix} \boldsymbol{0} \\ \boldsymbol{\beta} \end{pmatrix}.$$

Thus, we obtain

$$Px = x \Longrightarrow PT\begin{pmatrix}\alpha\\0\end{pmatrix} = T\begin{pmatrix}\alpha\\0\end{pmatrix} = T\Delta_r\begin{pmatrix}\alpha\\0\end{pmatrix},$$

$$Py = 0 \Longrightarrow PT\begin{pmatrix}0\\\beta\end{pmatrix} = \begin{pmatrix}0\\0\end{pmatrix} = T\Delta_r\begin{pmatrix}0\\\beta\end{pmatrix}.$$

Adding the two equations above, we obtain

$$PT\begin{pmatrix}\alpha\\\beta\end{pmatrix} = T\Delta_r\begin{pmatrix}\alpha\\\beta\end{pmatrix}.$$

Since $\begin{pmatrix}\alpha\\\beta\end{pmatrix}$ is an arbitrary vector in the n-dimensional space E^n, it follows that

$$PT = T\Delta_r \Longrightarrow P = T\Delta_r T^{-1}.$$

Furthermore, T can be an arbitrary nonsingular matrix since $V = \mathrm{Sp}(A)$ and $W = \mathrm{Sp}(B)$ such that $E^n = V \oplus W$ can be chosen arbitrarily.

(Sufficiency) P is a projection matrix, since $P^2 = P$, and $\mathrm{rank}(P) = r$ from Theorem 2.1. (Theorem 2.2 can also be used to prove the theorem above.) Q.E.D.

Lemma 2.2 Let P be a projection matrix. Then,

$$\mathrm{rank}(P) = \mathrm{tr}(P). \tag{2.9}$$

Proof. $\mathrm{rank}(P) = \mathrm{rank}(T\Delta_r T^{-1}) = \mathrm{rank}(\Delta_r) = \mathrm{tr}(T\Delta T^{-1}) = \mathrm{tr}(P)$. Q.E.D.

The following theorem holds.

Theorem 2.4 *Let P be a square matrix of order n. Then the following three statements are equivalent.*

$$P^2 = P, \tag{2.10}$$

$$\mathrm{rank}(P) + \mathrm{rank}(I_n - P) = n, \tag{2.11}$$

$$E^n = \mathrm{Sp}(P) \oplus \mathrm{Sp}(I_n - P). \tag{2.12}$$

Proof. (2.10) → (2.11): It is clear from $\mathrm{rank}(P) = \mathrm{tr}(P)$.

(2.11) → (2.12): Let $V = \text{Sp}(\boldsymbol{P})$ and $W = \text{Sp}(\boldsymbol{I}_n - \boldsymbol{P})$. Then, $\dim(V + W) = \dim(V) + \dim(W) - \dim(V \cap W)$. Since $\boldsymbol{x} = \boldsymbol{P}\boldsymbol{x} + (\boldsymbol{I}_n - \boldsymbol{P})\boldsymbol{x}$ for an arbitrary n-component vector $\boldsymbol{x}$, we have $E^n = V + W$. Hence, $\dim(V \cap W) = 0 \Longrightarrow V \cap W = \{\boldsymbol{0}\}$, establishing (2.12).

(2.12) → (2.10): Postmultiplying $\boldsymbol{I}_n = \boldsymbol{P} + (\boldsymbol{I}_n - \boldsymbol{P})$ by $\boldsymbol{P}$, we obtain $\boldsymbol{P} = \boldsymbol{P}^2 + (\boldsymbol{I}_n - \boldsymbol{P})\boldsymbol{P}$, which implies $\boldsymbol{P}(\boldsymbol{I}_n - \boldsymbol{P}) = (\boldsymbol{I}_n - \boldsymbol{P})\boldsymbol{P}$. On the other hand, we have $\boldsymbol{P}(\boldsymbol{I}_n - \boldsymbol{P}) = \boldsymbol{O}$ and $(\boldsymbol{I}_n - \boldsymbol{P})\boldsymbol{P} = \boldsymbol{O}$ because $\text{Sp}(\boldsymbol{P}(\boldsymbol{I}_n - \boldsymbol{P})) \subset \text{Sp}(\boldsymbol{P})$ and $\text{Sp}((\boldsymbol{I}_n - \boldsymbol{P})\boldsymbol{P}) \subset \text{Sp}(\boldsymbol{I}_n - \boldsymbol{P})$. Q.E.D.

Corollary

$$\boldsymbol{P}^2 = \boldsymbol{P} \Longleftrightarrow \text{Ker}(\boldsymbol{P}) = \text{Sp}(\boldsymbol{I}_n - \boldsymbol{P}). \tag{2.13}$$

Proof. (⇒): It is clear from Lemma 2.1.

(⇐): $\text{Ker}(\boldsymbol{P}) = \text{Sp}(\boldsymbol{I}_n - \boldsymbol{P}) \Leftrightarrow \boldsymbol{P}(\boldsymbol{I}_n - \boldsymbol{P}) = \boldsymbol{O} \Rightarrow \boldsymbol{P}^2 = \boldsymbol{P}$. Q.E.D.

2.2 Orthogonal Projection Matrices

Suppose we specify a subspace V in E^n. There are in general infinitely many ways to choose its complement subspace $V^c = W$. We will discuss some of them in Chapter 4. In this section, we consider the case in which V and W are orthogonal, that is, $W = V^\perp$.

Let $\boldsymbol{x}, \boldsymbol{y} \in E^n$, and let $\boldsymbol{x}$ and $\boldsymbol{y}$ be decomposed as $\boldsymbol{x} = \boldsymbol{x}_1 + \boldsymbol{x}_2$ and $\boldsymbol{y} = \boldsymbol{y}_1 + \boldsymbol{y}_2$, where $\boldsymbol{x}_1, \boldsymbol{y}_1 \in V$ and $\boldsymbol{x}_2, \boldsymbol{y}_2 \in W$. Let $\boldsymbol{P}$ denote the projection matrix onto V along $V^\perp$. Then, $\boldsymbol{x}_1 = \boldsymbol{P}\boldsymbol{x}$ and $\boldsymbol{y}_1 = \boldsymbol{P}\boldsymbol{y}$. Since $(\boldsymbol{x}_2, \boldsymbol{P}\boldsymbol{y}) = (\boldsymbol{y}_2, \boldsymbol{P}\boldsymbol{x}) = 0$, it must hold that

$$\begin{aligned}(\boldsymbol{x}, \boldsymbol{P}\boldsymbol{y}) &= (\boldsymbol{P}\boldsymbol{x} + \boldsymbol{x}_2, \boldsymbol{P}\boldsymbol{y}) = (\boldsymbol{P}\boldsymbol{x}, \boldsymbol{P}\boldsymbol{y}) \\ &= (\boldsymbol{P}\boldsymbol{x}, \boldsymbol{P}\boldsymbol{y} + \boldsymbol{y}_2) = (\boldsymbol{P}\boldsymbol{x}, \boldsymbol{y}) = (\boldsymbol{x}, \boldsymbol{P}'\boldsymbol{y})\end{aligned}$$

for any $\boldsymbol{x}$ and $\boldsymbol{y}$, implying

$$\boldsymbol{P}' = \boldsymbol{P}. \tag{2.14}$$

Theorem 2.5 *The necessary and sufficient condition for a square matrix $\boldsymbol{P}$ of order n to be an orthogonal projection matrix (an orthogonal projector) is given by*

$$\text{(i) } \boldsymbol{P}^2 = \boldsymbol{P} \text{ and (ii) } \boldsymbol{P}' = \boldsymbol{P}.$$

Proof. (Necessity) That $\boldsymbol{P}^2 = \boldsymbol{P}$ is clear from the definition of a projection matrix. That $\boldsymbol{P}' = \boldsymbol{P}$ is as shown above.

(Sufficiency) Let $\boldsymbol{x} = \boldsymbol{P}\boldsymbol{\alpha} \in \text{Sp}(\boldsymbol{P})$. Then, $\boldsymbol{P}\boldsymbol{x} = \boldsymbol{P}^2\boldsymbol{\alpha} = \boldsymbol{P}\boldsymbol{\alpha} = \boldsymbol{x}$. Let $\boldsymbol{y} \in \text{Sp}(\boldsymbol{P})^\perp$. Then, $\boldsymbol{P}\boldsymbol{y} = \boldsymbol{0}$ since $(\boldsymbol{P}\boldsymbol{x}, \boldsymbol{y}) = \boldsymbol{x}'\boldsymbol{P}'\boldsymbol{y} = \boldsymbol{x}'\boldsymbol{P}\boldsymbol{y} = 0$ must hold for an arbitrary $\boldsymbol{x}$. From Theorem 2.2, $\boldsymbol{P}$ is the projection matrix onto $\mathrm{Sp}(\boldsymbol{P})$ along $\mathrm{Sp}(\boldsymbol{P})^{\perp}$; that is, the orthogonal projection matrix onto $\mathrm{Sp}(\boldsymbol{P})$. Q.E.D.

Definition 2.2 *A projection matrix* $\boldsymbol{P}$ *such that* $\boldsymbol{P}^2 = \boldsymbol{P}$ *and* $\boldsymbol{P}' = \boldsymbol{P}$ *is called an orthogonal projection matrix (projector). Furthermore, the vector* $\boldsymbol{P}\boldsymbol{x}$ *is called the orthogonal projection of* $\boldsymbol{x}$*. The orthogonal projector* $\boldsymbol{P}$ *is in fact the projection matrix onto* $\mathrm{Sp}(\boldsymbol{P})$ *along* $\mathrm{Sp}(\boldsymbol{P})^{\perp}$*, but it is usually referred to as the orthogonal projector onto* $\mathrm{Sp}(\boldsymbol{P})$. See Figure 2.3.

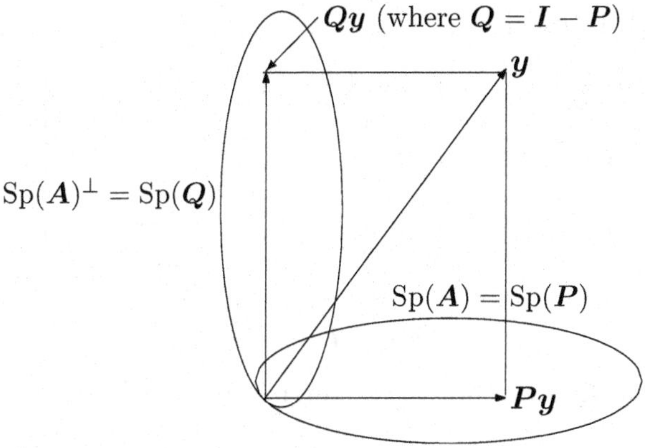

Figure 2.3: Orthogonal projection.

Note A projection matrix that does not satisfy $\boldsymbol{P}' = \boldsymbol{P}$ is called an oblique projector as opposed to an orthogonal projector.

Theorem 2.6 *Let* $\boldsymbol{A} = [\boldsymbol{a}_1, \boldsymbol{a}_2, \cdots, \boldsymbol{a}_m]$*, where* $\boldsymbol{a}_1, \boldsymbol{a}_2, \cdots, \boldsymbol{a}_m$ *are linearly independent. Then the orthogonal projector onto* $V = \mathrm{Sp}(\boldsymbol{A})$ *spanned by* $\boldsymbol{a}_1, \boldsymbol{a}_2, \cdots, \boldsymbol{a}_m$ *is given by*

$$\boldsymbol{P} = \boldsymbol{A}(\boldsymbol{A}'\boldsymbol{A})^{-1}\boldsymbol{A}'. \tag{2.15}$$

Proof. Let $\boldsymbol{x}_1 \in \mathrm{Sp}(\boldsymbol{A})$. From $\boldsymbol{x}_1 = \boldsymbol{A}\boldsymbol{\alpha}$, we obtain $\boldsymbol{P}\boldsymbol{x}_1 = \boldsymbol{x}_1 = \boldsymbol{A}\boldsymbol{\alpha} = \boldsymbol{A}(\boldsymbol{A}'\boldsymbol{A})^{-1}\boldsymbol{A}'\boldsymbol{x}_1$. On the other hand, let $\boldsymbol{x}_2 \in \mathrm{Sp}(\boldsymbol{A})^{\perp}$. Then, $\boldsymbol{A}'\boldsymbol{x}_2 = \boldsymbol{0} \Longrightarrow \boldsymbol{A}(\boldsymbol{A}'\boldsymbol{A})^{-1}\boldsymbol{A}'\boldsymbol{x}_2 = \boldsymbol{0}$. Let $\boldsymbol{x} = \boldsymbol{x}_1 + \boldsymbol{x}_2$. From $\boldsymbol{P}\boldsymbol{x}_2 = \boldsymbol{0}$, we obtain $\boldsymbol{P}\boldsymbol{x} = \boldsymbol{A}(\boldsymbol{A}'\boldsymbol{A})^{-1}\boldsymbol{A}'\boldsymbol{x}$, and (2.15) follows because $\boldsymbol{x}$ is arbitrary.

Let $\boldsymbol{Q} = \boldsymbol{I}_n - \boldsymbol{P}$. Then $\boldsymbol{Q}$ is the orthogonal projector onto $\text{Sp}(\boldsymbol{A})^\perp$, the ortho-complement subspace of $\text{Sp}(\boldsymbol{A})$.

Example 2.3 Let $\mathbf{1}_n = (1, 1, \cdots, 1)'$ (the vector with n ones). Let $\boldsymbol{P}_M$ denote the orthogonal projector onto $V_M = \text{Sp}(\mathbf{1}_n)$. Then,

$$\boldsymbol{P}_M = \mathbf{1}_n(\mathbf{1}_n'\mathbf{1}_n)^{-1}\mathbf{1}_n' = \begin{bmatrix} \frac{1}{n} & \cdots & \frac{1}{n} \\ \vdots & \ddots & \vdots \\ \frac{1}{n} & \cdots & \frac{1}{n} \end{bmatrix}. \tag{2.16}$$

The orthogonal projector onto $V_M^\perp = \text{Sp}(\mathbf{1}_n)^\perp$, the ortho-complement subspace of $\text{Sp}(\mathbf{1}_n)$, is given by

$$\boldsymbol{I}_n - \boldsymbol{P}_M = \begin{bmatrix} 1-\frac{1}{n} & -\frac{1}{n} & \cdots & -\frac{1}{n} \\ -\frac{1}{n} & 1-\frac{1}{n} & \cdots & -\frac{1}{n} \\ \vdots & \vdots & \ddots & \vdots \\ -\frac{1}{n} & -\frac{1}{n} & \cdots & 1-\frac{1}{n} \end{bmatrix}. \tag{2.17}$$

Let

$$\boldsymbol{Q}_M = \boldsymbol{I}_n - \boldsymbol{P}_M. \tag{2.18}$$

Clearly, $\boldsymbol{P}_M$ and $\boldsymbol{Q}_M$ are both symmetric, and the following relation holds:

$$\boldsymbol{P}_M^2 = \boldsymbol{P}_M,\ \boldsymbol{Q}_M^2 = \boldsymbol{Q}_M, \text{ and } \boldsymbol{P}_M\boldsymbol{Q}_M = \boldsymbol{Q}_M\boldsymbol{P}_M = \boldsymbol{O}. \tag{2.19}$$

Note The matrix $\boldsymbol{Q}_M$ in (2.18) is sometimes written as $\boldsymbol{P}_M^\perp$.

Example 2.4 Let

$$\boldsymbol{x}_R = \begin{pmatrix} x_1 \\ x_2 \\ \vdots \\ x_n \end{pmatrix},\ \boldsymbol{x} = \begin{pmatrix} x_1 - \bar{x} \\ x_2 - \bar{x} \\ \vdots \\ x_n - \bar{x} \end{pmatrix}, \text{ where } \bar{x} = \frac{1}{n}\sum_{j=1}^n x_j.$$

Then,

$$\boldsymbol{x} = \boldsymbol{Q}_M \boldsymbol{x}_R, \tag{2.20}$$

and so

$$\sum_{j=1}^n (x_j - \bar{x})^2 = ||\boldsymbol{x}||^2 = \boldsymbol{x}'\boldsymbol{x} = \boldsymbol{x}_R'\boldsymbol{Q}_M\boldsymbol{x}_R.$$

The proof is omitted.

2.3 Subspaces and Projection Matrices

In this section, we consider the relationships between subspaces and projectors when the n-dimensional space E^n is decomposed into the sum of several subspaces.

2.3.1 Decomposition into a direct-sum of disjoint subspaces

Lemma 2.3 *When there exist two distinct ways of decomposing E^n,*

$$E^n = V_1 \oplus W_1 = V_2 \oplus W_2, \tag{2.21}$$

and if $V_1 \subset W_2$ or $V_2 \subset W_1$, the following relation holds:

$$E^n = (V_1 \oplus V_2) \oplus (W_1 \cap W_2). \tag{2.22}$$

Proof. When $V_1 \subset W_2$, Theorem 1.5 leads to the following relation:

$$V_1 + (W_1 \cap W_2) = (V_1 + W_1) \cap W_2 = E^n \cap W_2 = W_2.$$

Also from $V_1 \cap (W_1 \cap W_2) = (V_1 \cap W_1) \cap W_2 = \{\mathbf{0}\}$, we have $W_2 = V_1 \oplus (W_1 \cap W_2)$. Hence the following relation holds:

$$E^n = V_2 \oplus W_2 = V_2 \oplus V_1 \oplus (W_1 \cap W_2) = (V_1 \oplus V_2) \oplus (W_1 \cap W_2).$$

When $V_2 \subset W_2$, the same result follows by using $W_1 = V_2 \oplus (W_1 \cap W_2)$. Q.E.D.

Corollary *When $V_1 \subset V_2$ or $W_2 \subset W_1$,*

$$E^n = (V_1 \oplus W_2) \oplus (V_2 \cap W_1). \tag{2.23}$$

Proof. In the proof of Lemma 2.3, exchange the roles of W_2 and V_2. Q.E.D.

Theorem 2.7 *Let $\boldsymbol{P}_1$ and $\boldsymbol{P}_2$ denote the projection matrices onto V_1 along W_1 and onto V_2 along W_2, respectively. Then the following three statements are equivalent:*

(i) $\boldsymbol{P}_1 + \boldsymbol{P}_2$ *is the projector onto $V_1 \oplus V_2$ along $W_1 \cap W_2$.*

(ii) $\boldsymbol{P}_1\boldsymbol{P}_2 = \boldsymbol{P}_2\boldsymbol{P}_1 = \boldsymbol{O}$.

(iii) $V_1 \subset W_2$ and $V_2 \subset W_1$. *(In this case, V_1 and V_2 are disjoint spaces.)*

Proof. (i) → (ii): From $(\boldsymbol{P}_1+\boldsymbol{P}_2)^2 = \boldsymbol{P}_1+\boldsymbol{P}_2$, $\boldsymbol{P}_1^2 = \boldsymbol{P}_1$, and $\boldsymbol{P}_2^2 = \boldsymbol{P}_2$, we have $\boldsymbol{P}_1\boldsymbol{P}_2 = -\boldsymbol{P}_2\boldsymbol{P}_1$. Pre- and postmutiplying both sides by $\boldsymbol{P}_1$, we obtain $\boldsymbol{P}_1\boldsymbol{P}_2 = -\boldsymbol{P}_1\boldsymbol{P}_2\boldsymbol{P}_1$ and $\boldsymbol{P}_1\boldsymbol{P}_2\boldsymbol{P}_1 = -\boldsymbol{P}_2\boldsymbol{P}_1$, respectively, which imply $\boldsymbol{P}_1\boldsymbol{P}_2 = \boldsymbol{P}_2\boldsymbol{P}_1$. This and $\boldsymbol{P}_1\boldsymbol{P}_2 = -\boldsymbol{P}_2\boldsymbol{P}_1$ lead to $\boldsymbol{P}_1\boldsymbol{P}_2 = \boldsymbol{P}_2\boldsymbol{P}_1 = \boldsymbol{O}$.

(ii) $\rightarrow$ (iii): For an arbitrary vector $\boldsymbol{x} \in V_1$, $\boldsymbol{P}_1\boldsymbol{x} = \boldsymbol{x}$ because $\boldsymbol{P}_1\boldsymbol{x} \in V_1$. Hence, $\boldsymbol{P}_2\boldsymbol{P}_1\boldsymbol{x} = \boldsymbol{P}_2\boldsymbol{x} = \boldsymbol{0}$, which implies $\boldsymbol{x} \in W_2$, and so $V_1 \subset W_2$. On the other hand, when $\boldsymbol{x} \in V_2$, it follows that $\boldsymbol{P}_2\boldsymbol{x} \in V_2$, and so $\boldsymbol{P}_1\boldsymbol{P}_2\boldsymbol{x} = \boldsymbol{P}_1\boldsymbol{x} = \boldsymbol{0}$, implying $\boldsymbol{x} \in W_2$. We thus have $V_2 \subset W_2$.

(iii) $\rightarrow$ (ii): For $\boldsymbol{x} \in E^n$, $\boldsymbol{P}_1\boldsymbol{x} \in V_1$, which implies $(\boldsymbol{I}_n - \boldsymbol{P}_2)\boldsymbol{P}_1\boldsymbol{x} = \boldsymbol{P}_1\boldsymbol{x}$, which holds for any $\boldsymbol{x}$. Thus, $(\boldsymbol{I}_n - \boldsymbol{P}_2)\boldsymbol{P}_1 = \boldsymbol{P}_1$, implying $\boldsymbol{P}_1\boldsymbol{P}_2 = \boldsymbol{O}$. We also have $\boldsymbol{x} \in E^n \Rightarrow \boldsymbol{P}_2\boldsymbol{x} \in V_2 \Rightarrow (\boldsymbol{I}_n - \boldsymbol{P}_1)\boldsymbol{P}_2\boldsymbol{x} = \boldsymbol{P}_2\boldsymbol{x}$, which again holds for any $\boldsymbol{x}$, which implies $(\boldsymbol{I}_n - \boldsymbol{P}_1)\boldsymbol{P}_2 = \boldsymbol{P}_2 \Rightarrow \boldsymbol{P}_1\boldsymbol{P}_2 = \boldsymbol{O}$. Similarly, $\boldsymbol{P}_2\boldsymbol{P}_1 = \boldsymbol{O}$.

(ii) $\rightarrow$ (i): An arbitrary vector $\boldsymbol{x} \in (V_1 \oplus V_2)$ can be decomposed into $\boldsymbol{x} = \boldsymbol{x}_1 + \boldsymbol{x}_2$, where $\boldsymbol{x}_1 \in V_1$ and $\boldsymbol{x}_2 \in V_2$. From $\boldsymbol{P}_1\boldsymbol{x}_2 = \boldsymbol{P}_1\boldsymbol{P}_2\boldsymbol{x} = \boldsymbol{0}$ and $\boldsymbol{P}_2\boldsymbol{x}_1 = \boldsymbol{P}_2\boldsymbol{P}_1\boldsymbol{x} = \boldsymbol{0}$, we have $(\boldsymbol{P}_1 + \boldsymbol{P}_2)\boldsymbol{x} = (\boldsymbol{P}_1 + \boldsymbol{P}_2)(\boldsymbol{x}_1 + \boldsymbol{x}_2) = \boldsymbol{P}_1\boldsymbol{x}_1 + \boldsymbol{P}_2\boldsymbol{x}_2 = \boldsymbol{x}_1 + \boldsymbol{x}_2 = \boldsymbol{x}$. On the other hand, by noting that $\boldsymbol{P}_1 = \boldsymbol{P}_1(\boldsymbol{I}_n - \boldsymbol{P}_2)$ and $\boldsymbol{P}_2 = \boldsymbol{P}_2(\boldsymbol{I}_n - \boldsymbol{P}_1)$ for any $\boldsymbol{x} \in (W_1 \cap W_2)$, we have $(\boldsymbol{P}_1 + \boldsymbol{P}_2)\boldsymbol{x} = \boldsymbol{P}_1(\boldsymbol{I}_n - \boldsymbol{P}_2)\boldsymbol{x} + \boldsymbol{P}_2(\boldsymbol{I}_n - \boldsymbol{P}_1)\boldsymbol{x} = \boldsymbol{0}$. Since $V_1 \subset W_2$ and $V_2 \subset W_1$, the decomposition on the right-hand side of (2.22) holds. Hence, we know $\boldsymbol{P}_1 + \boldsymbol{P}_2$ is the projector onto $V_1 \oplus V_2$ along $W_1 \cap W_2$ by Theorem 2.2. Q.E.D.

Note In the theorem above, $\boldsymbol{P}_1\boldsymbol{P}_2 = \boldsymbol{O}$ in (ii) does not imply $\boldsymbol{P}_2\boldsymbol{P}_1 = \boldsymbol{O}$. $\boldsymbol{P}_1\boldsymbol{P}_2 = \boldsymbol{O}$ corresponds with $V_2 \subset W_1$, and $\boldsymbol{P}_2\boldsymbol{P}_1 = \boldsymbol{O}$ with $V_1 \subset W_2$ in (iii). It should be clear that $V_1 \subset W_2 \Longleftrightarrow V_2 \subset W_1$ does not hold.

Theorem 2.8 *Given the decompositions of E^n in (2.21), the following three statements are equivalent:*

(i) $\boldsymbol{P}_2 - \boldsymbol{P}_1$ *is the projector onto* $V_2 \cap W_1$ *along* $V_1 \oplus W_2$.

(ii) $\boldsymbol{P}_1\boldsymbol{P}_2 = \boldsymbol{P}_2\boldsymbol{P}_1 = \boldsymbol{P}_1$.

(iii) $V_1 \subset V_2$ and $W_2 \subset W_1$.

Proof. (i) $\rightarrow$ (ii): $(\boldsymbol{P}_2 - \boldsymbol{P}_1)^2 = \boldsymbol{P}_2 - \boldsymbol{P}_1$ implies $2\boldsymbol{P}_1 = \boldsymbol{P}_1\boldsymbol{P}_2 + \boldsymbol{P}_2\boldsymbol{P}_1$. Pre- and postmultiplying both sides by $\boldsymbol{P}_2$, we obtain $\boldsymbol{P}_2\boldsymbol{P}_1 = \boldsymbol{P}_2\boldsymbol{P}_1\boldsymbol{P}_2$ and $\boldsymbol{P}_1\boldsymbol{P}_2 = \boldsymbol{P}_2\boldsymbol{P}_1\boldsymbol{P}_2$, respectively, which imply $\boldsymbol{P}_1\boldsymbol{P}_2 = \boldsymbol{P}_2\boldsymbol{P}_1 = \boldsymbol{P}_1$.

(ii) $\rightarrow$ (iii): For $\forall \boldsymbol{x} \in E^n$, $\boldsymbol{P}_1\boldsymbol{x} \in V_1$, which implies $\boldsymbol{P}_1\boldsymbol{x} = \boldsymbol{P}_2\boldsymbol{P}_1\boldsymbol{x} \in V_2$, which in turn implies $V_1 \subset V_2$. Let $\boldsymbol{Q}_j = \boldsymbol{I}_n - \boldsymbol{P}_j$ $(j = 1, 2)$. Then, $\boldsymbol{P}_1\boldsymbol{P}_2 = \boldsymbol{P}_1$ implies $\boldsymbol{Q}_1\boldsymbol{Q}_2 = \boldsymbol{Q}_2$, and so $\boldsymbol{Q}_2\boldsymbol{x} \in W_2$, which implies $\boldsymbol{Q}_2\boldsymbol{x} = \boldsymbol{Q}_1\boldsymbol{Q}_2\boldsymbol{x} \in W_1$, which in turn implies $W_2 \subset W_1$.

(iii) → (ii): From $V_1 \subset V_2$, for $\forall \boldsymbol{x} \in E^n$, $\boldsymbol{P}_1\boldsymbol{x} \in V_1 \subset V_2 \Rightarrow \boldsymbol{P}_2(\boldsymbol{P}_1\boldsymbol{x}) = \boldsymbol{P}_1\boldsymbol{x} \Rightarrow \boldsymbol{P}_2\boldsymbol{P}_1 = \boldsymbol{P}_1$. On the other hand, from $W_2 \subset W_1$, $\boldsymbol{Q}_2\boldsymbol{x} \in W_2 \subset W_1$ for $\forall \boldsymbol{x} \in E^n \Rightarrow \boldsymbol{Q}_1\boldsymbol{Q}_2\boldsymbol{x} = \boldsymbol{Q}_2\boldsymbol{x} \Rightarrow \boldsymbol{Q}_1\boldsymbol{Q}_2\boldsymbol{Q}_2 \Rightarrow (\boldsymbol{I}_n - \boldsymbol{P}_1)(\boldsymbol{I}_n - \boldsymbol{P}_2) = (\boldsymbol{I}_n - \boldsymbol{P}_2) \Rightarrow \boldsymbol{P}_1\boldsymbol{P}_2 = \boldsymbol{P}_1$.

(ii) → (i): For $\boldsymbol{x} \in (V_2 \cap W_1)$, it holds that $(\boldsymbol{P}_2 - \boldsymbol{P}_1)\boldsymbol{x} = \boldsymbol{Q}_1\boldsymbol{P}_2\boldsymbol{x} = \boldsymbol{Q}_1\boldsymbol{x} = \boldsymbol{x}$. On the other hand, let $\boldsymbol{x} = \boldsymbol{y} + \boldsymbol{z}$, where $\boldsymbol{y} \in V_1$ and $\boldsymbol{z} \in W_2$. Then, $(\boldsymbol{P}_2 - \boldsymbol{P}_1)\boldsymbol{x} = (\boldsymbol{P}_2 - \boldsymbol{P}_1)\boldsymbol{y} + (\boldsymbol{P}_2 - \boldsymbol{P}_1)\boldsymbol{z} = \boldsymbol{P}_2\boldsymbol{Q}_1\boldsymbol{y} + \boldsymbol{Q}_1\boldsymbol{P}_2\boldsymbol{z} = \boldsymbol{0}$. Hence, $\boldsymbol{P}_2 - \boldsymbol{P}_1$ is the projector onto $V_2 \cap W_1$ along $V_1 \oplus W_2$. Q.E.D.

Note As in Theorem 2.7, $\boldsymbol{P}_1\boldsymbol{P}_2 = \boldsymbol{P}_1$ does not necessarily imply $\boldsymbol{P}_2\boldsymbol{P}_1 = \boldsymbol{P}_1$. Note that $\boldsymbol{P}_1\boldsymbol{P}_2 = \boldsymbol{P}_1 \Longleftrightarrow W_2 \subset W_1$, and $\boldsymbol{P}_2\boldsymbol{P}_1 = \boldsymbol{P}_1 \Longleftrightarrow V_1 \subset V_2$.

Theorem 2.9 *When the decompositions in (2.21) and (2.22) hold, and if*

$$\boldsymbol{P}_1\boldsymbol{P}_2 = \boldsymbol{P}_2\boldsymbol{P}_1, \tag{2.24}$$

then $\boldsymbol{P}_1\boldsymbol{P}_2$ (or $\boldsymbol{P}_2\boldsymbol{P}_1$) is the projector onto $V_1 \cap V_2$ along $W_1 + W_2$.

Proof. $\boldsymbol{P}_1\boldsymbol{P}_2 = \boldsymbol{P}_2\boldsymbol{P}_1$ implies $(\boldsymbol{P}_1\boldsymbol{P}_2)^2 = \boldsymbol{P}_1\boldsymbol{P}_2\boldsymbol{P}_1\boldsymbol{P}_2 = \boldsymbol{P}_1^2\boldsymbol{P}_2^2 = \boldsymbol{P}_1\boldsymbol{P}_2$, indicating that $\boldsymbol{P}_1\boldsymbol{P}_2$ is a projection matrix. On the other hand, let $\boldsymbol{x} \in V_1 \cap V_2$. Then, $\boldsymbol{P}_1(\boldsymbol{P}_2\boldsymbol{x}) = \boldsymbol{P}_1\boldsymbol{x} = \boldsymbol{x}$. Furthermore, let $\boldsymbol{x} \in W_1 + W_2$ and $\boldsymbol{x} = \boldsymbol{x}_1 + \boldsymbol{x}_2$, where $\boldsymbol{x}_1 \in W_1$ and $\boldsymbol{x}_2 \in W_2$. Then, $\boldsymbol{P}_1\boldsymbol{P}_2\boldsymbol{x} = \boldsymbol{P}_1\boldsymbol{P}_2\boldsymbol{x}_1 + \boldsymbol{P}_1\boldsymbol{P}_2\boldsymbol{x}_2 = \boldsymbol{P}_2\boldsymbol{P}_1\boldsymbol{x}_1 + \boldsymbol{0} = \boldsymbol{0}$. Since $E^n = (V_1 \cap V_2) \oplus (W_1 \oplus W_2)$ by the corollary to Lemma 2.3, we know that $\boldsymbol{P}_1\boldsymbol{P}_2$ is the projector onto $V_1 \cap V_2$ along $W_1 \oplus W_2$. Q.E.D.

Note Using the theorem above, (ii) → (i) in Theorem 2.7 can also be proved as follows: From $\boldsymbol{P}_1\boldsymbol{P}_2 = \boldsymbol{O}$

$$\boldsymbol{Q}_1\boldsymbol{Q}_2 = (\boldsymbol{I}_n - \boldsymbol{P}_1)(\boldsymbol{I}_n - \boldsymbol{P}_2) = \boldsymbol{I}_n - \boldsymbol{P}_1 - \boldsymbol{P}_2 = \boldsymbol{Q}_2\boldsymbol{Q}_1.$$

Hence, $\boldsymbol{Q}_1\boldsymbol{Q}_2$ is the projector onto $W_1 \cap W_2$ along $V_1 \oplus V_2$, and $\boldsymbol{P}_1 + \boldsymbol{P}_2 = \boldsymbol{I}_n - \boldsymbol{Q}_1\boldsymbol{Q}_2$ is the projector onto $V_1 \oplus V_2$ along $W_1 \cap W_2$.

If we take $W_1 = V_1^{\perp}$ and $W_2 = V_2^{\perp}$ in the theorem above, $\boldsymbol{P}_1$ and $\boldsymbol{P}_2$ become orthogonal projectors.

Theorem 2.10 *Let $\boldsymbol{P}_1$ and $\boldsymbol{P}_2$ be the orthogonal projectors onto V_1 and V_2, respectively. Then the following three statements are equivalent:*

(i) $\boldsymbol{P}_1 + \boldsymbol{P}_2$ *is the orthogonal projector onto* $V_1 \dot{\oplus} V_2$.

(ii) $\boldsymbol{P}_1\boldsymbol{P}_2 = \boldsymbol{P}_2\boldsymbol{P}_1 = \boldsymbol{O}$.

(iii) V_1 *and* V_2 *are orthogonal.*

Theorem 2.11 *The following three statements are equivalent:*

(i) $\boldsymbol{P}_2 - \boldsymbol{P}_1$ *is the orthogonal projector onto* $V_2 \cap V_1^{\perp}$.

(ii) $\boldsymbol{P}_1\boldsymbol{P}_2 = \boldsymbol{P}_2\boldsymbol{P}_1 = \boldsymbol{P}_1$.

(iii) $V_1 \subset V_2$.

The two theorems above can be proved by setting $W_1 = V_1^{\perp}$ and $W_2 = V_2^{\perp}$ in Theorems 2.7 and 2.8.

Theorem 2.12 *The necessary and sufficient condition for $\boldsymbol{P}_1\boldsymbol{P}_2$ to be the orthogonal projector onto $V_1 \cap V_2$ is (2.24).*

Proof. Sufficiency is clear from Theorem 2.9. Necessity follows from $\boldsymbol{P}_1\boldsymbol{P}_2 = (\boldsymbol{P}_1\boldsymbol{P}_2)'$, which implies $\boldsymbol{P}_1\boldsymbol{P}_2 = \boldsymbol{P}_2\boldsymbol{P}_1$ since $\boldsymbol{P}_1\boldsymbol{P}_2$ is an orthogonal projector. Q.E.D.

We next present a theorem concerning projection matrices when E^n is expressed as a direct-sum of m subspaces, namely

$$E^n = V_1 \oplus V_2 \oplus \cdots \oplus V_m. \tag{2.25}$$

Theorem 2.13 *Let $\boldsymbol{P}_i$ $(i = 1, \cdots, m)$ be square matrices that satisfy*

$$\boldsymbol{P}_1 + \boldsymbol{P}_2 + \cdots + \boldsymbol{P}_m = \boldsymbol{I}_n. \tag{2.26}$$

Then the following three statements are equivalent:

$$\boldsymbol{P}_i\boldsymbol{P}_j = \boldsymbol{O} \;\; (i \neq j). \tag{2.27}$$

$$\boldsymbol{P}_i^2 = \boldsymbol{P}_i \;\; (i = 1, \cdots m). \tag{2.28}$$

$$\text{rank}(\boldsymbol{P}_1) + \text{rank}(\boldsymbol{P}_2) + \cdots + \text{rank}(\boldsymbol{P}_m) = n. \tag{2.29}$$

Proof. (i) → (ii): Multiply (2.26) by $\boldsymbol{P}_i$.

(ii) → (iii): Use $\text{rank}(\boldsymbol{P}_i) = \text{tr}(\boldsymbol{P}_i)$ when $\boldsymbol{P}_i^2 = \boldsymbol{P}_i$. Then,

$$\sum_{i=1}^{m} \text{rank}(\boldsymbol{P}_i) = \sum_{i=1}^{m} \text{tr}(\boldsymbol{P}_i) = \text{tr}\left(\sum_{i=1}^{m} \boldsymbol{P}_i\right) = \text{tr}(\boldsymbol{I}_n) = n.$$

(iii) → (i), (ii): Let $V_i = \text{Sp}(\boldsymbol{P}_i)$. From $\text{rank}(\boldsymbol{P}_i) = \dim(V_i)$, we obtain $\dim(V_1) + \dim(V_2) + \cdots \dim(V_m) = n$; that is, E^n is decomposed into the sum of m disjoint subspaces as in (2.26). By postmultiplying (2.26) by $\boldsymbol{P}_i$, we obtain

$$\boldsymbol{P}_1\boldsymbol{P}_i + \boldsymbol{P}_2\boldsymbol{P}_i + \cdots + \boldsymbol{P}_i(\boldsymbol{P}_i - \boldsymbol{I}_n) + \cdots + \boldsymbol{P}_m\boldsymbol{P}_i = \boldsymbol{O}.$$

Since $\text{Sp}(\boldsymbol{P}_1), \text{Sp}(\boldsymbol{P}_2), \cdots, \text{Sp}(\boldsymbol{P}_m)$ are disjoint, (2.27) and (2.28) hold from Theorem 1.4. Q.E.D.

Note $\boldsymbol{P}_i$ in Theorem 2.13 is a projection matrix. Let $E^n = V_1 \oplus \cdots \oplus V_r$, and let

$$V_{(i)} = V_1 \oplus \cdots \oplus V_{i-1} \oplus V_{i+1} \oplus \cdots \oplus V_r. \tag{2.30}$$

Then, $E^n = V_i \oplus V_{(i)}$. Let $\boldsymbol{P}_{i\cdot(i)}$ denote the projector onto V_i along $V_{(i)}$. This matrix coincides with the $\boldsymbol{P}_i$ that satisfies the four equations given in (2.26) through (2.29).

The following relations hold.

Corollary 1

$$\boldsymbol{P}_{1\cdot(1)} + \boldsymbol{P}_{2\cdot(2)} + \cdots + \boldsymbol{P}_{m\cdot(m)} = \boldsymbol{I}_n, \tag{2.31}$$

$$\boldsymbol{P}_{i\cdot(i)}^2 = \boldsymbol{P}_{i\cdot(i)} \;\; (i = 1, \cdots, m), \tag{2.32}$$

$$\boldsymbol{P}_{i\cdot(i)}\boldsymbol{P}_{j\cdot(j)} = \boldsymbol{O} \;\; (i \neq j). \tag{2.33}$$

Corollary 2 *Let $\boldsymbol{P}_{(i)\cdot i}$ denote the projector onto $V_{(i)}$ along V_i. Then the following relation holds:*

$$\boldsymbol{P}_{(i)\cdot i} = \boldsymbol{P}_{1\cdot(1)} + \cdots + \boldsymbol{P}_{i-1\cdot(i-1)} + \boldsymbol{P}_{i+1\cdot(i+1)} + \cdots + \boldsymbol{P}_{m\cdot(m)}. \tag{2.34}$$

Proof. The proof is straightforward by noting $\boldsymbol{P}_{i\cdot(i)} + \boldsymbol{P}_{(i)\cdot i} = \boldsymbol{I}_n$. Q.E.D.

Note The projection matrix $\boldsymbol{P}_{i\cdot(i)}$ onto V_i along $V_{(i)}$ is uniquely determined. Assume that there are two possible representations, $\boldsymbol{P}_{i\cdot(i)}$ and $\boldsymbol{P}^*_{i\cdot(i)}$. Then,

$$\boldsymbol{P}_{1\cdot(1)} + \boldsymbol{P}_{2\cdot(2)} + \cdots + \boldsymbol{P}_{m\cdot(m)} = \boldsymbol{P}^*_{1\cdot(1)} + \boldsymbol{P}^*_{2\cdot(2)} + \cdots + \boldsymbol{P}^*_{m\cdot(m)},$$

from which

$$(\boldsymbol{P}_{1\cdot(1)} - \boldsymbol{P}^*_{1\cdot(1)}) + (\boldsymbol{P}_{2\cdot(2)} - \boldsymbol{P}^*_{2\cdot(2)}) + \cdots + (\boldsymbol{P}_{m\cdot(m)} - \boldsymbol{P}^*_{m\cdot(m)}) = \boldsymbol{O}.$$

Each term in the equation above belongs to one of the respective subspaces V_1, V_2, $\cdots, V_m$, which are mutually disjoint. Hence, from Theorem 1.4, we obtain $\boldsymbol{P}_{i\cdot(i)} = \boldsymbol{P}^*_{i\cdot(i)}$. This indicates that when a direct-sum of E^n is given, an identity matrix $\boldsymbol{I}_n$ of order n is decomposed accordingly, and the projection matrices that constitute the decomposition are uniquely determined.

The following theorem due to Khatri (1968) generalizes Theorem 2.13.

Theorem 2.14 *Let $\boldsymbol{P}_i$ denote a square matrix of order n such that*

$$\boldsymbol{P} = \boldsymbol{P}_1 + \boldsymbol{P}_2 + \cdots + \boldsymbol{P}_m. \tag{2.35}$$

Consider the following four propositions:

(i) $\boldsymbol{P}_i^2 = \boldsymbol{P}_i \quad (i = 1, \cdots m)$,

(ii) $\boldsymbol{P}_i\boldsymbol{P}_j = \boldsymbol{O} \quad (i \neq j)$, *and* $\text{rank}(\boldsymbol{P}_i^2) = \text{rank}(\boldsymbol{P}_i)$,

(iii) $\boldsymbol{P}^2 = \boldsymbol{P}$,

(iv) $\text{rank}(\boldsymbol{P}) = \text{rank}(\boldsymbol{P}_1) + \cdots + \text{rank}(\boldsymbol{P}_m)$.

All other propositions can be derived from any two of (i), (ii), *and* (iii), *and* (i) *and* (ii) *can be derived from* (iii) *and* (iv).

Proof. That (i) and (ii) imply (iii) is obvious. To show that (ii) and (iii) imply (iv), we may use

$$\boldsymbol{P}^2 = \boldsymbol{P}_1^2 + \boldsymbol{P}_2^2 + \cdots + \boldsymbol{P}_m^2 \text{ and } \boldsymbol{P}^2 = \boldsymbol{P},$$

which follow from (2.35).

(ii), (iii) → (i): Postmultiplying (2.35) by $\boldsymbol{P}_i$, we obtain $\boldsymbol{P}\boldsymbol{P}_i = \boldsymbol{P}_i^2$, from which it follows that $\boldsymbol{P}_i^3 = \boldsymbol{P}_i^2$. On the other hand, $\text{rank}(\boldsymbol{P}_i^2) = \text{rank}(\boldsymbol{P}_i)$ implies that there exists $\boldsymbol{W}$ such that $\boldsymbol{P}_i^2\boldsymbol{W}_i = \boldsymbol{P}_i$. Hence, $\boldsymbol{P}_i^3 = \boldsymbol{P}_i^2 \Rightarrow \boldsymbol{P}_i^3\boldsymbol{W}_i = \boldsymbol{P}_i^2\boldsymbol{W}_i \Rightarrow \boldsymbol{P}_i(\boldsymbol{P}_i^2\boldsymbol{W}_i) = \boldsymbol{P}_i^2\boldsymbol{W} \Rightarrow \boldsymbol{P}_i^2 = \boldsymbol{P}_i$.

(iii), (iv) → (i), (ii): We have $\text{Sp}(\boldsymbol{P}) \oplus \text{Sp}(\boldsymbol{I}_n - \boldsymbol{P}) = E^n$ from $\boldsymbol{P}^2 = \boldsymbol{P}$. Hence, by postmultiplying the identity

$$\boldsymbol{P}_1 + \boldsymbol{P}_2 + \cdots + \boldsymbol{P}_m + (\boldsymbol{I}_n - \boldsymbol{P}) = \boldsymbol{I}_n$$

by $\boldsymbol{P}$, we obtain $\boldsymbol{P}_i^2 = \boldsymbol{P}_i$, and $\boldsymbol{P}_i\boldsymbol{P}_j = \boldsymbol{O}$ $(i \neq j)$. Q.E.D.

Next we consider the case in which subspaces have inclusion relationships like the following.

Theorem 2.15 *Let*

$$E^n = V_k \supset V_{k-1} \supset \cdots \supset V_2 \supset V_1 = \{\boldsymbol{0}\},$$

and let W_i denote a complement subspace of V_i. Let $\boldsymbol{P}_i$ be the orthogonal projector onto V_i along W_i, and let $\boldsymbol{P}_i^* = \boldsymbol{P}_i - \boldsymbol{P}_{i-1}$, where $\boldsymbol{P}_0 = \boldsymbol{O}$ and $\boldsymbol{P}_k = \boldsymbol{I}_n$. Then the following relations hold:

(i) $\boldsymbol{I}_n = \boldsymbol{P}_1^* + \boldsymbol{P}_2^* + \cdots + \boldsymbol{P}_k^*$.

(ii) $(\boldsymbol{P}_i^*)^2 = \boldsymbol{P}_i^*$.

(iii) $\boldsymbol{P}_i^*\boldsymbol{P}_j^* = \boldsymbol{P}_j^*\boldsymbol{P}_i^* = \boldsymbol{O}$ $(i \neq j)$.

(iv) *$\boldsymbol{P}_i$ is the projector onto $V_i \cap W_{i-1}$ along $V_{i-1} \oplus W_i$.*

Proof. (i): Obvious. (ii): Use $\boldsymbol{P}_i\boldsymbol{P}_{i-1} = \boldsymbol{P}_{i-1}\boldsymbol{P}_i = \boldsymbol{P}_{i-1}$. (iii): It follows from $(\boldsymbol{P}_i^*)^2 = \boldsymbol{P}_i^*$ that $\text{rank}(\boldsymbol{P}_i^*) = \text{tr}(\boldsymbol{P}_i^*) = \text{tr}(\boldsymbol{P}_i - \boldsymbol{P}_{i-1}) = \text{tr}(\boldsymbol{P}_i) - \text{tr}(\boldsymbol{P}_{i-1})$. Hence, $\sum_{i=1}^k \text{rank}(\boldsymbol{P}_i^*) = \text{tr}(\boldsymbol{P}_k) - \text{tr}(\boldsymbol{P}_0) = n$, from which $\boldsymbol{P}_i^*\boldsymbol{P}_j^* = \boldsymbol{O}$ follows by Theorem 2.13. (iv): Clear from Theorem 2.8(i). Q.E.D.

Note The theorem above does not presuppose that $\boldsymbol{P}_i$ is an orthogonal projector. However, if $W_i = V_i^\perp$, $\boldsymbol{P}_i$ and $\boldsymbol{P}_i^*$ are orthogonal projectors. The latter, in particular, is the orthogonal projector onto $V_i \cap V_{i-1}^\perp$.

2.3.2 Decomposition into nondisjoint subspaces

In this section, we present several theorems indicating how projectors are decomposed when the corresponding subspaces are not necessarily disjoint. We elucidate their meaning in connection with the commutativity of projectors.

We first consider the case in which there are two direct-sum decompositions of E^n, namely

$$E^n = V_1 \oplus W_1 = V_2 \oplus W_2,$$

as given in (2.21). Let $V_{12} = V_1 \cap V_2$ denote the product space between V_1 and V_2, and let V_3 denote a complement subspace to $V_1 + V_2$ in E^n. Furthermore, let $\boldsymbol{P}_{1+2}$ denote the projection matrix onto $V_{1+2} = V_1 + V_2$ along V_3, and let $\boldsymbol{P}_j$ $(j = 1, 2)$ represent the projection matrix onto V_j $(j = 1, 2)$ along W_j $(j = 1, 2)$. Then the following theorem holds.

Theorem 2.16 (i) *The necessary and sufficient condition for* $\boldsymbol{P}_{1+2} = \boldsymbol{P}_1 + \boldsymbol{P}_2 - \boldsymbol{P}_1\boldsymbol{P}_2$ *is*

$$(V_{1+2} \cap W_2) \subset (V_1 \oplus V_3). \tag{2.36}$$

(ii) *The necessary and sufficient condition for* $\boldsymbol{P}_{1+2} = \boldsymbol{P}_1 + \boldsymbol{P}_2 - \boldsymbol{P}_2\boldsymbol{P}_1$ *is*

$$(V_{1+2} \cap W_1) \subset (V_2 \oplus V_3). \tag{2.37}$$

Proof. (i): Since $V_{1+2} \supset V_1$ and $V_{1+2} \supset V_2$, $\boldsymbol{P}_{1+2} - \boldsymbol{P}_1$ is the projector onto $V_{1+2} \cap W_1$ along $V_1 \oplus V_3$ by Theorem 2.8. Hence, $\boldsymbol{P}_{1+2}\boldsymbol{P}_1 = \boldsymbol{P}_1$ and $\boldsymbol{P}_{1+2}\boldsymbol{P}_2 = \boldsymbol{P}_2$. Similarly, $\boldsymbol{P}_{1+2} - \boldsymbol{P}_2$ is the projector onto $V_{1+2} \cap W_2$ along $V_2 \oplus V_3$. Hence, by Theorem 2.8,

$$\boldsymbol{P}_{1+2} - \boldsymbol{P}_1 - \boldsymbol{P}_2 + \boldsymbol{P}_1\boldsymbol{P}_2 = \boldsymbol{O} \Longleftrightarrow (\boldsymbol{P}_{1+2} - \boldsymbol{P}_1)(\boldsymbol{P}_{1+2} - \boldsymbol{P}_2) = \boldsymbol{O}.$$

Furthermore,

$$(\boldsymbol{P}_{1+2} - \boldsymbol{P}_1)(\boldsymbol{P}_{1+2} - \boldsymbol{P}_2) = \boldsymbol{O} \Longleftrightarrow (V_{1+2} \cap W_2) \subset (V_1 \oplus V_3).$$

(ii): Similarly, $\boldsymbol{P}_{1+2} - \boldsymbol{P}_1 - \boldsymbol{P}_2 + \boldsymbol{P}_2\boldsymbol{P}_1 = \boldsymbol{O} \Longleftrightarrow (\boldsymbol{P}_{1+2} - \boldsymbol{P}_2)(\boldsymbol{P}_{1+2} - \boldsymbol{P}_1) = \boldsymbol{O} \Longleftrightarrow (V_{1+2} \cap W_1) \subset (V_2 \oplus V_3)$. Q.E.D.

Corollary *Assume that the decomposition (2.21) holds. The necessary and sufficient condition for* $\boldsymbol{P}_1\boldsymbol{P}_2 = \boldsymbol{P}_2\boldsymbol{P}_1$ *is that both (2.36) and (2.37) hold.*

The following theorem can readily be derived from the theorem above.

Theorem 2.17 *Let* $E^n = (V_1 + V_2) \oplus V_3$, $V_1 = V_{11} \oplus V_{12}$, *and* $V_2 = V_{22} \oplus V_{12}$, *where* $V_{12} = V_1 \cap V_2$. *Let* $\boldsymbol{P}^*_{1+2}$ *denote the projection matrix onto* $V_1 + V_2$ *along* V_3, *and let* $\boldsymbol{P}^*_1$ *and* $\boldsymbol{P}^*_2$ *denote the projectors onto* V_1 *along* $V_3 \oplus V_{22}$ *and onto* V_2 *along* $V_3 \oplus V_{11}$, *respectively. Then,*

$$\boldsymbol{P}^*_1\boldsymbol{P}^*_2 = \boldsymbol{P}^*_2\boldsymbol{P}^*_1 \tag{2.38}$$

and

$$\boldsymbol{P}^*_{1+2} = \boldsymbol{P}^*_1 + \boldsymbol{P}^*_2 - \boldsymbol{P}^*_1\boldsymbol{P}^*_2. \tag{2.39}$$

Proof. Since $V_{11} \subset V_1$ and $V_{22} \subset V_2$, we obtain

$$V_{1+2} \cap W_2 = V_{11} \subset (V_1 \oplus V_3) \text{ and } V_{1+2} \cap W_1 = V_{22} \subset (V_2 \oplus V_3)$$

by setting $W_1 = V_{22} \oplus V_3$ and $W_2 = V_{11} \oplus V_3$ in Theorem 2.16.
Another proof. Let $\boldsymbol{y} = \boldsymbol{y}_1 + \boldsymbol{y}_2 + \boldsymbol{y}_{12} + \boldsymbol{y}_3 \in E^n$, where $\boldsymbol{y}_1 \in V_{11}$, $\boldsymbol{y}_2 \in V_{22}$, $\boldsymbol{y}_{12} \in V_{12}$, and $\boldsymbol{y}_3 \in V_3$. Then it suffices to show that $(\boldsymbol{P}^*_1\boldsymbol{P}^*_2)\boldsymbol{y} = (\boldsymbol{P}^*_2\boldsymbol{P}^*_1)\boldsymbol{y}$. Q.E.D.

Let $\boldsymbol{P}_j$ $(j = 1, 2)$ denote the projection matrix onto V_j along W_j. Assume that $E^n = V_1 \oplus W_1 \oplus V_3 = V_2 \oplus W_2 \oplus V_3$ and $V_1 + V_2 = V_{11} \oplus V_{22} \oplus V_{12}$ hold. However, $W_1 = V_{22}$ may not hold, even if $V_1 = V_{11} \oplus V_{12}$. That is, (2.38) and (2.39) hold only when we set $W_1 = V_{22}$ and $W_2 = V_{11}$.

Theorem 2.18 *Let $\boldsymbol{P}_1$ and $\boldsymbol{P}_2$ be the orthogonal projectors onto V_1 and V_2, respectively, and let $\boldsymbol{P}_{1+2}$ denote the orthogonal projector onto V_{1+2}. Let $V_{12} = V_1 \cap V_2$. Then the following three statements are equivalent:*

(i) $\boldsymbol{P}_1\boldsymbol{P}_2 = \boldsymbol{P}_2\boldsymbol{P}_1$.

(ii) $\boldsymbol{P}_{1+2} = \boldsymbol{P}_1 + \boldsymbol{P}_2 - \boldsymbol{P}_1\boldsymbol{P}_2$.

(iii) $V_{11} = V_1 \cap V_{12}^\perp$ *and* $V_{22} = V_2 \cap V_{12}^\perp$ *are orthogonal.*

Proof. (i) → (ii): Obvious from Theorem 2.16.

(ii) → (iii): $\boldsymbol{P}_{1+2} = \boldsymbol{P}_1 + \boldsymbol{P}_2 - \boldsymbol{P}_1\boldsymbol{P}_2 \Rightarrow (\boldsymbol{P}_{1+2} - \boldsymbol{P}_1)(\boldsymbol{P}_{1+2} - \boldsymbol{P}_2) = (\boldsymbol{P}_{1+2} - \boldsymbol{P}_2)(\boldsymbol{P}_{1+2} - \boldsymbol{P}_1) = \boldsymbol{O} \Rightarrow V_{11}$ and V_{22} are orthogonal.

(iii) → (i): Set $V_3 = (V_1 + V_2)^\perp$ in Theorem 2.17. Since V_{11} and V_{22}, and V_1 and V_{22}, are orthogonal, the result follows. Q.E.D.

When $\boldsymbol{P}_1$, $\boldsymbol{P}_2$, and $\boldsymbol{P}_{1+2}$ are orthogonal projectors, the following corollary holds.

Corollary $\boldsymbol{P}_{1+2} = \boldsymbol{P}_1 + \boldsymbol{P}_2 - \boldsymbol{P}_1\boldsymbol{P}_2 \Longleftrightarrow \boldsymbol{P}_1\boldsymbol{P}_2 = \boldsymbol{P}_2\boldsymbol{P}_1$.

2.3.3 Commutative projectors

In this section, we focus on orthogonal projectors and discuss the meaning of Theorem 2.18 and its corollary. We also generalize the results to the case in which there are three or more subspaces.

Theorem 2.19 *Let* $\boldsymbol{P}_j$ *denote the orthogonal projector onto* V_j*. If* $\boldsymbol{P}_1\boldsymbol{P}_2 = \boldsymbol{P}_2\boldsymbol{P}_1$*,* $\boldsymbol{P}_1\boldsymbol{P}_3 = \boldsymbol{P}_3\boldsymbol{P}_1$*, and* $\boldsymbol{P}_2\boldsymbol{P}_3 = \boldsymbol{P}_3\boldsymbol{P}_2$*, the following relations hold:*

$$V_1 + (V_2 \cap V_3) = (V_1 + V_2) \cap (V_1 + V_3), \tag{2.40}$$

$$V_2 + (V_1 \cap V_3) = (V_1 + V_2) \cap (V_2 + V_3), \tag{2.41}$$

$$V_3 + (V_1 \cap V_2) = (V_1 + V_3) \cap (V_2 + V_3). \tag{2.42}$$

Proof. Let $\boldsymbol{P}_{1+(2\cap 3)}$ denote the orthogonal projector onto $V_1 + (V_2 \cap V_3)$. Then the orthogonal projector onto $V_2 \cap V_3$ is given by $\boldsymbol{P}_2\boldsymbol{P}_3$ (or by $\boldsymbol{P}_3\boldsymbol{P}_2$). Since $\boldsymbol{P}_1\boldsymbol{P}_2 = \boldsymbol{P}_2\boldsymbol{P}_1 \Rightarrow \boldsymbol{P}_1\boldsymbol{P}_2\boldsymbol{P}_3 = \boldsymbol{P}_2\boldsymbol{P}_3\boldsymbol{P}_1$, we obtain

$$\boldsymbol{P}_{1+(2\cap 3)} = \boldsymbol{P}_1 + \boldsymbol{P}_2\boldsymbol{P}_3 - \boldsymbol{P}_1\boldsymbol{P}_2\boldsymbol{P}_3$$

by Theorem 2.18. On the other hand, from $\boldsymbol{P}_1\boldsymbol{P}_2 = \boldsymbol{P}_2\boldsymbol{P}_1$ and $\boldsymbol{P}_1\boldsymbol{P}_3 = \boldsymbol{P}_3\boldsymbol{P}_1$, the orthogonal projectors onto $V_1 + V_2$ and $V_1 + V_3$ are given by

$$\boldsymbol{P}_{1+2} = \boldsymbol{P}_1 + \boldsymbol{P}_2 - \boldsymbol{P}_1\boldsymbol{P}_2 \text{ and } \boldsymbol{P}_{1+3} = \boldsymbol{P}_1 + \boldsymbol{P}_3 - \boldsymbol{P}_1\boldsymbol{P}_3,$$

respectively, and so $\boldsymbol{P}_{1+2}\boldsymbol{P}_{1+3} = \boldsymbol{P}_{1+3}\boldsymbol{P}_{1+2}$ holds. Hence, the orthogonal projector onto $(V_1 + V_2) \cap (V_1 + V_3)$ is given by

$$(\boldsymbol{P}_1 + \boldsymbol{P}_2 - \boldsymbol{P}_1\boldsymbol{P}_2)(\boldsymbol{P}_1 + \boldsymbol{P}_3 - \boldsymbol{P}_1\boldsymbol{P}_3) = \boldsymbol{P}_1 + \boldsymbol{P}_2\boldsymbol{P}_3 - \boldsymbol{P}_1\boldsymbol{P}_2\boldsymbol{P}_3,$$

which implies $\boldsymbol{P}_{1+(2\cap 3)} = \boldsymbol{P}_{1+2}\boldsymbol{P}_{1+3}$. Since there is a one-to-one correspondence between projectors and subspaces, (2.40) holds.

Relations (2.41) and (2.42) can be similarly proven by noting that $(\boldsymbol{P}_1 + \boldsymbol{P}_2 - \boldsymbol{P}_1\boldsymbol{P}_2)(\boldsymbol{P}_2 + \boldsymbol{P}_3 - \boldsymbol{P}_2\boldsymbol{P}_3) = \boldsymbol{P}_2 + \boldsymbol{P}_1\boldsymbol{P}_3 - \boldsymbol{P}_1\boldsymbol{P}_2\boldsymbol{P}_3$ and $(\boldsymbol{P}_1 + \boldsymbol{P}_3 - \boldsymbol{P}_1\boldsymbol{P}_3)(\boldsymbol{P}_2 + \boldsymbol{P}_3 - \boldsymbol{P}_2\boldsymbol{P}_3) = \boldsymbol{P}_3 + \boldsymbol{P}_1\boldsymbol{P}_2 - \boldsymbol{P}_1\boldsymbol{P}_2\boldsymbol{P}_3$, respectively.

Q.E.D.

The three identities from (2.40) to (2.42) indicate the distributive law of subspaces, which holds only if the commutativity of orthogonal projectors holds.

We now present a theorem on the decomposition of the orthogonal projectors defined on the sum space $V_1 + V_2 + V_3$ of V_1, V_2, and V_3.

Theorem 2.20 *Let* $\boldsymbol{P}_{1+2+3}$ *denote the orthogonal projector onto* $V_1 + V_2 + V_3$*, and let* $\boldsymbol{P}_1$*,* $\boldsymbol{P}_2$*, and* $\boldsymbol{P}_3$ *denote the orthogonal projectors onto* V_1*,* V_2*, and* V_3*, respectively. Then a sufficient condition for the decomposition*

$$\boldsymbol{P}_{1+2+3} = \boldsymbol{P}_1 + \boldsymbol{P}_2 + \boldsymbol{P}_3 - \boldsymbol{P}_1\boldsymbol{P}_2 - \boldsymbol{P}_2\boldsymbol{P}_3 - \boldsymbol{P}_3\boldsymbol{P}_1 + \boldsymbol{P}_1\boldsymbol{P}_2\boldsymbol{P}_3 \tag{2.43}$$

to hold is

$$\boldsymbol{P}_1\boldsymbol{P}_2 = \boldsymbol{P}_2\boldsymbol{P}_1,\ \ \boldsymbol{P}_2\boldsymbol{P}_3 = \boldsymbol{P}_3\boldsymbol{P}_2,\ \textit{and}\ \boldsymbol{P}_1\boldsymbol{P}_3 = \boldsymbol{P}_3\boldsymbol{P}_1. \tag{2.44}$$

Proof. $\boldsymbol{P}_1\boldsymbol{P}_2 = \boldsymbol{P}_2\boldsymbol{P}_1 \Rightarrow \boldsymbol{P}_{1+2} = \boldsymbol{P}_1 + \boldsymbol{P}_2 - \boldsymbol{P}_1\boldsymbol{P}_2$ and $\boldsymbol{P}_2\boldsymbol{P}_3 = \boldsymbol{P}_3\boldsymbol{P}_2 \Rightarrow \boldsymbol{P}_{2+3} = \boldsymbol{P}_2 + \boldsymbol{P}_3 - \boldsymbol{P}_2\boldsymbol{P}_3$. We therefore have $\boldsymbol{P}_{1+2}\boldsymbol{P}_{2+3} = \boldsymbol{P}_{2+3}\boldsymbol{P}_{1+2}$. We also have $\boldsymbol{P}_{1+2+3} = \boldsymbol{P}_{(1+2)+(1+3)}$, from which it follows that

$$\begin{aligned}\boldsymbol{P}_{1+2+3} &= \boldsymbol{P}_{(1+2)+(1+3)} = \boldsymbol{P}_{1+2} + \boldsymbol{P}_{1+3} - \boldsymbol{P}_{1+2}\boldsymbol{P}_{1+3}\\ &= (\boldsymbol{P}_1 + \boldsymbol{P}_2 - \boldsymbol{P}_1\boldsymbol{P}_2) + (\boldsymbol{P}_1 + \boldsymbol{P}_3 - \boldsymbol{P}_1\boldsymbol{P}_3)\\ &\qquad\qquad - (\boldsymbol{P}_2\boldsymbol{P}_3 + \boldsymbol{P}_1 - \boldsymbol{P}_1\boldsymbol{P}_2\boldsymbol{P}_3)\\ &= \boldsymbol{P}_1 + \boldsymbol{P}_2 + \boldsymbol{P}_3 - \boldsymbol{P}_1\boldsymbol{P}_2 - \boldsymbol{P}_2\boldsymbol{P}_3 - \boldsymbol{P}_1\boldsymbol{P}_3 + \boldsymbol{P}_1\boldsymbol{P}_2\boldsymbol{P}_3.\end{aligned}$$

An alternative proof. From $\boldsymbol{P}_1\boldsymbol{P}_{2+3} = \boldsymbol{P}_{2+3}\boldsymbol{P}_1$, we have $\boldsymbol{P}_{1+2+3} = \boldsymbol{P}_1 + \boldsymbol{P}_{2+3} - \boldsymbol{P}_1\boldsymbol{P}_{2+3}$. If we substitute $\boldsymbol{P}_{2+3} = \boldsymbol{P}_2 + \boldsymbol{P}_3 - \boldsymbol{P}_2\boldsymbol{P}_3$ into this equation, we obtain (2.43). Q.E.D.

Assume that (2.44) holds, and let

$$\boldsymbol{P}_{\tilde{1}} = \boldsymbol{P}_1 - \boldsymbol{P}_1\boldsymbol{P}_2 - \boldsymbol{P}_1\boldsymbol{P}_3 + \boldsymbol{P}_1\boldsymbol{P}_2\boldsymbol{P}_3,$$

$$\boldsymbol{P}_{\tilde{2}} = \boldsymbol{P}_2 - \boldsymbol{P}_2\boldsymbol{P}_3 - \boldsymbol{P}_1\boldsymbol{P}_2 + \boldsymbol{P}_1\boldsymbol{P}_2\boldsymbol{P}_3,$$

$$\boldsymbol{P}_{\tilde{3}} = \boldsymbol{P}_3 - \boldsymbol{P}_1\boldsymbol{P}_3 - \boldsymbol{P}_2\boldsymbol{P}_3 + \boldsymbol{P}_1\boldsymbol{P}_2\boldsymbol{P}_3,$$

$$\boldsymbol{P}_{12(3)} = \boldsymbol{P}_1\boldsymbol{P}_2 - \boldsymbol{P}_1\boldsymbol{P}_2\boldsymbol{P}_3,$$

$$P_{13(2)} = \boldsymbol{P}_1\boldsymbol{P}_3 - \boldsymbol{P}_1\boldsymbol{P}_2\boldsymbol{P}_3,$$

$$\boldsymbol{P}_{23(1)} = \boldsymbol{P}_2\boldsymbol{P}_3 - \boldsymbol{P}_1\boldsymbol{P}_2\boldsymbol{P}_3,$$

and

$$\boldsymbol{P}_{123} = \boldsymbol{P}_1\boldsymbol{P}_2\boldsymbol{P}_3.$$

Then,

$$\boldsymbol{P}_{1+2+3} = \boldsymbol{P}_{\tilde{1}} + \boldsymbol{P}_{\tilde{2}} + \boldsymbol{P}_{\tilde{3}} + \boldsymbol{P}_{12(3)} + \boldsymbol{P}_{13(2)} + \boldsymbol{P}_{23(1)} + \boldsymbol{P}_{123}. \tag{2.45}$$

Additionally, all matrices on the right-hand side of (2.45) are orthogonal projectors, which are also all mutually orthogonal.

Note Since $\boldsymbol{P}_{\tilde{1}} = \boldsymbol{P}_1(\boldsymbol{I}_n - \boldsymbol{P}_{2+3})$, $\boldsymbol{P}_{\tilde{2}} = \boldsymbol{P}_2(\boldsymbol{I}_n - \boldsymbol{P}_{1+3})$, $\boldsymbol{P}_{\tilde{3}} = \boldsymbol{P}_3(\boldsymbol{I} - \boldsymbol{P}_{1+2})$, $\boldsymbol{P}_{12(3)} = \boldsymbol{P}_1\boldsymbol{P}_2(\boldsymbol{I}_n - \boldsymbol{P}_3)$, $\boldsymbol{P}_{13(2)} = \boldsymbol{P}_1\boldsymbol{P}_3(\boldsymbol{I}_n - \boldsymbol{P}_2)$, and $\boldsymbol{P}_{23(1)} = \boldsymbol{P}_2\boldsymbol{P}_3(\boldsymbol{I}_n - \boldsymbol{P}_1)$, the decomposition of the projector $\boldsymbol{P}_{1\cup 2\cup 3}$ corresponds with the decomposition of the subspace $V_1 + V_2 + V_3$

$$V_1 + V_2 + V_3 = V_{\tilde{1}} \dot{\oplus} V_{\tilde{2}} \dot{\oplus} V_{\tilde{3}} \dot{\oplus} V_{12(3)} \dot{\oplus} V_{13(2)} \dot{\oplus} V_{23(1)} \dot{\oplus} V_{123}, \tag{2.46}$$

where $V_{\tilde{1}} = V_1 \cap (V_2 + V_3)^\perp$, $V_{\tilde{2}} = V_2 \cap (V_1 + V_3)^\perp$, $V_{\tilde{3}} = V_3 \cap (V_1 + V_2)^\perp$, $V_{12(3)} = V_1 \cap V_2 \cap V_3^\perp$, $V_{13(2)} = V_1 \cap V_2^\perp \cap V_3$, $V_{23(1)} = V_1^\perp \cap V_2 \cap V_3$, and $V_{123} = V_1 \cap V_2 \cap V_3$.

Theorem 2.20 can be generalized as follows.

Corollary *Let $V = V_1 + V_2 + \cdots + V_s$ $(s \geq 2)$. Let $\boldsymbol{P}_V$ denote the orthogonal projector onto V, and let $\boldsymbol{P}_j$ denote the orthogonal projector onto V_j. A sufficient condition for*

$$\boldsymbol{P}_V = \sum_{j=1}^{s} \boldsymbol{P}_j - \sum_{i<j} \boldsymbol{P}_i \boldsymbol{P}_j + \sum_{i<j<k} \boldsymbol{P}_i \boldsymbol{P}_j \boldsymbol{P}_k + \cdots + (-1)^{s-1} \boldsymbol{P}_1 \boldsymbol{P}_2 \boldsymbol{P}_3 \cdots \boldsymbol{P}_s \tag{2.47}$$

to hold is

$$\boldsymbol{P}_i \boldsymbol{P}_j = \boldsymbol{P}_j \boldsymbol{P}_i \ \ (i \neq j). \tag{2.48}$$

2.3.4 Noncommutative projectors

We now consider the case in which two subspaces V_1 and V_2 and the corresponding projectors $\boldsymbol{P}_1$ and $\boldsymbol{P}_2$ are given but $\boldsymbol{P}_1 \boldsymbol{P}_2 = \boldsymbol{P}_2 \boldsymbol{P}_1$ does not necessarily hold. Let $\boldsymbol{Q}_j = \boldsymbol{I}_n - \boldsymbol{P}_j$ $(j = 1, 2)$. Then the following lemma holds.

Lemma 2.4

$$\begin{aligned} V_1 + V_2 &= \mathrm{Sp}(\boldsymbol{P}_1) \oplus \mathrm{Sp}(\boldsymbol{Q}_1 \boldsymbol{P}_2) \quad &(2.49) \\ &= \mathrm{Sp}(\boldsymbol{Q}_2 \boldsymbol{P}_1) \oplus \mathrm{Sp}(\boldsymbol{P}_2). \quad &(2.50) \end{aligned}$$

Proof. $[\boldsymbol{P}_1, \boldsymbol{Q}_1 \boldsymbol{P}_2]$ and $[\boldsymbol{Q}_2 \boldsymbol{P}_1, \boldsymbol{P}_2]$ can be expressed as

$$[\boldsymbol{P}_1, \boldsymbol{Q}_1 \boldsymbol{P}_2] = [\boldsymbol{P}_1, \boldsymbol{P}_2] \begin{bmatrix} \boldsymbol{I}_n & -\boldsymbol{P}_2 \\ \boldsymbol{O} & \boldsymbol{I}_n \end{bmatrix} = [\boldsymbol{P}_1, \boldsymbol{P}_2] \boldsymbol{S}$$

and

$$[\boldsymbol{Q}_2 \boldsymbol{P}_1, \boldsymbol{P}_2] = [\boldsymbol{P}_1, \boldsymbol{P}_2] \begin{bmatrix} \boldsymbol{I}_n & \boldsymbol{O} \\ -\boldsymbol{P}_1 & \boldsymbol{I}_n \end{bmatrix} = [\boldsymbol{P}_1, \boldsymbol{P}_2] \boldsymbol{T}.$$

Since $\boldsymbol{S}$ and $\boldsymbol{T}$ are nonsingular, we have

$$\text{rank}(\boldsymbol{P}_1, \boldsymbol{P}_2) = \text{rank}(\boldsymbol{P}_1, \boldsymbol{Q}_1\boldsymbol{P}_2) = \text{rank}(\boldsymbol{Q}_2\boldsymbol{P}_1, \boldsymbol{P}_1),$$

which implies

$$V_1 + V_2 = \text{Sp}(\boldsymbol{P}_1, \boldsymbol{Q}_1\boldsymbol{P}_2) = \text{Sp}(\boldsymbol{Q}_2\boldsymbol{P}_1, \boldsymbol{P}_2).$$

Furthermore, let $\boldsymbol{P}_1\boldsymbol{x} + \boldsymbol{Q}_1\boldsymbol{P}_2\boldsymbol{y} = \boldsymbol{0}$. Premultiplying both sides by $\boldsymbol{P}_1$, we obtain $\boldsymbol{P}_1\boldsymbol{x} = \boldsymbol{0}$ (since $\boldsymbol{P}_1\boldsymbol{Q}_1 = \boldsymbol{O}$), which implies $\boldsymbol{Q}_1\boldsymbol{P}_2\boldsymbol{y} = \boldsymbol{0}$. Hence, $\text{Sp}(\boldsymbol{P}_1)$ and $\text{Sp}(\boldsymbol{Q}_1\boldsymbol{P}_2)$ give a direct-sum decomposition of $V_1 + V_2$, and so do $\text{Sp}(\boldsymbol{Q}_2\boldsymbol{P}_1)$ and $\text{Sp}(\boldsymbol{P}_2)$. Q.E.D.

The following theorem follows from Lemma 2.4.

Theorem 2.21 *Let $E^n = (V_1 + V_2) \oplus W$. Furthermore, let*

$$V_{2[1]} = \{\boldsymbol{x}|\boldsymbol{x} = \boldsymbol{Q}_1\boldsymbol{y}, \boldsymbol{y} \in V_2\} \tag{2.51}$$

and

$$V_{1[2]} = \{\boldsymbol{x}|\boldsymbol{x} = \boldsymbol{Q}_2\boldsymbol{y}, \boldsymbol{y} \in V_1\}. \tag{2.52}$$

Let $\boldsymbol{Q}_j = \boldsymbol{I}_n - \boldsymbol{P}_j$ $(j = 1, 2)$, where $\boldsymbol{P}_j$ is the orthogonal projector onto V_j, and let $\boldsymbol{P}^*$, $\boldsymbol{P}_1^*$, $\boldsymbol{P}_2^*$, $\boldsymbol{P}_{1[2]}$, and $\boldsymbol{P}_{2[1]}$ denote the projectors onto $V_1 + V_2$ along W, onto V_1 along $V_{2[1]} \oplus W$, onto V_2 along $V_{1[2]} \oplus W$, onto $V_{1[2]}$ along $V_2 \oplus W$, and onto $V_{2[1]}$ along $V_1 \oplus W$, respectively. Then,

$$\boldsymbol{P}^* = \boldsymbol{P}_1^* + \boldsymbol{P}_{2[1]}^* \tag{2.53}$$

or

$$\boldsymbol{P}^* = \boldsymbol{P}_{1[2]}^* + \boldsymbol{P}_2^* \tag{2.54}$$

holds.

Note When $W = (V_1 + V_2)^\perp$, $\boldsymbol{P}_j^*$ is the orthogonal projector onto V_j, while $\boldsymbol{P}_{j[i]}^*$ is the orthogonal projector onto $V_j[i]$.

Corollary *Let $\boldsymbol{P}$ denote the orthogonal projector onto $V = V_1 \oplus V_2$, and let $\boldsymbol{P}_j$ $(j = 1, 2)$ be the orthogonal projectors onto V_j. If V_i and V_j are orthogonal, the following equation holds:*

$$\boldsymbol{P} = \boldsymbol{P}_1 + \boldsymbol{P}_2. \tag{2.55}$$

2.4 Norm of Projection Vectors

We now present theorems concerning the norm of the projection vector $\boldsymbol{Px}$ ($\boldsymbol{x} \in E^n$) obtained by projecting $\boldsymbol{x}$ onto $\text{Sp}(\boldsymbol{P})$ along $\text{Ker}(\boldsymbol{P})$ by $\boldsymbol{P}$.

Lemma 2.5 $\boldsymbol{P}' = \boldsymbol{P}$ *and* $\boldsymbol{P}^2 = \boldsymbol{P} \Longleftrightarrow \boldsymbol{P}'\boldsymbol{P} = \boldsymbol{P}$.

(The proof is trivial and hence omitted.)

Theorem 2.22 *Let* $\boldsymbol{P}$ *denote a projection matrix (i.e.,* $\boldsymbol{P}^2 = \boldsymbol{P}$*). The necessary and sufficient condition to have*

$$||\boldsymbol{Px}|| \le ||\boldsymbol{x}|| \tag{2.56}$$

for an arbitrary vector $\boldsymbol{x}$ *is*

$$\boldsymbol{P}' = \boldsymbol{P}. \tag{2.57}$$

Proof. (Sufficiency) Let $\boldsymbol{x}$ be decomposed as $\boldsymbol{x} = \boldsymbol{Px} + (\boldsymbol{I}_n - \boldsymbol{P})\boldsymbol{x}$. We have $(\boldsymbol{Px})'(\boldsymbol{I}_n - \boldsymbol{P})\boldsymbol{x} = \boldsymbol{x}'(\boldsymbol{P}' - \boldsymbol{P}'\boldsymbol{P})\boldsymbol{x} = 0$ because $\boldsymbol{P}' = \boldsymbol{P} \Rightarrow \boldsymbol{P}'\boldsymbol{P} = \boldsymbol{P}'$ from Lemma 2.5. Hence,

$$||\boldsymbol{x}||^2 = ||\boldsymbol{Px}||^2 + ||(\boldsymbol{I}_n - \boldsymbol{P})\boldsymbol{x}||^2 \ge ||\boldsymbol{Px}||^2.$$

(Necessity) By assumption, we have $\boldsymbol{x}'(\boldsymbol{I}_n - \boldsymbol{P}'\boldsymbol{P})\boldsymbol{x} \ge 0$, which implies $\boldsymbol{I}_n - \boldsymbol{P}'\boldsymbol{P}$ is *nnd* with all nonnegative eigenvalues. Let $\lambda_1, \lambda_2, \cdots, \lambda_n$ denote the eigenvalues of $\boldsymbol{P}'\boldsymbol{P}$. Then, $1 - \lambda_j \ge 0$ or $0 \ge \lambda_j \ge 1$ $(j = 1, \cdots, n)$. Hence, $\sum_{j=1}^n \lambda_j^2 \le \sum_{j=1}^n \lambda_j$, which implies $\text{tr}(\boldsymbol{P}'\boldsymbol{P})^2 \le \text{tr}(\boldsymbol{P}'\boldsymbol{P})$.

On the other hand, we have

$$(\text{tr}(\boldsymbol{P}'\boldsymbol{P}))^2 = (\text{tr}(\boldsymbol{PP}'\boldsymbol{P}))^2 \le \text{tr}(\boldsymbol{P}'\boldsymbol{P})\text{tr}(\boldsymbol{P}'\boldsymbol{P})^2$$

from the generalized Schwarz inequality (set $\boldsymbol{A}' = \boldsymbol{P}$ and $\boldsymbol{B} = \boldsymbol{P}'\boldsymbol{P}$ in (1.19)) and $\boldsymbol{P}^2 = \boldsymbol{P}$. Hence, $\text{tr}(\boldsymbol{P}'\boldsymbol{P}) \le \text{tr}(\boldsymbol{P}'\boldsymbol{P})^2 \Rightarrow \text{tr}(\boldsymbol{P}'\boldsymbol{P}) = \text{tr}(\boldsymbol{P}'\boldsymbol{P})^2$, from which it follows that $\text{tr}\{(\boldsymbol{P} - \boldsymbol{P}'\boldsymbol{P})'(\boldsymbol{P} - \boldsymbol{P}'\boldsymbol{P})\} = \text{tr}\{\boldsymbol{P}'\boldsymbol{P} - \boldsymbol{P}'\boldsymbol{P} - \boldsymbol{P}'\boldsymbol{P} + (\boldsymbol{P}'\boldsymbol{P})^2\} = \text{tr}\{\boldsymbol{P}'\boldsymbol{P} - (\boldsymbol{P}'\boldsymbol{P})^2\} = 0$. Thus, $\boldsymbol{P} = \boldsymbol{P}'\boldsymbol{P} \Rightarrow \boldsymbol{P}' = \boldsymbol{P}$. Q.E.D.

Corollary *Let* $\boldsymbol{M}$ *be a symmetric pd matrix, and define the (squared) norm of* $\boldsymbol{x}$ *by*

$$||\boldsymbol{x}||_M^2 = \boldsymbol{x}'\boldsymbol{Mx}. \tag{2.58}$$

The necessary and sufficient condition for a projection matrix $\boldsymbol{P}$ *(satisfying* $\boldsymbol{P}^2 = \boldsymbol{P}$*) to satisfy*

$$||\boldsymbol{P}\boldsymbol{x}||^2_M \leq ||\boldsymbol{x}||^2_M \tag{2.59}$$

for an arbitrary n-component vector $\boldsymbol{x}$ *is given by*

$$(\boldsymbol{M}\boldsymbol{P})' = \boldsymbol{M}\boldsymbol{P}. \tag{2.60}$$

Proof. Let $\boldsymbol{M} = \boldsymbol{U}\boldsymbol{\Delta}^2\boldsymbol{U}'$ be the spectral decomposition of $\boldsymbol{M}$, and let $\boldsymbol{M}^{1/2} = \boldsymbol{\Delta}\boldsymbol{U}'$. Then, $\boldsymbol{M}^{-1/2} = \boldsymbol{U}\boldsymbol{\Delta}^{-1}$. Define $\boldsymbol{y} = \boldsymbol{M}^{1/2}\boldsymbol{x}$, and let $\tilde{\boldsymbol{P}} = \boldsymbol{M}^{1/2}\boldsymbol{P}\boldsymbol{M}^{-1/2}$. Then, $\tilde{\boldsymbol{P}}^2 = \tilde{\boldsymbol{P}}$, and (2.58) can be rewritten as $||\tilde{\boldsymbol{P}}\boldsymbol{y}||^2 \leq ||\boldsymbol{y}||^2$. By Theorem 2.22, the necessary and sufficient condition for (2.59) to hold is given by

$$\tilde{\boldsymbol{P}}^2 = \tilde{\boldsymbol{P}} \Longrightarrow (\boldsymbol{M}^{1/2}\boldsymbol{P}\boldsymbol{M}^{-1/2})' = \boldsymbol{M}^{1/2}\boldsymbol{P}\boldsymbol{M}^{-1/2}, \tag{2.61}$$

leading to (2.60). Q.E.D.

Note The theorem above implies that with an oblique projector $\boldsymbol{P}$ ($\boldsymbol{P}^2 = \boldsymbol{P}$, but $\boldsymbol{P}' \neq \boldsymbol{P}$) it is possible to have $||\boldsymbol{P}\boldsymbol{x}|| \geq ||\boldsymbol{x}||$. For example, let

$$\boldsymbol{P} = \begin{bmatrix} 1 & 1 \\ 0 & 0 \end{bmatrix} \text{ and } \boldsymbol{x} = \begin{pmatrix} 1 \\ 1 \end{pmatrix}.$$

Then, $||\boldsymbol{P}\boldsymbol{x}|| = 2$ and $||\boldsymbol{x}|| = \sqrt{2}$.

Theorem 2.23 *Let* $\boldsymbol{P}_1$ *and* $\boldsymbol{P}_2$ *denote the orthogonal projectors onto* V_1 *and* V_2*, respectively. Then, for an arbitrary* $\boldsymbol{x} \in E^n$*, the following relations hold:*

$$||\boldsymbol{P}_2\boldsymbol{P}_1\boldsymbol{x}|| \leq ||\boldsymbol{P}_1\boldsymbol{x}|| \leq ||\boldsymbol{x}|| \tag{2.62}$$

and, if $V_2 \subset V_1$,

$$||\boldsymbol{P}_2\boldsymbol{x}|| \leq ||\boldsymbol{P}_1\boldsymbol{x}||. \tag{2.63}$$

Proof. (2.62): Replace $\boldsymbol{x}$ by $\boldsymbol{P}_1\boldsymbol{x}$ in Theorem 2.22.

(2.63): By Theorem 2.11, we have $\boldsymbol{P}_1\boldsymbol{P}_2 = \boldsymbol{P}_2$, from which (2.63) follows immediately.

Let $\boldsymbol{x}_1, \boldsymbol{x}_2, \cdots, \boldsymbol{x}_p$ represent p n-component vectors in E^n, and define $\boldsymbol{X} = [\boldsymbol{x}_1, \boldsymbol{x}_2, \cdots, \boldsymbol{x}_p]$. From (1.15) and $\boldsymbol{P} = \boldsymbol{P}'\boldsymbol{P}$, the following identity holds:

$$||\boldsymbol{P}\boldsymbol{x}_1||^2 + ||\boldsymbol{P}\boldsymbol{x}_2||^2 + \cdots + ||\boldsymbol{P}\boldsymbol{x}_p||^2 = \text{tr}(\boldsymbol{X}'\boldsymbol{P}\boldsymbol{X}). \tag{2.64}$$

The above identity and Theorem 2.23 lead to the following corollary.

Corollary

(i) *If* $V_2 \subset V_1$, $\mathrm{tr}(\boldsymbol{X}'\boldsymbol{P}_2\boldsymbol{X}) \leq \mathrm{tr}(\boldsymbol{X}'\boldsymbol{P}_1\boldsymbol{X}) \leq \mathrm{tr}(\boldsymbol{X}'\boldsymbol{X})$.

(ii) *Let* $\boldsymbol{P}$ *denote an orthogonal projector onto an arbitrary subspace in* E^n. *If* $V_1 \supset V_2$,

$$\mathrm{tr}(\boldsymbol{P}_1\boldsymbol{P}) \geq \mathrm{tr}(\boldsymbol{P}_2\boldsymbol{P}).$$

Proof. (i): Obvious from Theorem 2.23. (ii): We have $\mathrm{tr}(\boldsymbol{P}_j\boldsymbol{P}) = \mathrm{tr}(\boldsymbol{P}_j\boldsymbol{P}^2)$ $= \mathrm{tr}(\boldsymbol{P}\boldsymbol{P}_j\boldsymbol{P})$ $(j = 1, 2)$, and $(\boldsymbol{P}_1 - \boldsymbol{P}_2)^2 = \boldsymbol{P}_1 - \boldsymbol{P}_2$, so that

$$\mathrm{tr}(\boldsymbol{P}\boldsymbol{P}_1\boldsymbol{P}) - \mathrm{tr}(\boldsymbol{P}\boldsymbol{P}_2\boldsymbol{P}) = \mathrm{tr}(\boldsymbol{S}\boldsymbol{S}') \geq 0,$$

where $\boldsymbol{S} = (\boldsymbol{P}_1 - \boldsymbol{P}_2)\boldsymbol{P}$. It follows that $\mathrm{tr}(\boldsymbol{P}_1\boldsymbol{P}) \geq \mathrm{tr}(\boldsymbol{P}_2\boldsymbol{P})$.

Q.E.D.

We next present a theorem on the trace of two orthogonal projectors.

Theorem 2.24 *Let* $\boldsymbol{P}_1$ *and* $\boldsymbol{P}_2$ *be orthogonal projectors of order* n. *Then the following relations hold:*

$$\mathrm{tr}(\boldsymbol{P}_1\boldsymbol{P}_2) = \mathrm{tr}(\boldsymbol{P}_2\boldsymbol{P}_1) \leq \min(\mathrm{tr}(\boldsymbol{P}_1), \mathrm{tr}(\boldsymbol{P}_2)). \tag{2.65}$$

Proof. We have $\mathrm{tr}(\boldsymbol{P}_1) - \mathrm{tr}(\boldsymbol{P}_1\boldsymbol{P}_2) = \mathrm{tr}(\boldsymbol{P}_1(\boldsymbol{I}_n - \boldsymbol{P}_2)) = \mathrm{tr}(\boldsymbol{P}_1\boldsymbol{Q}_2) =$ $\mathrm{tr}(\boldsymbol{P}_1\boldsymbol{Q}_2\boldsymbol{P}_1) = \mathrm{tr}(\boldsymbol{S}'\boldsymbol{S}) \geq 0$, where $\boldsymbol{S} = \boldsymbol{Q}_2\boldsymbol{P}_1$, establishing $\mathrm{tr}(\boldsymbol{P}_1) \geq$ $\mathrm{tr}(\boldsymbol{P}_1\boldsymbol{P}_2)$. Similarly, (2.65) follows from $\mathrm{tr}(\boldsymbol{P}_2) \geq \mathrm{tr}(\boldsymbol{P}_1\boldsymbol{P}_2) = \mathrm{tr}(\boldsymbol{P}_2\boldsymbol{P}_1)$.

Q.E.D.

Note From (1.19), we obtain

$$\mathrm{tr}(\boldsymbol{P}_1\boldsymbol{P}_2) \leq \sqrt{\mathrm{tr}(\boldsymbol{P}_1)\mathrm{tr}(\boldsymbol{P}_2)}. \tag{2.66}$$

However, (2.65) is more general than (2.66) because $\sqrt{\mathrm{tr}(\boldsymbol{P}_1)\mathrm{tr}(\boldsymbol{P}_2)} \geq \min(\mathrm{tr}(\boldsymbol{P}_1),$ $\mathrm{tr}(\boldsymbol{P}_2))$.

2.5 Matrix Norm and Projection Matrices

Let $\boldsymbol{A} = [a_{ij}]$ be an n by p matrix. We define its Euclidean norm (also called the Frobenius norm) by

$$||\boldsymbol{A}|| = \{\text{tr}(\boldsymbol{A}'\boldsymbol{A})\}^{1/2} = \sqrt{\sum_{i=1}^{n}\sum_{j=1}^{p} a_{ij}^2}. \tag{2.67}$$

Then the following four relations hold.

Lemma 2.6

$$||\boldsymbol{A}|| \geq 0. \tag{2.68}$$

$$||\boldsymbol{CA}|| \leq ||\boldsymbol{C}|| \cdot ||\boldsymbol{A}||, \tag{2.69}$$

Let both $\boldsymbol{A}$ *and* $\boldsymbol{B}$ *be* n *by* p *matrices. Then,*

$$||\boldsymbol{A} + \boldsymbol{B}|| \leq ||\boldsymbol{A}|| + ||\boldsymbol{B}||. \tag{2.70}$$

Let $\boldsymbol{U}$ *and* $\boldsymbol{V}$ *be orthogonal matrices of orders* n *and* p*, respectively. Then*

$$||\boldsymbol{UAV}|| = ||\boldsymbol{A}||. \tag{2.71}$$

Proof. Relations (2.68) and (2.69) are trivial. Relation (2.70) follows immediately from (1.20). Relation (2.71) is obvious from

$$\text{tr}(\boldsymbol{V}'\boldsymbol{A}'\boldsymbol{U}'\boldsymbol{UAV}) = \text{tr}(\boldsymbol{A}'\boldsymbol{AVV}') = \text{tr}(\boldsymbol{A}'\boldsymbol{A}).$$

Q.E.D.

Note Let $\boldsymbol{M}$ be a symmetric *nnd* matrix of order n. Then the norm defined in (2.67) can be generalized as

$$||\boldsymbol{A}||_M = \{\text{tr}(\boldsymbol{A}'\boldsymbol{MA})\}^{1/2}. \tag{2.72}$$

This is called the norm of $\boldsymbol{A}$ with respect to $\boldsymbol{M}$ (sometimes called a metric matrix). Properties analogous to those given in Lemma 2.6 hold for this generalized norm.

There are other possible definitions of the norm of $\boldsymbol{A}$. For example,

(i) $||\boldsymbol{A}||_1 = \max_j \sum_{i=1}^{n} |a_{ij}|$,
(ii) $||\boldsymbol{A}||_2 = \mu_1(\boldsymbol{A})$, where $\mu_1(\boldsymbol{A})$ is the largest singular value of $\boldsymbol{A}$ (see Chapter 5), and
(iii) $||\boldsymbol{A}||_3 = \max_i \sum_{j=1}^{p} |a_{ij}|$.

All of these norms satisfy (2.68), (2.69), and (2.70). (However, only $||\boldsymbol{A}||_2$ satisfies (2.71).)

Lemma 2.7 *Let* $\boldsymbol{P}$ *and* $\tilde{\boldsymbol{P}}$ *denote orthogonal projectors of orders* n *and* p*, respectively. Then,*

$$||\boldsymbol{PA}|| \leq ||\boldsymbol{A}|| \tag{2.73}$$

(the equality holds if and only if $\boldsymbol{PA} = \boldsymbol{A}$*) and*

$$||\boldsymbol{A}\tilde{\boldsymbol{P}}|| \leq ||\boldsymbol{A}|| \tag{2.74}$$

(the equality holds if and only if $\boldsymbol{A}\tilde{\boldsymbol{P}} = \boldsymbol{A}$*).*

Proof. (2.73): Square both sides and subtract the right-hand side from the left. Then,

$$\begin{aligned} \mathrm{tr}(\boldsymbol{A}'\boldsymbol{A}) - \mathrm{tr}(\boldsymbol{A}'\boldsymbol{PA}) &= \mathrm{tr}\{\boldsymbol{A}'(\boldsymbol{I}_n - \boldsymbol{P})\boldsymbol{A}\} \\ &= \mathrm{tr}(\boldsymbol{A}'\boldsymbol{QA}) = \mathrm{tr}(\boldsymbol{QA})'(\boldsymbol{QA}) \geq 0 \ \ (\text{where } \boldsymbol{Q} = \boldsymbol{I}_n - \boldsymbol{P}). \end{aligned}$$

The equality holds when $\boldsymbol{QA} = \boldsymbol{O} \Longleftrightarrow \boldsymbol{PA} = \boldsymbol{A}$.

(2.74): This can be proven similarly by noting that $||\boldsymbol{A}\tilde{\boldsymbol{P}}||^2 = \mathrm{tr}(\tilde{\boldsymbol{P}}\boldsymbol{A}'\boldsymbol{A}\tilde{\boldsymbol{P}}) = \mathrm{tr}(\boldsymbol{A}\tilde{\boldsymbol{P}}\boldsymbol{A}') = ||\tilde{\boldsymbol{P}}\boldsymbol{A}'||^2$. The equality holds when $\tilde{\boldsymbol{Q}}\boldsymbol{A}' = \boldsymbol{O} \Longleftrightarrow \tilde{\boldsymbol{P}}\boldsymbol{A}' = \boldsymbol{A}' \Longleftrightarrow \boldsymbol{A}\tilde{\boldsymbol{P}} = \boldsymbol{A}$, where $\tilde{\boldsymbol{Q}} = \boldsymbol{I}_n - \tilde{\boldsymbol{P}}$. Q.E.D.

The two lemmas above lead to the following theorem.

Theorem 2.25 *Let* $\boldsymbol{A}$ *be an* n *by* p *matrix,* $\boldsymbol{B}$ *and* $\boldsymbol{Y}$ n *by* r *matrices, and* $\boldsymbol{C}$ *and* $\boldsymbol{X}$ r *by* p *matrices. Then,*

$$||\boldsymbol{A} - \boldsymbol{BX}|| \geq ||(\boldsymbol{I}_n - \boldsymbol{P}_B)\boldsymbol{A}||, \tag{2.75}$$

where $\boldsymbol{P}_B$ *is the orthogonal projector onto* $\mathrm{Sp}(\boldsymbol{B})$*. The equality holds if and only if* $\boldsymbol{BX} = \boldsymbol{P}_B\boldsymbol{A}$*. We also have*

$$||\boldsymbol{A} - \boldsymbol{YC}|| \geq ||\boldsymbol{A}(\boldsymbol{I}_p - \boldsymbol{P}_{C'})||, \tag{2.76}$$

where $\boldsymbol{P}_{C'}$ *is the orthogonal projector onto* $\mathrm{Sp}(\boldsymbol{C}')$*. The equality holds if and only if* $\boldsymbol{YC} = \boldsymbol{AP}_{C'}$*. We also have*

$$||\boldsymbol{A} - \boldsymbol{BX} - \boldsymbol{YC}|| \geq ||(\boldsymbol{I}_n - \boldsymbol{P}_B)\boldsymbol{A}(\boldsymbol{I}_p - \boldsymbol{P}_{C'})||. \tag{2.77}$$

The equality holds if and only if

$$\boldsymbol{P}_B(\boldsymbol{A} - \boldsymbol{YC}) = \boldsymbol{BX} \text{ and } (\boldsymbol{I}_n - \boldsymbol{P}_B)\boldsymbol{AP}_{C'} = (\boldsymbol{I}_n - \boldsymbol{P}_B)\boldsymbol{YC} \tag{2.78}$$

or

$$(\boldsymbol{A}-\boldsymbol{B}\boldsymbol{X})\boldsymbol{P}_{C'}=\boldsymbol{Y}\boldsymbol{C} \text{ and } \boldsymbol{P}_B\boldsymbol{A}(\boldsymbol{I}_p-\boldsymbol{P}_{C'})=\boldsymbol{B}\boldsymbol{X}(\boldsymbol{I}_n-\boldsymbol{P}_{C'}). \quad (2.79)$$

Proof. (2.75): We have $(\boldsymbol{I}_n-\boldsymbol{P}_B)(\boldsymbol{A}-\boldsymbol{B}\boldsymbol{X})=\boldsymbol{A}-\boldsymbol{B}\boldsymbol{X}-\boldsymbol{P}_B\boldsymbol{A}+\boldsymbol{B}\boldsymbol{X}=(\boldsymbol{I}_n-\boldsymbol{P}_B)\boldsymbol{A}$. Since $\boldsymbol{I}_n-\boldsymbol{P}_B$ is an orthogonal projector, we have $||\boldsymbol{A}-\boldsymbol{B}\boldsymbol{X}|| \geq ||(\boldsymbol{I}_n-\boldsymbol{P}_B)(\boldsymbol{A}-\boldsymbol{B}\boldsymbol{X})||=||(\boldsymbol{I}_n-\boldsymbol{P}_B)\boldsymbol{A}||$ by (2.73) in Lemma 2.7. The equality holds when $(\boldsymbol{I}_n-\boldsymbol{P}_B)(\boldsymbol{A}-\boldsymbol{B}\boldsymbol{X})=\boldsymbol{A}-\boldsymbol{B}\boldsymbol{X}$, namely $\boldsymbol{P}_B\boldsymbol{A}=\boldsymbol{B}\boldsymbol{X}$.

(2.76): It suffices to use $(\boldsymbol{A}-\boldsymbol{Y}\boldsymbol{C})(\boldsymbol{I}_p-\boldsymbol{P}_{C'})=\boldsymbol{A}(\boldsymbol{I}_p-\boldsymbol{P}_{C'})$ and (2.74) in Lemma 2.7. The equality holds when $(\boldsymbol{A}-\boldsymbol{Y}\boldsymbol{C})(\boldsymbol{I}_p-\boldsymbol{P}_{C'})=\boldsymbol{A}-\boldsymbol{Y}\boldsymbol{C}$ holds, which implies $\boldsymbol{Y}\boldsymbol{C}=\boldsymbol{A}\boldsymbol{P}_{C'}$.

(2.77): $||\boldsymbol{A}-\boldsymbol{B}\boldsymbol{X}-\boldsymbol{Y}\boldsymbol{C}|| \geq ||(\boldsymbol{I}_n-\boldsymbol{P}_B)(\boldsymbol{A}-\boldsymbol{Y}\boldsymbol{C})|| \geq ||(\boldsymbol{I}_n-\boldsymbol{P}_B)\boldsymbol{A}(\boldsymbol{I}_p-\boldsymbol{P}_{C'})||$ or $||\boldsymbol{A}-\boldsymbol{B}\boldsymbol{X}-\boldsymbol{Y}\boldsymbol{C}|| \geq ||(\boldsymbol{A}-\boldsymbol{B}\boldsymbol{X})(\boldsymbol{I}_p-\boldsymbol{P}_{C'})|| \geq ||(\boldsymbol{I}_p-\boldsymbol{P}_B)\boldsymbol{A}(\boldsymbol{I}_p-\boldsymbol{P}_{C'})||$. The first equality condition (2.78) follows from the first relation above, and the second equality condition (2.79) follows from the second relation above. Q.E.D.

Note Relations (2.75), (2.76), and (2.77) can also be shown by the least squares method. Here we show this only for (2.77). We have

$$\begin{aligned}||\boldsymbol{A}-\boldsymbol{B}\boldsymbol{X}-\boldsymbol{Y}\boldsymbol{C}||^2 &= \text{tr}\{(\boldsymbol{A}-\boldsymbol{B}\boldsymbol{X}-\boldsymbol{Y}\boldsymbol{C})'(\boldsymbol{A}-\boldsymbol{B}\boldsymbol{X}-\boldsymbol{Y}\boldsymbol{C})\}\\ &= \text{tr}(\boldsymbol{A}-\boldsymbol{Y}\boldsymbol{C})'(\boldsymbol{A}-\boldsymbol{Y}\boldsymbol{C})-2\text{tr}(\boldsymbol{B}\boldsymbol{X})'(\boldsymbol{A}-\boldsymbol{Y}\boldsymbol{C})+\text{tr}(\boldsymbol{B}\boldsymbol{X})'(\boldsymbol{B}\boldsymbol{X})\end{aligned}$$

to be minimized. Differentiating the criterion above by $\boldsymbol{X}$ and setting the result to zero, we obtain $\boldsymbol{B}'(\boldsymbol{A}-\boldsymbol{Y}\boldsymbol{C})=\boldsymbol{B}'\boldsymbol{B}\boldsymbol{X}$. Premultiplying this equation by $\boldsymbol{B}(\boldsymbol{B}'\boldsymbol{B})^{-1}$, we obtain $\boldsymbol{P}_B(\boldsymbol{A}-\boldsymbol{Y}\boldsymbol{C})=\boldsymbol{B}\boldsymbol{X}$. Furthermore, we may expand the criterion above as

$$\text{tr}(\boldsymbol{A}-\boldsymbol{B}\boldsymbol{X})'(\boldsymbol{A}-\boldsymbol{B}\boldsymbol{X})-2\text{tr}(\boldsymbol{Y}\boldsymbol{C}(\boldsymbol{A}-\boldsymbol{B}\boldsymbol{X})')+\text{tr}(\boldsymbol{Y}\boldsymbol{C})(\boldsymbol{Y}\boldsymbol{C})'.$$

Differentiating this criterion with respect to $\boldsymbol{Y}$ and setting the result equal to zero, we obtain $\boldsymbol{C}(\boldsymbol{A}-\boldsymbol{B}\boldsymbol{X})=\boldsymbol{C}\boldsymbol{C}'\boldsymbol{Y}'$ or $(\boldsymbol{A}-\boldsymbol{B}\boldsymbol{X})\boldsymbol{C}'=\boldsymbol{Y}\boldsymbol{C}\boldsymbol{C}'$. Postmultiplying the latter by $(\boldsymbol{C}\boldsymbol{C}')^{-1}\boldsymbol{C}'$, we obtain $(\boldsymbol{A}-\boldsymbol{B}\boldsymbol{X})\boldsymbol{P}_{C'}=\boldsymbol{Y}\boldsymbol{C}$. Substituting this into $\boldsymbol{P}_B(\boldsymbol{A}-\boldsymbol{Y}\boldsymbol{C})=\boldsymbol{B}\boldsymbol{X}$, we obtain $\boldsymbol{P}_B\boldsymbol{A}(\boldsymbol{I}_p-\boldsymbol{P}_{C'})=\boldsymbol{B}\boldsymbol{X}(\boldsymbol{I}_p-\boldsymbol{P}_{C'})$ after some simplification. If, on the other hand, $\boldsymbol{B}\boldsymbol{X}=\boldsymbol{P}_B(\boldsymbol{A}-\boldsymbol{Y}\boldsymbol{C})$ is substituted into $(\boldsymbol{A}-\boldsymbol{B}\boldsymbol{X})\boldsymbol{P}_{C'}=\boldsymbol{Y}\boldsymbol{C}$, we obtain $(\boldsymbol{I}_n-\boldsymbol{P}_B)\boldsymbol{A}\boldsymbol{P}_{C'}=(\boldsymbol{I}_n-\boldsymbol{P}_B)\boldsymbol{Y}\boldsymbol{C}$. (In the derivation above, the regular inverses can be replaced by the respective generalized inverses. See the next chapter.)

2.6 General Form of Projection Matrices

The projectors we have been discussing so far are based on Definition 2.1, namely square matrices that satisfy $\boldsymbol{P}^2 = \boldsymbol{P}$ (idempotency). In this section, we introduce a generalized form of projection matrices that do not necessarily satisfy $\boldsymbol{P}^2 = \boldsymbol{P}$, based on Rao (1974) and Rao and Yanai (1979).

Definition 2.3 *Let $V \subset E^n$ (but $V \neq E^n$) be decomposed as a direct-sum of m subspaces, namely $V = V_1 \oplus V_2 \oplus \cdots \oplus V_m$. A square matrix $\boldsymbol{P}_j^*$ of order n that maps an arbitrary vector $\boldsymbol{y}$ in V into V_j is called the projection matrix onto V_j along $V_{(j)} = V_1 \oplus \cdots \oplus V_{j-1} \oplus V_{j+1} \oplus \cdots \oplus V_m$ if and only if*

$$\boldsymbol{P}_j^* \boldsymbol{x} = \boldsymbol{x} \quad \forall \boldsymbol{x} \in V_j \ \ (j = 1, \cdots, m) \tag{2.80}$$

and

$$\boldsymbol{P}_j^* \boldsymbol{x} = \boldsymbol{0} \quad \forall \boldsymbol{x} \in V_{(j)} \ \ (j = 1, \cdots, m). \tag{2.81}$$

Let $\boldsymbol{x}_j \in V_j$. Then any $\boldsymbol{x} \in V$ can be expressed as

$$\boldsymbol{x} = \boldsymbol{x}_1 + \boldsymbol{x}_2 + \cdots + \boldsymbol{x}_m = (\boldsymbol{P}_1^* + \boldsymbol{P}_2^* + \cdots \boldsymbol{P}_m^*)\boldsymbol{x}.$$

Premultiplying the equation above by $\boldsymbol{P}_j^*$, we obtain

$$\boldsymbol{P}_i^* \boldsymbol{P}_j^* \boldsymbol{x} = \boldsymbol{0} \ \ (i \neq j) \ \text{ and } \ (\boldsymbol{P}_j^*)^2 \boldsymbol{x} = \boldsymbol{P}_j^* \boldsymbol{x} \ \ (i = 1, \cdots, m) \tag{2.82}$$

since $\text{Sp}(\boldsymbol{P}_1), \text{Sp}(\boldsymbol{P}_2), \cdots, \text{Sp}(\boldsymbol{P}_m)$ are mutually disjoint. However, $\boldsymbol{V}$ does not cover the entire E^n ($\boldsymbol{x} \in V \neq E^n$), so (2.82) does not imply $(\boldsymbol{P}_j^*)^2 = \boldsymbol{P}_j^*$ or $\boldsymbol{P}_i^* \boldsymbol{P}_j^* = \boldsymbol{O}$ $(i \neq j)$.

Let V_1 and $V_2 \in E^3$ denote the subspaces spanned by $\boldsymbol{e}_1 = (0, 0, 1)'$ and $\boldsymbol{e}_2 = (0, 1, 0)'$, respectively. Suppose

$$\boldsymbol{P}^* = \begin{bmatrix} a & 0 & 0 \\ b & 0 & 0 \\ c & 0 & 1 \end{bmatrix}.$$

Then, $\boldsymbol{P}^* \boldsymbol{e}_1 = \boldsymbol{e}_1$ and $\boldsymbol{P}^* \boldsymbol{e}_2 = \boldsymbol{0}$, so that $\boldsymbol{P}^*$ is the projector onto V_1 along V_2 according to Definition 2.3. However, $(\boldsymbol{P}^*)^2 \neq \boldsymbol{P}^*$ except when $a = b = 0$, or $a = 1$ and $c = 0$. That is, when V does not cover the entire space E^n, the projector $\boldsymbol{P}_j^*$ in the sense of Definition 2.3 is not idempotent. However, by specifying a complement subspace of V, we can construct an idempotent matrix from $\boldsymbol{P}_j^*$ as follows.

Theorem 2.26 *Let P_j^* $(j = 1, \cdots, m)$ denote the projector in the sense of Definition 2.3, and let P denote the projector onto V along V_{m+1}, where $V = V_1 \oplus V_2 \oplus \cdots \oplus V_m$ is a subspace in E^n and where V_{m+1} is a complement subspace to V. Then,*

$$P_j = P_j^* P \ (j = 1, \cdots m) \text{ and } P_{m+1} = I_n - P \tag{2.83}$$

are projectors (in the sense of Definition 2.1) onto V_j $(j = 1, \cdots, m+1)$ along $V_{(j)}^* = V_1 \oplus \cdots \oplus V_{j-1} \oplus V_{j+1} \oplus \cdots \oplus V_m \oplus V_{m+1}$.

Proof. Let $x \in V$. If $x \in V_j$ $(j = 1, \cdots, m)$, we have $P_j^* P x = P_j^* x = x$. On the other hand, if $x \in V_i$ $(i \neq j, i = 1, \cdots, m)$, we have $P_j^* P x = P_j^* x = 0$. Furthermore, if $x \in V_{m+1}$, we have $P_j^* P x = 0$ $(j = 1, \cdots, m)$. On the other hand, if $x \in V$, we have $P_{m+1} x = (I_n - P) x = x - x = 0$, and if $x \in V_{m+1}$, $P_{m+1} x = (I_n - P) x = x - 0 = x$. Hence, by Theorem 2.2, P_j $(j = 1, \cdots, m+1)$ is the projector onto V_j along $V_{(j)}$. Q.E.D.

2.7 Exercises for Chapter 2

1. Let $\tilde{A} = \begin{bmatrix} A_1 & O \\ O & A_2 \end{bmatrix}$ and $A = \begin{bmatrix} A_1 \\ A_2 \end{bmatrix}$. Show that $P_{\tilde{A}} P_A = P_A$.

2. Let P_A and P_B denote the orthogonal projectors onto Sp(A) and Sp(B), respectively. Show that the necessary and sufficient condition for $\text{Sp}(A) = \{\text{Sp}(A) \cap \text{Sp}(B)\} \dot{\oplus} \{\text{Sp}(A) \cap \text{Sp}(B)^\perp\}$ is $P_A P_B = P_B P_A$.

3. Let P be a square matrix of order n such that $P^2 = P$, and suppose

$$||Px|| = ||x||$$

for any n-component vector x. Show the following:
(i) When $x \in (\text{Ker}(P))^\perp$, $Px = x$.
(ii) $P' = P$.

4. Let $\text{Sp}(A) = \text{Sp}(A_1) \dot{\oplus} \cdots \dot{\oplus} \text{Sp}(A_m)$, and let P_j $(j = 1, \cdots, m)$ denote the projector onto Sp(A_j). For $\forall x \in E^n$:
(i) Show that

$$||x||^2 \geq ||P_1 x||^2 + ||P_2 x||^2 + \cdots + ||P_m x||^2. \tag{2.84}$$

(Also, show that the equality holds if and only if $\text{Sp}(A) = E^n$.)
(ii) Show that Sp(A_i) and Sp(A_j) $(i \neq j)$ are orthogonal if $\text{Sp}(A) = \text{Sp}(A_1) \oplus \text{Sp}(A_2) \oplus \cdots \oplus \text{Sp}(A_m)$ and the inequality in (i) above holds.
(iii) Let $P_{[j]} = P_1 + P_2 + \cdots + P_j$. Show that

$$||P_{[m]} x|| \geq ||P_{[m-1]} x|| \geq \cdots \geq ||P_{[2]} x|| \geq ||P_{[1]} x||.$$

5. Let $E^n = V_1 \oplus W_1 = V_2 \oplus W_2 = V_3 \oplus W_3$, and let $\boldsymbol{P}_j$ denote the projector onto V_j $(j = 1, 2, 3)$ along W_j. Show the following:
(i) Let $\boldsymbol{P}_i\boldsymbol{P}_j = \boldsymbol{O}$ for $i \neq j$. Then, $\boldsymbol{P}_1 + \boldsymbol{P}_2 + \boldsymbol{P}_3$ is the projector onto $V_1 + V_2 + V_3$ along $W_1 \cap W_2 \cap W_3$.
(ii) Let $\boldsymbol{P}_1\boldsymbol{P}_2 = \boldsymbol{P}_2\boldsymbol{P}_1$, $\boldsymbol{P}_1\boldsymbol{P}_3 = \boldsymbol{P}_3\boldsymbol{P}_1$, and $\boldsymbol{P}_2\boldsymbol{P}_3 = \boldsymbol{P}_3\boldsymbol{P}_2$. Then $\boldsymbol{P}_1\boldsymbol{P}_2\boldsymbol{P}_3$ is the projector onto $V_1 \cap V_2 \cap V_3$ along $W_1 + W_2 + W_3$.
(iii) Suppose that the three identities in (ii) hold, and let $\boldsymbol{P}_{1+2+3}$ denote the projection matrix onto $V_1 + V_2 + V_3$ along $W_1 \cap W_2 \cap W_3$. Show that

$$\boldsymbol{P}_{1+2+3} = \boldsymbol{P}_1 + \boldsymbol{P}_2 + \boldsymbol{P}_3 - \boldsymbol{P}_1\boldsymbol{P}_2 - \boldsymbol{P}_2\boldsymbol{P}_3 - \boldsymbol{P}_1\boldsymbol{P}_3 + \boldsymbol{P}_1\boldsymbol{P}_2\boldsymbol{P}_3.$$

6. Show that

$$\boldsymbol{Q}_{[A,B]} = \boldsymbol{Q}_A\boldsymbol{Q}_{Q_AB},$$

where $\boldsymbol{Q}_{[A,B]}$, $\boldsymbol{Q}_A$, and $\boldsymbol{Q}_{Q_AB}$ are the orthogonal projectors onto the null space of $[\boldsymbol{A}, \boldsymbol{B}]$, onto the null space of $\boldsymbol{A}$, and onto the null space of $\boldsymbol{Q}_A\boldsymbol{B}$, respectively.

7. (a) Show that

$$\boldsymbol{P}_X = \boldsymbol{P}_{XA} + \boldsymbol{P}_{X(X'X)^{-1}B},$$

where $\boldsymbol{P}_X$, $\boldsymbol{P}_{XA}$, and $\boldsymbol{P}_{X(X'X)^{-1}B}$ are the orthogonal projectors onto $\text{Sp}(\boldsymbol{X})$, $\text{Sp}(\boldsymbol{X}\boldsymbol{A})$, and $\text{Sp}(\boldsymbol{X}(\boldsymbol{X}'\boldsymbol{X})^{-1}\boldsymbol{B})$, respectively, and $\boldsymbol{A}$ and $\boldsymbol{B}$ are such that $\text{Ker}(\boldsymbol{A}') = \text{Sp}(\boldsymbol{B})$.
(b) Use the decomposition above to show that

$$\boldsymbol{P}_{[X_1,X_2]} = \boldsymbol{P}_{X_1} + \boldsymbol{P}_{Q_{X_1}X_2},$$

where $\boldsymbol{X} = [\boldsymbol{X}_1, \boldsymbol{X}_2]$, $\boldsymbol{P}_{Q_{X_1}X_2}$ is the orthogonal projector onto $\text{Sp}(\boldsymbol{Q}_{X_1}\boldsymbol{X}_2)$, and $\boldsymbol{Q}_{X_1} = \boldsymbol{I} - \boldsymbol{X}_1(\boldsymbol{X}_1'\boldsymbol{X}_1)^{-1}\boldsymbol{X}_1'$.

8. Let $E^n = V_1 \oplus W_1 = V_2 \oplus W_2$, and let $\boldsymbol{P}_1 = \boldsymbol{P}_{V_1 \cdot W_1}$ and $\boldsymbol{P}_2 = \boldsymbol{P}_{V_2 \cdot W_2}$ be two projectors (not necessarily orthogonal) of the same size. Show the following:
(a) The necessary and sufficient condition for $\boldsymbol{P}_1\boldsymbol{P}_2$ to be a projector is $V_{12} \subset V_2 \oplus (W_1 \cap W_2)$, where $V_{12} = \text{Sp}(\boldsymbol{P}_1\boldsymbol{P}_2)$ (Brown and Page, 1970).
(b) The condition in (a) is equivalent to $V_2 \subset V_1 \oplus (W_1 \cap V_2) \oplus (W_1 \cap W_2)$ (Werner, 1992).

9. Let $\boldsymbol{A}$ and $\boldsymbol{B}$ be n by a $(n \geq a)$ and n by b $(n \geq b)$ matrices, respectively. Let $\boldsymbol{P}_A$ and $\boldsymbol{P}_B$ be the orthogonal projectors defined by $\boldsymbol{A}$ and $\boldsymbol{B}$, and let $\boldsymbol{Q}_A$ and $\boldsymbol{Q}_B$ be their orthogonal complements. Show that the following six statements are equivalent: (1) $\boldsymbol{P}_A\boldsymbol{P}_B = \boldsymbol{P}_B\boldsymbol{P}_A$, (2) $\boldsymbol{A}'\boldsymbol{B} = \boldsymbol{A}'\boldsymbol{P}_B\boldsymbol{P}_A\boldsymbol{B}$, (3) $(\boldsymbol{P}_A\boldsymbol{P}_B)^2 = \boldsymbol{P}_A\boldsymbol{P}_B$, (4) $\boldsymbol{P}_{[A,B]} = \boldsymbol{P}_A + \boldsymbol{P}_B - \boldsymbol{P}_A\boldsymbol{P}_B$, (5) $\boldsymbol{A}'\boldsymbol{Q}_B\boldsymbol{Q}_A\boldsymbol{B} = \boldsymbol{O}$, and (6) $\text{rank}(\boldsymbol{Q}_A\boldsymbol{B}) = \text{rank}(\boldsymbol{B}) - \text{rank}(\boldsymbol{A}'\boldsymbol{B})$.

Chapter 3

Generalized Inverse Matrices

3.1 Definition through Linear Transformations

Let $\boldsymbol{A}$ be a square matrix of order n. If it is nonsingular, then $\text{Ker}(\boldsymbol{A}) = \{\boldsymbol{0}\}$ and, as mentioned earlier, the solution vector $\boldsymbol{x}$ in the equation $\boldsymbol{y} = \boldsymbol{A}\boldsymbol{x}$ is determined uniquely as $\boldsymbol{x} = \boldsymbol{A}^{-1}\boldsymbol{y}$. Here, $\boldsymbol{A}^{-1}$ is called the inverse (matrix) of $\boldsymbol{A}$ defining the inverse transformation from $\boldsymbol{y} \in E^n$ to $\boldsymbol{x} \in E^m$, whereas the matrix $\boldsymbol{A}$ represents a transformation from $\boldsymbol{x}$ to $\boldsymbol{y}$. When $\boldsymbol{A}$ is n by m, $\boldsymbol{A}\boldsymbol{x} = \boldsymbol{y}$ has a solution if and only if $\boldsymbol{y} \in \text{Sp}(\boldsymbol{A})$. Even then, if $\text{Ker}(\boldsymbol{A}) \neq \{\boldsymbol{0}\}$, there are many solutions to the equation $\boldsymbol{A}\boldsymbol{x} = \boldsymbol{y}$ due to the existence of $\boldsymbol{x}_0$ ($\neq \boldsymbol{0}$) such that $\boldsymbol{A}\boldsymbol{x}_0 = \boldsymbol{0}$, so that $\boldsymbol{A}(\boldsymbol{x} + \boldsymbol{x}_0) = \boldsymbol{y}$. If $\boldsymbol{y} \notin \text{Sp}(\boldsymbol{A})$, there is no solution vector to the equation $\boldsymbol{A}\boldsymbol{x} = \boldsymbol{y}$.

Assume that $\boldsymbol{y} \in \text{Sp}(\boldsymbol{A})$. Consider a linear transformation $\boldsymbol{G}$ such that $\boldsymbol{x} = \boldsymbol{G}\boldsymbol{y}$ is a solution to the (linear) equation $\boldsymbol{A}\boldsymbol{x} = \boldsymbol{y}$. The existence of such a transformation can be verified as follows. Let $\text{rank}(\boldsymbol{A}) = \dim(\text{Sp}(\boldsymbol{A})) = r$, and let $\boldsymbol{y}_1, \cdots, \boldsymbol{y}_r$ represent the basis vectors for $\text{Sp}(\boldsymbol{A})$. Then there exists an $\boldsymbol{x}_i$ such that $\boldsymbol{A}\boldsymbol{x}_i = \boldsymbol{y}_i$ ($i = 1, \cdots, r$). Let an arbitrary vector $\boldsymbol{y} \in \text{Sp}(\boldsymbol{A})$ be represented as $\boldsymbol{y} = c_1\boldsymbol{y}_1 + \cdots + c_r\boldsymbol{y}_r$, and consider the transformation of $\boldsymbol{y}$ into $\boldsymbol{x} = c_1\boldsymbol{x}_1 + \cdots + c_r\boldsymbol{x}_r$. This is a linear transformation and satisfies

$$\boldsymbol{A}\boldsymbol{x} = c_1\boldsymbol{A}\boldsymbol{x}_1 + \cdots + c_r\boldsymbol{A}\boldsymbol{x}_r = c_1\boldsymbol{y}_1 + \cdots + c_r\boldsymbol{y}_r = \boldsymbol{y}.$$

Definition 3.1 *Let $\boldsymbol{A}$ be an n by m matrix, and assume that $\boldsymbol{y} \in \text{Sp}(\boldsymbol{A})$. If a solution to the linear equation $\boldsymbol{A}\boldsymbol{x} = \boldsymbol{y}$ can be expressed as $\boldsymbol{x} = \boldsymbol{A}^{-}\boldsymbol{y}$, an m by n matrix $\boldsymbol{A}^{-}$ is called a generalized inverse (g-inverse) matrix of $\boldsymbol{A}$.*

Theorem 3.1 *The necessary and sufficient condition for an m by n matrix* $\boldsymbol{A}^-$ *to be a generalized inverse matrix of* $\boldsymbol{A}$ *is given by*

$$\boldsymbol{A}\boldsymbol{A}^-\boldsymbol{A} = \boldsymbol{A}. \tag{3.1}$$

Proof. (Necessity) Let $\boldsymbol{x} = \boldsymbol{A}^-\boldsymbol{y}$ denote a solution to $\boldsymbol{A}\boldsymbol{x} = \boldsymbol{y}$. Since $\boldsymbol{y} \in \text{Sp}(\boldsymbol{A})$ can be expressed as $\boldsymbol{y} = \boldsymbol{A}\boldsymbol{\alpha}$ for some $\boldsymbol{\alpha}$, $\boldsymbol{A}\boldsymbol{x} = \boldsymbol{A}\boldsymbol{A}^-\boldsymbol{y} = \boldsymbol{A}\boldsymbol{A}^-\boldsymbol{A}\boldsymbol{\alpha} = \boldsymbol{A}\boldsymbol{\alpha} = \boldsymbol{y}$, which implies $\boldsymbol{A}\boldsymbol{A}^-\boldsymbol{A} = \boldsymbol{A}$.

(Sufficiency) $\boldsymbol{A}\boldsymbol{A}^-\boldsymbol{A} = \boldsymbol{A} \Rightarrow \boldsymbol{A}\boldsymbol{A}^-\boldsymbol{A}\boldsymbol{\alpha} = \boldsymbol{A}\boldsymbol{\alpha}$. Define $\boldsymbol{y} = \boldsymbol{A}\boldsymbol{\alpha}$. Then, $\boldsymbol{A}\boldsymbol{A}^-\boldsymbol{y} = \boldsymbol{y}$, from which a solution vector $\boldsymbol{x} = \boldsymbol{A}^-\boldsymbol{y}$ is obtained. Q.E.D.

Property (3.1) was presented by Rao (1962) as the most comprehensive property of a generalized inverse matrix and is often used as its definition. Clearly, when $\boldsymbol{A}$ is square and nonsingular, the regular inverse $\boldsymbol{A}^{-1}$ of $\boldsymbol{A}$ satisfies the property (3.1). This means that the regular inverse is a special case of a generalized inverse. As is clear from the definition, generalized inverse matrices can be defined even if $\boldsymbol{A}$ is not square.

Note Let a denote an arbitrary real number. A b that satisfies

$$aba = a$$

is given by $b = a^{-1}$ when $a \neq 0$ and by $b = k$ when $a = 0$, where k is any real number. The equation above is a special case of (3.1), and a b that satisfies this equation might be called a generalized reciprocal.

The defining property of a generalized inverse matrix given in (3.1) indicates that, when $\boldsymbol{y} \in \text{Sp}(\boldsymbol{A})$, a linear transformation from $\boldsymbol{y}$ to $\boldsymbol{x} \in E^m$ is given by $\boldsymbol{A}^-$. However, even when $\boldsymbol{y} \notin \text{Sp}(\boldsymbol{A})$, $\boldsymbol{A}^-$ can be defined as a transformation from $\boldsymbol{y}$ to $\boldsymbol{x}$ as follows.

Let $V = \text{Sp}(\boldsymbol{A})$, and let $\tilde{W} = \text{Ker}(\boldsymbol{A})$ denote the null space of $\boldsymbol{A}$. Furthermore, let W and $\tilde{V}$ denote complement subspaces of V and $\tilde{W}$, respectively. Then,

$$E^n = V \oplus W \text{ and } E^m = \tilde{V} \oplus \tilde{W}. \tag{3.2}$$

Let $\boldsymbol{y} = \boldsymbol{y}_1 + \boldsymbol{y}_2$ be a decomposition of an arbitrary vector $\boldsymbol{y} \in E^n$, where $\boldsymbol{y}_1 \in V$ and $\boldsymbol{y}_2 \in W$, and let $\boldsymbol{x} = \boldsymbol{x}_1 + \boldsymbol{x}_2$ be a decomposition of $\boldsymbol{x} \in E^m$, where $\boldsymbol{x}_1 \in \tilde{V}$ and $\boldsymbol{x}_2 \in \tilde{W}$. The transformation that maps $\boldsymbol{y}$ to $\boldsymbol{x}$ by mapping $\boldsymbol{y}_1$ to $\boldsymbol{x}_1$ and $\boldsymbol{y}_2$ to $\boldsymbol{x}_2$ is a linear transformation from E^n to E^m.

We have $\boldsymbol{Ax} = \boldsymbol{A}(\boldsymbol{x}_1+\boldsymbol{x}_2) = \boldsymbol{Ax}_1 = \boldsymbol{y}_1 \in V = \mathrm{Sp}(\boldsymbol{A})$. This transformation from V to $\tilde{V}$ is one-to-one, and so is the inverse transformation from $\tilde{V}$ to V. Hence, this inverse transformation from $\tilde{V}$ to V is uniquely determined. Let this inverse transformation be denoted by $\boldsymbol{x}_1 = \phi^-_{\tilde{V}}(\boldsymbol{y}_1)$. We then arbitrarily choose a linear transformation from $\tilde{W}$ to W in such a way that $\boldsymbol{x}_2 = \phi^-_M(\boldsymbol{y}_2)$. We define a transformation ϕ^- that maps $\boldsymbol{y} \in E^n$ to $\boldsymbol{x} \in E^m$ by

$$\boldsymbol{x} = \Phi^-_{\tilde{V}}(\boldsymbol{y}_1) + \phi^-_M(\boldsymbol{y}_2) = \phi^-(\boldsymbol{y}). \tag{3.3}$$

We define the matrix representation of this linear transformation ϕ^-, namely $\boldsymbol{A}^-$, as a generalized inverse matrix of $\boldsymbol{A}$. As is clear from this definition, there is some arbitrariness in the choice of $\boldsymbol{A}^-$ due to the arbitrariness in the choice of W, $\tilde{V}$, and Φ^-_M. (See Figure 3.1.)

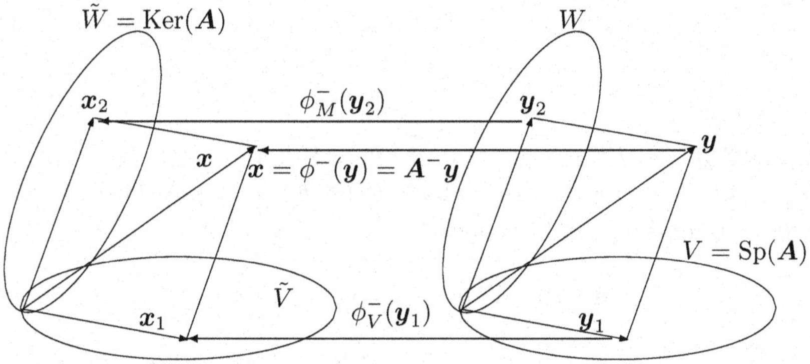

Figure 3.1: Geometric representation of a generalized inverse $\boldsymbol{A}^-$. V and $\tilde{W}$ are determined uniquely by $\boldsymbol{A}$, but W and $\tilde{V}$ are arbitrary except that they satisfy (3.2). There is also some arbitrariness in the choice of ϕ^-_M.

Lemma 3.1 *If $\boldsymbol{y}_1 \in V$ and $\boldsymbol{y}_2 \in W$,*

$$\phi^-_{\tilde{V}}(\boldsymbol{y}_1) = \boldsymbol{A}^-\boldsymbol{y}_1 \text{ and } \Phi^-_M(\boldsymbol{y}_2) = \boldsymbol{A}^-\boldsymbol{y}_2. \tag{3.4}$$

Proof. Substitute $\boldsymbol{y}_1 = \boldsymbol{y}_1+\boldsymbol{0}$ and $\boldsymbol{y}_2 = \boldsymbol{0}+\boldsymbol{y}_2$ in (3.3). Q.E.D.

Conversely, the following statement holds.

Theorem 3.2 *Let $\boldsymbol{A}^-$ be a generalized inverse of $\boldsymbol{A}$, and let $V = \mathrm{Sp}(\boldsymbol{A})$ and $\tilde{W} = \mathrm{Ker}(\boldsymbol{A})$. Then there exist decompositions $E^n = V \oplus W$ and*

$E^m = \tilde{V} \oplus \tilde{W}$. Let $\boldsymbol{y} \in E^n$ be decomposed as $\boldsymbol{y} = \boldsymbol{y}_1 + \boldsymbol{y}_2$, where $\boldsymbol{y}_1 \in V$ and $\boldsymbol{y}_2 \in W$. Furthermore, let

$$\boldsymbol{x} = \boldsymbol{A}^- \boldsymbol{y} = \boldsymbol{x}_1 + \boldsymbol{x}_2 \ (\textit{where}\ \boldsymbol{x}_1 \in \tilde{V},\ \boldsymbol{x}_2 \in \tilde{W}). \tag{3.5}$$

Then,

$$\boldsymbol{x}_1 = \boldsymbol{A}^- \boldsymbol{y}_1 \ \textit{and}\ \boldsymbol{x}_2 = \boldsymbol{A}^- \boldsymbol{y}_2. \tag{3.6}$$

Proof. Let $E^n = V \oplus W$ be an arbitrary direct-sum decomposition of E^n. Let $\mathrm{Sp}(\boldsymbol{A}_{\tilde{V}}^-) = \tilde{V}$ denote the image of V by $\phi_{\tilde{V}}^-$. Since $\boldsymbol{y} \in \mathrm{Sp}(\boldsymbol{A})$ for any $\boldsymbol{y}$ such that $\boldsymbol{y} = \boldsymbol{y}_1 + \boldsymbol{y}_2$, where $\boldsymbol{y}_1 \in V$ and $\boldsymbol{y}_2 \in W$, we have $\boldsymbol{A}^-\boldsymbol{y}_1 = \boldsymbol{x}_1 \in \tilde{V}$ and $\boldsymbol{A}\boldsymbol{x}_1 = \boldsymbol{y}_1$. Also, if $\boldsymbol{y}_1 \neq \boldsymbol{0}$, then $\boldsymbol{y}_1 = \boldsymbol{A}\boldsymbol{x}_1 \neq \boldsymbol{0}$, and so $\boldsymbol{x}_1 \notin \tilde{W}$ or $\tilde{V} \cap \tilde{W} = \{\boldsymbol{0}\}$. Furthermore, if $\boldsymbol{x}_1$ and $\tilde{\boldsymbol{x}}_1 \in V$ but $\boldsymbol{x}_1 \neq \tilde{\boldsymbol{x}}_1$, then $\boldsymbol{x}_1 - \tilde{\boldsymbol{x}}_1 \notin \tilde{W}$, so that $\boldsymbol{A}(\boldsymbol{x}_1 - \tilde{\boldsymbol{x}}_1) \neq \boldsymbol{0}$, which implies $\boldsymbol{A}\boldsymbol{x}_1 \neq \boldsymbol{A}\tilde{\boldsymbol{x}}_1$. Hence, the correspondence between V and $\tilde{V}$ is one-to-one. Because $\dim(\tilde{V}) = \dim(V)$ implies $\dim(\tilde{W}) = m - \mathrm{rank}(\boldsymbol{A})$, we obtain $\tilde{V} \oplus \tilde{W} = E^m$. Q.E.D.

Theorem 3.3 *Let $E^n = V \oplus W$ and $E^m = \tilde{V} \oplus \tilde{W}$, where $V = \mathrm{Sp}(\boldsymbol{A})$ and $W = \mathrm{Ker}(\boldsymbol{A})$. Let an arbitrary vector $\boldsymbol{y} \in E^n$ be decomposed as $\boldsymbol{y} = \boldsymbol{y}_1 + \boldsymbol{y}_2$, where $\boldsymbol{y}_1 \in V$ and $\boldsymbol{y}_2 \in W$. Suppose*

$$\boldsymbol{A}^-\boldsymbol{y} = \boldsymbol{A}^-\boldsymbol{y}_1 + \boldsymbol{A}^-\boldsymbol{y}_2 = \boldsymbol{x}_1 + \boldsymbol{x}_2 \tag{3.7}$$

holds, where $\boldsymbol{x}_1 \in \tilde{V}$ and $\boldsymbol{x}_2 \in \tilde{W}$. Then the following three statements are equivalent:

(i) *$\boldsymbol{A}^-$ is a generalized inverse of $\boldsymbol{A}$.*

(ii) *$\boldsymbol{A}\boldsymbol{A}^-$ is the projector onto V along W.*

(iii) *$\boldsymbol{A}^-\boldsymbol{A}$ is the projector onto $\tilde{V}$ along $\tilde{W}$.*

Proof. (i) → (ii): Since $\boldsymbol{A}^-$ is a generalized inverse of $\boldsymbol{A}$, we have $\boldsymbol{A}^-\boldsymbol{y}_1 = \boldsymbol{x}_1$ and $\boldsymbol{A}^-\boldsymbol{y}_2 = \boldsymbol{x}_2$ by Theorem 3.2. Premultiplying (3.7) by $\boldsymbol{A}$ and taking (3.6) into account, we obtain

$$\boldsymbol{A}\boldsymbol{A}^-\boldsymbol{y}_1 = \boldsymbol{A}\boldsymbol{x}_1 = \boldsymbol{y}_1 \text{ and } \boldsymbol{A}\boldsymbol{A}^-\boldsymbol{y}_2 = \boldsymbol{A}\boldsymbol{x}_2 = \boldsymbol{0},$$

establishing (ii) by Theorem 2.2.

(ii) → (iii): $\boldsymbol{A}\boldsymbol{x}_1 = \boldsymbol{y}_1 \Rightarrow \boldsymbol{A}^-\boldsymbol{A}\boldsymbol{x}_1 = \boldsymbol{A}^-\boldsymbol{y}_1 = \boldsymbol{x}_1$. On the other hand, for $\boldsymbol{x}_2 \in \tilde{W}$, we have $\boldsymbol{A}\boldsymbol{x}_2 = \boldsymbol{0} \Rightarrow \boldsymbol{A}^-\boldsymbol{A}\boldsymbol{x}_2 = \boldsymbol{0}$, establishing (iii) by Theorem 2.2.

(iii) $\to$ (i): Decompose $\boldsymbol{y} = \boldsymbol{y}_1 + \boldsymbol{y}_2$, where $\boldsymbol{y}_1 \in V$ and $\boldsymbol{y}_2 \in W$. Then,

$$\boldsymbol{A}^- \boldsymbol{y} = \boldsymbol{A}^- \boldsymbol{y}_1 + \boldsymbol{A}^- \boldsymbol{y}_2 = \boldsymbol{x}_1 + \boldsymbol{x}_2,$$

where $\boldsymbol{x}_1 \in \tilde{V}$ and $\boldsymbol{x}_2 \in \tilde{W}$. Hence, $\boldsymbol{A}^- \boldsymbol{A}\boldsymbol{x}_1 = \boldsymbol{x}_1 \Rightarrow \boldsymbol{A}^- \boldsymbol{y}_1 = \boldsymbol{x}_1$ and so $\boldsymbol{A}^- \boldsymbol{y}_2 = \boldsymbol{x}_2$. From the properties of a generalized inverse matrix shown in Lemma 3.1 and Theorem 3.2, it is clear that $\boldsymbol{A}^-$ is a generalized inverse of $\boldsymbol{A}$. Q.E.D.

3.2 General Properties

We examine various properties of a generalized inverse matrix $\boldsymbol{A}^-$ that satisfies (3.1).

3.2.1 Properties of generalized inverse matrices

Theorem 3.4 *Let $\boldsymbol{H} = \boldsymbol{A}\boldsymbol{A}^-$, and let $\boldsymbol{F} = \boldsymbol{A}^-\boldsymbol{A}$. Then the following relations hold:*

$$\boldsymbol{H}^2 = \boldsymbol{H} \text{ and } \boldsymbol{F}^2 = \boldsymbol{F}, \tag{3.8}$$

$$\text{rank}(\boldsymbol{H}) = \text{rank}(\boldsymbol{F}) = \text{rank}(\boldsymbol{A}), \tag{3.9}$$

$$\text{rank}(\boldsymbol{A}^-) \geq \text{rank}(\boldsymbol{A}), \tag{3.10}$$

$$\text{rank}(\boldsymbol{A}^-\boldsymbol{A}\boldsymbol{A}^-) = \text{rank}(\boldsymbol{A}). \tag{3.11}$$

Proof. (3.8): Clear from the definition of generalized inverses.

(3.9): $\text{rank}(\boldsymbol{A}) \geq \text{rank}(\boldsymbol{A}\boldsymbol{A}^-) = \text{rank}(\boldsymbol{H})$, and $\text{rank}(\boldsymbol{A}) = \text{rank}(\boldsymbol{A}\boldsymbol{A}^-\boldsymbol{A}) = \text{rank}(\boldsymbol{H}\boldsymbol{A}) \leq \text{rank}(\boldsymbol{H})$, from which it follows that $\text{rank}(\boldsymbol{A}) = \text{rank}(\boldsymbol{H})$. $\text{rank}(\boldsymbol{F}) = \text{rank}(\boldsymbol{A})$ can be similarly proven.

(3.10): $\text{rank}(\boldsymbol{A}) = \text{rank}(\boldsymbol{A}\boldsymbol{A}^-\boldsymbol{A}) \leq \text{rank}(\boldsymbol{A}\boldsymbol{A}^-) \leq \text{rank}(\boldsymbol{A}^-)$.

(3.11): $\text{rank}(\boldsymbol{A}^-\boldsymbol{A}\boldsymbol{A}) \leq \text{rank}(\boldsymbol{A}^-\boldsymbol{A})$. We also have $\text{rank}(\boldsymbol{A}^-\boldsymbol{A}\boldsymbol{A}^-) \geq \text{rank}(\boldsymbol{A}^-\boldsymbol{A}\boldsymbol{A}^-\boldsymbol{A}) = \text{rank}(\boldsymbol{A}^-\boldsymbol{A})$, so that $\text{rank}(\boldsymbol{A}^-\boldsymbol{A}\boldsymbol{A}^-) = \text{rank}(\boldsymbol{A}^-\boldsymbol{A}) = \text{rank}(\boldsymbol{A})$. Q.E.D.

Example 3.1 Find a generalized inverse of $\boldsymbol{A} = \begin{bmatrix} 1 & 1 \\ 1 & 1 \end{bmatrix}$.

Solution. Let $\boldsymbol{A}^- = \begin{bmatrix} a & b \\ c & d \end{bmatrix}$. From

$$\begin{bmatrix} 1 & 1 \\ 1 & 1 \end{bmatrix} \begin{bmatrix} a & b \\ c & d \end{bmatrix} \begin{bmatrix} 1 & 1 \\ 1 & 1 \end{bmatrix} = \begin{bmatrix} 1 & 1 \\ 1 & 1 \end{bmatrix},$$

we must have $a+b+c+d=1$. Hence,

$$\boldsymbol{A}^- = \begin{bmatrix} a & b \\ c & 1-a-b-c \end{bmatrix},$$

where a, b, and c are arbitrary.

Note As is clear from the example above, the generalized inverse $\boldsymbol{A}^-$ of $\boldsymbol{A}$ is in general not uniquely determined. When $\boldsymbol{A}^-$ is not unique, the set of generalized inverses of $\boldsymbol{A}$ is sometimes denoted as $\{\boldsymbol{A}^-\}$. For example, let $\boldsymbol{A} = \begin{bmatrix} 1 & 1 \\ 1 & 1 \end{bmatrix}$, $\boldsymbol{A}_1 = \begin{bmatrix} \frac{1}{4} & \frac{1}{4} \\ \frac{1}{4} & \frac{1}{4} \end{bmatrix}$, and $\boldsymbol{A}_2 = \begin{bmatrix} 2 & 1 \\ -1 & -1 \end{bmatrix}$. Then, $\boldsymbol{A}_1, \boldsymbol{A}_2 \in \{\boldsymbol{A}^-\}$.

We next derive several basic theorems regarding $\boldsymbol{A}^-$.

Theorem 3.5 *The following relations hold for a generalized inverse $\boldsymbol{A}^-$ of $\boldsymbol{A}$:*

$$\{(\boldsymbol{A}^-)'\} = \{(\boldsymbol{A}')^-\}, \tag{3.12}$$

$$\boldsymbol{A}(\boldsymbol{A}'\boldsymbol{A})^-\boldsymbol{A}'\boldsymbol{A} = \boldsymbol{A}, \tag{3.13}$$

$$(\boldsymbol{A}(\boldsymbol{A}'\boldsymbol{A})^-\boldsymbol{A}')' = \boldsymbol{A}(\boldsymbol{A}'\boldsymbol{A})^-\boldsymbol{A}'. \tag{3.14}$$

Proof. (3.12): $\boldsymbol{A}\boldsymbol{A}^-\boldsymbol{A} = \boldsymbol{A} \Rightarrow \boldsymbol{A}'(\boldsymbol{A}^-)'\boldsymbol{A}' = \boldsymbol{A}'$. Hence, $\{(\boldsymbol{A}^-)'\} \subset \{(\boldsymbol{A}')^-\}$. On the other hand, $\boldsymbol{A}'(\boldsymbol{A}')^-\boldsymbol{A}' = \boldsymbol{A}'$, and so $((\boldsymbol{A}')^-)' \in \{\boldsymbol{A}^-\} \Rightarrow \{(\boldsymbol{A}')^-\} \subset \{(\boldsymbol{A}^-)'\}$. Thus, $\{(\boldsymbol{A}^-)'\} = \{(\boldsymbol{A}')^-\}$.

(3.13): Let $\boldsymbol{G} = (\boldsymbol{I}_n - \boldsymbol{A}(\boldsymbol{A}'\boldsymbol{A})^-\boldsymbol{A}')\boldsymbol{A} = \boldsymbol{A}(\boldsymbol{I}_n - (\boldsymbol{A}'\boldsymbol{A})^-\boldsymbol{A}'\boldsymbol{A})$. Then,

$$\boldsymbol{G}'\boldsymbol{G} = (\boldsymbol{I}_n - (\boldsymbol{A}'\boldsymbol{A})^-\boldsymbol{A}'\boldsymbol{A})'(\boldsymbol{A}'\boldsymbol{A} - \boldsymbol{A}'\boldsymbol{A}(\boldsymbol{A}'\boldsymbol{A})^-\boldsymbol{A}'\boldsymbol{A}) = \boldsymbol{O}.$$

Hence, $\boldsymbol{G} = \boldsymbol{O}$, leading to (3.13).

(3.14): Let $\boldsymbol{G}$ denote a generalized inverse of $\boldsymbol{A}'\boldsymbol{A}$. Then $\boldsymbol{G}'$ is also a generalized inverse of $\boldsymbol{A}'\boldsymbol{A}$, and $\boldsymbol{S} = (\boldsymbol{G}+\boldsymbol{G}')/2$ is a symmetric generalized inverse of $\boldsymbol{A}'\boldsymbol{A}$. Let $\boldsymbol{H} = \boldsymbol{A}\boldsymbol{S}\boldsymbol{A}' - \boldsymbol{A}(\boldsymbol{A}'\boldsymbol{A})^-\boldsymbol{A}'$. Then, using (3.13), we obtain

$$\begin{aligned} \boldsymbol{H}'\boldsymbol{H} &= (\boldsymbol{A}\boldsymbol{S}\boldsymbol{A}' - \boldsymbol{A}(\boldsymbol{A}'\boldsymbol{A})^-\boldsymbol{A}')'(\boldsymbol{A}\boldsymbol{S}\boldsymbol{A}' - \boldsymbol{A}(\boldsymbol{A}'\boldsymbol{A})^-\boldsymbol{A}') \\ &= (\boldsymbol{A}\boldsymbol{S} - \boldsymbol{A}(\boldsymbol{A}'\boldsymbol{A})^-)'(\boldsymbol{A}'\boldsymbol{A}\boldsymbol{S}\boldsymbol{A}' - \boldsymbol{A}'\boldsymbol{A}(\boldsymbol{A}'\boldsymbol{A})^-\boldsymbol{A}') = \boldsymbol{O}. \end{aligned}$$

Hence, $\boldsymbol{H} = \boldsymbol{O}$, leading to (3.14). Q.E.D.

Corollary *Let*

$$P_A = A(A'A)^- A' \tag{3.15}$$

and

$$P_{A'} = A'(AA')^- A. \tag{3.16}$$

Then P_A *and* $P_{A'}$ *are the orthogonal projectors onto* Sp(A) *and* Sp(A').

Note If Sp(A) = Sp($\tilde{A}$), then $P_A = P_{\tilde{A}}$. This implies that P_A only depends on Sp(A) but not the basis vectors spanning Sp(A). Hence, P_A would have been more accurately denoted as $P_{Sp(A)}$. However, to avoid notational clutter, we retain the notation P_A.

3.2.2 Representation of subspaces by generalized inverses

We start with the following lemma.

Lemma 3.2 *Let* A^- *denote an arbitrary generalized inverse of* A. *Then,*

$$V = \text{Sp}(A) = \text{Sp}(AA^-). \tag{3.17}$$

Proof. That $\text{Sp}(A) \supset \text{Sp}(AA^-)$ is clear. On the other hand, from rank($A \times A^-) \geq \text{rank}(AA^-A) = \text{rank}(A)$, we have $\text{Sp}(AA^-) \supset \text{Sp}(A) \Rightarrow \text{Sp}(A) = \text{Sp}(AA^-)$. Q.E.D.

Theorem 3.6 *Using a generalized inverse* A *of* A^-, *we can express any complement subspace* W *of* $V = \text{Sp}(A)$ *as*

$$W = \text{Sp}(I_n - AA^-). \tag{3.18}$$

Proof. (Sufficiency) Let $AA^-x + (I_n - AA^-)y = 0$. Premultiplying both sides by AA^-, we obtain $AA^-x = 0$, which implies $(I_n - AA^-)y = 0$. On the other hand, let $P = AA^-$. Then, $P^2 = P$, and so $\text{rank}(AA^-) + \text{rank}(I_n - AA^-) = n$. Hence, $E^n = V \oplus W$.

(Necessity) Let $P = AA^-$. Then $P^2 = P$. From Lemma 2.1, the null (annihilation) space of P is given by $\text{Sp}(I_n - P)$. Hence, $\text{Sp}(P) \cap \text{Sp}(I_n - P) = \{0\}$, and $\text{Sp}(I_n - P)$ gives a general expression for a complement subspace of $\text{Sp}(P)$, establishing (3.18). Q.E.D.

Like Lemma 2.1, the following theorem is extremely useful in understanding generalized inverses in relation to linear transformations.

Lemma 3.3

$$\mathrm{Ker}(\boldsymbol{A}) = \mathrm{Ker}(\boldsymbol{A}^-\boldsymbol{A}), \tag{3.19}$$

$$\mathrm{Ker}(\boldsymbol{A}) = \mathrm{Sp}(\boldsymbol{I}_n - \boldsymbol{A}^-\boldsymbol{A}), \tag{3.20}$$

and a complement space of $\tilde{W} = \mathrm{Ker}(\boldsymbol{A})$ *is given by*

$$\tilde{V} = \mathrm{Sp}(\boldsymbol{A}^-\boldsymbol{A}), \tag{3.21}$$

where $\boldsymbol{A}^-$ *is a generalized inverse of* $\boldsymbol{A}$.

Proof. (3.19): $\boldsymbol{Ax} = \boldsymbol{0} \Rightarrow \boldsymbol{A}^-\boldsymbol{Ax} = \boldsymbol{0} \Rightarrow \mathrm{Ker}(\boldsymbol{A}) \subset \mathrm{Ker}(\boldsymbol{A}^-\boldsymbol{A})$. On the other hand, $\boldsymbol{A}^-\boldsymbol{Ax} = \boldsymbol{0} \Rightarrow \boldsymbol{AA}^-\boldsymbol{Ax} = \boldsymbol{Ax} = \boldsymbol{0} \Rightarrow \mathrm{Ker}(\boldsymbol{A}^-\boldsymbol{A}) \subset \mathrm{Ker}(\boldsymbol{A})$. Hence, $\mathrm{Ker}(\boldsymbol{A}) = \mathrm{Ker}(\boldsymbol{AA}^-)$.

(3.20): Use (3.19) and (2.4) in Lemma 2.1.

(3.21): Note that $(\boldsymbol{I}_m - \boldsymbol{A}^-\boldsymbol{A})^2 = \boldsymbol{I}_m - \boldsymbol{A}^-\boldsymbol{A}$. From Theorem 3.6, we obtain $\{\mathrm{Ker}(\boldsymbol{A})\}^c = \mathrm{Sp}(\boldsymbol{I}_m - (\boldsymbol{I}_m - \boldsymbol{A}^-\boldsymbol{A})) = \mathrm{Sp}(\boldsymbol{A}^-\boldsymbol{A})$. Q.E.D.

From Theorem 3.6 and Lemma 3.3, we obtain the following theorem.

Theorem 3.7 *Let* $\boldsymbol{A}$ *be an* m *by* n *matrix. Then,*

$$\mathrm{Sp}(\boldsymbol{AA}^-) \oplus \mathrm{Sp}(\boldsymbol{I}_n - \boldsymbol{AA}^-) = E^n, \tag{3.22}$$

$$\mathrm{Sp}(\boldsymbol{A}^-\boldsymbol{A}) \oplus \mathrm{Sp}(\boldsymbol{I}_m - \boldsymbol{A}^-\boldsymbol{A}) = E^m. \tag{3.23}$$

Proof. Clear from $\mathrm{Ker}(\boldsymbol{AA}^-) = \mathrm{Sp}(\boldsymbol{I}_n - \boldsymbol{AA}^-)$ and $\mathrm{Ker}(\boldsymbol{A}^-\boldsymbol{A}) = \mathrm{Sp}(\boldsymbol{I}_m - \boldsymbol{A}^-\boldsymbol{A})$. Q.E.D.

Note Equation (3.22) corresponds to $E^n = V \oplus W$, and (3.23) corresponds to $E^m = \tilde{V} \oplus \tilde{W}$. A complement subspace $W = \mathrm{Sp}(\boldsymbol{I}_n - \boldsymbol{AA}^-)$ of $V = \mathrm{Sp}(\boldsymbol{A}) = \mathrm{Sp}(\boldsymbol{AA}^-)$ in E^n is not uniquely determined. However, the null space (kernel) of $\boldsymbol{A}$, $\tilde{W} = \mathrm{Sp}(\boldsymbol{I}_m - \boldsymbol{A}^-\boldsymbol{A}) = \mathrm{Sp}(\boldsymbol{I}_m - \boldsymbol{A}'(\boldsymbol{AA}')^-\boldsymbol{A}) = \mathrm{Sp}(\boldsymbol{A}')^\perp$, is uniquely determined, although a complement subspace of $\tilde{W}$, namely $\tilde{V} = \mathrm{Sp}(\boldsymbol{A}^-\boldsymbol{A})$, is not uniquely determined. (See Example 3.2.)

Note Equation (3.23) means

$$\mathrm{rank}(\boldsymbol{A}^-\boldsymbol{A}) + \mathrm{rank}(\boldsymbol{I}_m - \boldsymbol{A}^-\boldsymbol{A}) = m$$

and that (1.55) in Theorem 1.9 holds from $\text{rank}(\boldsymbol{A}^-\boldsymbol{A}) = \text{rank}(\boldsymbol{A})$ and $\text{rank}(\boldsymbol{I}_m - \boldsymbol{A}^-\boldsymbol{A}) = \dim(\text{Sp}(\boldsymbol{I}_m - \boldsymbol{A}^-\boldsymbol{A})) = \dim(\text{Ker}(\boldsymbol{A}))$.

Example 3.2 Let $\boldsymbol{A} = \begin{bmatrix} 1 & 1 \\ 1 & 1 \end{bmatrix}$. Find (i) $W = \text{Sp}(\boldsymbol{I}_2 - \boldsymbol{A}\boldsymbol{A}^-)$, (ii) $\tilde{W} = \text{Sp}(\boldsymbol{I}_2 - \boldsymbol{A}^-\boldsymbol{A})$, and (iii) $\tilde{V} = \text{Sp}(\boldsymbol{A}^-\boldsymbol{A})$.

Solution (i): From Example 3.1,

$$\boldsymbol{A}^- = \begin{bmatrix} a & b \\ c & 1-a-b-c \end{bmatrix}.$$

Hence,

$$\begin{aligned} \boldsymbol{I}_2 - \boldsymbol{A}\boldsymbol{A}^- &= \begin{bmatrix} 1 & 0 \\ 0 & 1 \end{bmatrix} - \begin{bmatrix} 1 & 1 \\ 1 & 1 \end{bmatrix} \begin{bmatrix} a & b \\ c & 1-a-b-c \end{bmatrix} \\ &= \begin{bmatrix} 1 & 0 \\ 0 & 1 \end{bmatrix} - \begin{bmatrix} a+c & 1-a-c \\ a+c & 1-a-b-c \end{bmatrix} \\ &= \begin{bmatrix} 1-a-c & -(1-a-c) \\ -(a+c) & a+c \end{bmatrix}. \end{aligned}$$

Let $x = 1-(a+c)$. Then $W = \text{Sp}(\boldsymbol{I}_2 - \boldsymbol{A}\boldsymbol{A}^-)$ is the unidimensional space spanned by vector $(x, x-1)'$. (Since x can take any value, $\text{Sp}(\boldsymbol{I}_2 - \boldsymbol{A}\boldsymbol{A}^-)$ is not uniquely determined.)

(ii): We have

$$\begin{aligned} \boldsymbol{I}_2 - \boldsymbol{A}^-\boldsymbol{A} &= \begin{bmatrix} 1-a-b & -(a+b) \\ -(1-a-b) & a+b \end{bmatrix} \\ &= \begin{bmatrix} 1 & -1 \\ -1 & 1 \end{bmatrix} \begin{bmatrix} 1-a-b & 0 \\ 0 & a+b \end{bmatrix}. \end{aligned}$$

Hence, $\tilde{W} = \text{Sp}(\boldsymbol{I}_2 - \boldsymbol{A}^-\boldsymbol{A})$ is the unidimensional space $Y = -X$ spanned by $(1, -1)'$, which is uniquely determined.

(iii): We have

$$\begin{aligned} \boldsymbol{A}^-\boldsymbol{A} &= \begin{bmatrix} a & b \\ c & 1-a-b-c \end{bmatrix} \begin{bmatrix} 1 & 1 \\ 1 & 1 \end{bmatrix} \\ &= \begin{bmatrix} a+b & a+b \\ 1-a-b & 1-a-b \end{bmatrix}. \end{aligned}$$

Let $a + b = x$. Then $\text{Sp}(\boldsymbol{A}^-\boldsymbol{A})$ is generated by the two-component vector $(x, 1-x)'$. Since x can take any value, it is not uniquely determined.

Note $\text{Sp}(\boldsymbol{A})$ is spanned by $(1,1)'$, and so it is represented by a line $Y = X$ passing through the origin. Its complement subspace is a line connecting (0,0) and an arbitrary point $P_1(X, X-1)$ on $Y = X - 1$ (Figure 3.2).

Note Since $\tilde{W} = \text{Ker}(\boldsymbol{A}) = \{(1,-1)'\}$, $\tilde{V} = \text{Sp}(\boldsymbol{A}^-\boldsymbol{A})$ is represented by a line connecting the origin and an arbitrary point $P_2(X, 1-X)$ on the line $Y = 1 - X$ (Figure 3.3).

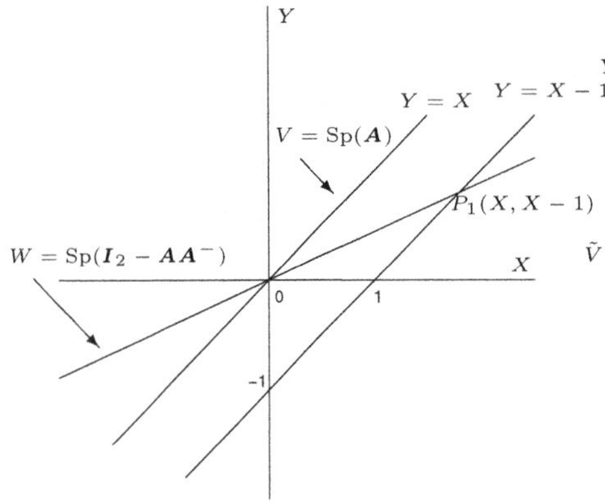

Figure 3.2: Representation of $E^2 = V \oplus W$ by a line.

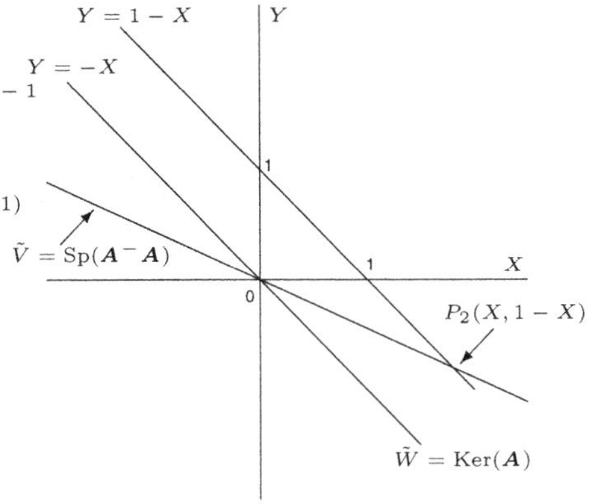

Figure 3.3: Representation of $E^2 = \tilde{V} \oplus \tilde{W}$ by a line.

3.2.3 Generalized inverses and linear equations

We use theorems in the previous section to represent solutions to linear equations in terms of generalized inverse matrices.

Theorem 3.8 *Let* $\boldsymbol{A}\boldsymbol{x} = \boldsymbol{b}$, *and suppose* $\boldsymbol{b} \in \text{Sp}(\boldsymbol{A})$. *Then,*

$$\boldsymbol{x} = \boldsymbol{A}^-\boldsymbol{b} + (\boldsymbol{I}_m - \boldsymbol{A}^-\boldsymbol{A})\boldsymbol{z}, \tag{3.24}$$

where $\boldsymbol{z}$ *is an arbitrary* m*-component vector.*

Proof. Let $\boldsymbol{b} \in \text{Sp}(\boldsymbol{A})$ and $\boldsymbol{x}_1 = \boldsymbol{A}^-\boldsymbol{b}$. Then, $\boldsymbol{A}\boldsymbol{x}_1 = \boldsymbol{b}$. On the other hand, from (3.20), a solution to $\boldsymbol{A}\boldsymbol{x}_0 = \boldsymbol{0}$ is given by $\boldsymbol{x}_0 = (\boldsymbol{I}_m - \boldsymbol{A}^-\boldsymbol{A})\boldsymbol{z}$. Equation

(3.24) is obtained by $\boldsymbol{x} = \boldsymbol{x}_1 + \boldsymbol{x}_0$. Conversely, it is clear that (3.24) satisfies $\boldsymbol{A}\boldsymbol{x} = \boldsymbol{b}$. Q.E.D.

Corollary *The necessary and sufficient condition for* $\boldsymbol{A}\boldsymbol{x} = \boldsymbol{b}$ *to have a solution is*

$$\boldsymbol{A}\boldsymbol{A}^{-}\boldsymbol{b} = \boldsymbol{b}. \tag{3.25}$$

Proof. The sufficiency is obvious. The necessity can be shown by substituting $\boldsymbol{A}\boldsymbol{x} = \boldsymbol{b}$ into $\boldsymbol{A}\boldsymbol{A}^{-}\boldsymbol{A}\boldsymbol{x} = \boldsymbol{A}\boldsymbol{x}$. Q.E.D.

The corollary above can be generalized as follows.

Theorem 3.9 *The necessary and sufficient condition for*

$$\boldsymbol{A}\boldsymbol{X}\boldsymbol{B} = \boldsymbol{C} \tag{3.26}$$

to have a solution is

$$\boldsymbol{A}\boldsymbol{A}^{-}\boldsymbol{C}\boldsymbol{B}^{-}\boldsymbol{B} = \boldsymbol{C}. \tag{3.27}$$

Proof. The sufficiency can be shown by setting $\boldsymbol{X} = \boldsymbol{A}^{-}\boldsymbol{C}\boldsymbol{B}^{-}$ in (3.26). The necessity can be shown by pre- and postmultiplying $\boldsymbol{A}\boldsymbol{X}\boldsymbol{B} = \boldsymbol{C}$ by $\boldsymbol{A}\boldsymbol{A}^{-}$ and $\boldsymbol{B}^{-}\boldsymbol{B}$, respectively, to obtain $\boldsymbol{A}\boldsymbol{A}^{-}\boldsymbol{A}\boldsymbol{X}\boldsymbol{B}\boldsymbol{B}^{-}\boldsymbol{B} = \boldsymbol{A}\boldsymbol{X}\boldsymbol{B} = \boldsymbol{A}\boldsymbol{A}^{-}\boldsymbol{C}\boldsymbol{B}^{-}\boldsymbol{B}$. Q.E.D.

Note Let $\boldsymbol{A}$, $\boldsymbol{B}$, and $\boldsymbol{C}$ be n by p, q by r, and n by r matrices, respectively. Then $\boldsymbol{X}$ is a p by q matrix. When $q = r$, and $\boldsymbol{B}$ is the identity matrix of order q, the necessary and sufficient condition for $\boldsymbol{A}\boldsymbol{X} = \boldsymbol{C}$ to have a general solution $\boldsymbol{X} = \boldsymbol{A}^{-}\boldsymbol{C} + (\boldsymbol{I}_p - \boldsymbol{A}^{-}\boldsymbol{A})\boldsymbol{Z}$, where $\boldsymbol{Z}$ is an arbitrary square matrix of order p, is given by $\boldsymbol{A}\boldsymbol{A}^{-}\boldsymbol{C} = \boldsymbol{C}$. When, on the other hand, $n = p$, and $\boldsymbol{A}$ is the identity matrix of order p, the necessary and sufficient condition for $\boldsymbol{X}\boldsymbol{B} = \boldsymbol{C}$ to have a general solution $\boldsymbol{X} = \boldsymbol{C}\boldsymbol{B}^{-} + \boldsymbol{Z}(\boldsymbol{I}_q - \boldsymbol{B}\boldsymbol{B}^{-})$, where $\boldsymbol{Z}$ is an arbitrary square matrix of order q, is given by $\boldsymbol{C}\boldsymbol{B}^{-}\boldsymbol{B} = \boldsymbol{C}$.

Clearly,

$$\boldsymbol{X} = \boldsymbol{A}^{-}\boldsymbol{C}\boldsymbol{B}^{-} \tag{3.28}$$

is a solution to (3.26). In addition,

$$\boldsymbol{X} = \boldsymbol{A}^{-}\boldsymbol{C}\boldsymbol{B}^{-} + (\boldsymbol{I}_p - \boldsymbol{A}^{-}\boldsymbol{A})\boldsymbol{Z}_1 + \boldsymbol{Z}_2(\boldsymbol{I}_q - \boldsymbol{B}\boldsymbol{B}^{-}) \tag{3.29}$$

also satisfies (3.26), which can be derived from

$$\boldsymbol{X}_1 = (\boldsymbol{I}_p - \boldsymbol{A}^- \boldsymbol{A})\boldsymbol{Z}_1 \text{ and } \boldsymbol{X}_2 = \boldsymbol{Z}_2(\boldsymbol{I}_q - \boldsymbol{B}\boldsymbol{B}^-),$$

which satisfy $\boldsymbol{A}\boldsymbol{X}_1 = \boldsymbol{O}$ and $\boldsymbol{X}_2\boldsymbol{B} = \boldsymbol{O}$, respectively. Furthermore,

$$\boldsymbol{X} = \boldsymbol{A}^-\boldsymbol{C}\boldsymbol{B}^- + \boldsymbol{Z} - \boldsymbol{A}^-\boldsymbol{A}\boldsymbol{Z}\boldsymbol{B}\boldsymbol{B}^- \tag{3.30}$$

also satisfies (3.26), which is obtained by setting $\boldsymbol{Z}_2 = \boldsymbol{A}^-\boldsymbol{A}\boldsymbol{Z}$ and $\boldsymbol{Z}_1 = \boldsymbol{Z}$ in (3.29). If we use $\boldsymbol{A}$ for both $\boldsymbol{B}$ and $\boldsymbol{C}$ in the equation above, we obtain the following theorem.

Theorem 3.10 *Let A^- denote a generalized inverse of an n by m matrix $\boldsymbol{A}$. Then,*

$$\boldsymbol{G} = \boldsymbol{A}^- + \boldsymbol{Z} - \boldsymbol{A}^-\boldsymbol{A}\boldsymbol{Z}\boldsymbol{A}\boldsymbol{A}^- \tag{3.31}$$

and

$$\boldsymbol{G} = \boldsymbol{A}^- + \boldsymbol{Z}_1(\boldsymbol{I}_n - \boldsymbol{A}\boldsymbol{A}^-) + (\boldsymbol{I}_m - \boldsymbol{A}^-\boldsymbol{A})\boldsymbol{Z}_2 \tag{3.32}$$

are both generalized inverses of $\boldsymbol{A}$, where $\boldsymbol{Z}$, $\boldsymbol{Z}_1$, and $\boldsymbol{Z}_2$ are arbitrary m by n matrices. (Proof omitted.)

We give a fundamental theorem on inclusion relations between subspaces and the corresponding generalized inverses.

Theorem 3.11

$$\text{Sp}(\boldsymbol{A}) \supset \text{Sp}(\boldsymbol{B}) \Longrightarrow \boldsymbol{A}\boldsymbol{A}^-\boldsymbol{B} = \boldsymbol{B} \tag{3.33}$$

and

$$\text{Sp}(\boldsymbol{A}') \supset \text{Sp}(\boldsymbol{B}') \Longrightarrow \boldsymbol{B}\boldsymbol{A}^-\boldsymbol{A} = \boldsymbol{B}. \tag{3.34}$$

Proof. (3.33): $\text{Sp}(\boldsymbol{A}) \supset \text{Sp}(\boldsymbol{B})$ implies that there exists a $\boldsymbol{W}$ such that $\boldsymbol{B} = \boldsymbol{A}\boldsymbol{W}$. Hence, $\boldsymbol{A}\boldsymbol{A}^-\boldsymbol{B} = \boldsymbol{A}\boldsymbol{A}^-\boldsymbol{A}\boldsymbol{W} = \boldsymbol{A}\boldsymbol{W} = \boldsymbol{B}$.

(3.34): We have $\boldsymbol{A}'(\boldsymbol{A}')^-\boldsymbol{B}' = \boldsymbol{B}'$ from (3.33). Transposing both sides, we obtain $\boldsymbol{B} = \boldsymbol{B}((\boldsymbol{A}')^-)'\boldsymbol{A}$, from which we obtain $\boldsymbol{B} = \boldsymbol{B}\boldsymbol{A}^-\boldsymbol{A}$ because $(\boldsymbol{A}')^- = (\boldsymbol{A}^-)'$ from (3.12) in Theorem 3.5. Q.E.D.

Theorem 3.12 *When* $\text{Sp}(\boldsymbol{A}+\boldsymbol{B}) \supset \text{Sp}(\boldsymbol{B})$ *and* $\text{Sp}(\boldsymbol{A}'+\boldsymbol{B}') \supset \text{Sp}(\boldsymbol{B}')$, *the following statements hold* (Rao and Mitra, 1971):

$$\boldsymbol{A}(\boldsymbol{A}+\boldsymbol{B})^-\boldsymbol{B} = \boldsymbol{B}(\boldsymbol{A}+\boldsymbol{B})^-\boldsymbol{A}, \tag{3.35}$$

$$A^- + B^- \in \{(A(A+B)^-B)^-\}, \tag{3.36}$$

and

$$\mathrm{Sp}(A) \cap \mathrm{Sp}(B) = \mathrm{Sp}(A(A+B)^-B). \tag{3.37}$$

Proof. (3.35): This is clear from the following relation:

$$\begin{aligned} A(A+B)^-B &= (A+B-B)(A+B)^-B \\ &= (A+B)(A+B)^-B - B(A+B)^-(A+B) \\ &\qquad\qquad\qquad\qquad\qquad + B(A+B)^-A \\ &= B - B + B(A+B)^-A = B(A+B)^-A. \end{aligned}$$

(3.36): Clear from

$$\begin{aligned} &A(A+B)^-B(A^- + B^-)A(A+B)^-B \\ &= (B(A+B)^-AA^- + A(A+B)^-BB^-)A(A+B)^-B \\ &= B(A+B)^-A(A+B)^-B + A(A+B)^-B(A+B)^-A \\ &= B(A+B)^-A(A+B)^-B + A(A+B)^-A(A+B)^-B \\ &= (A+B)(A+B)^-A(A+B)^-B = A(A+B)^-B. \end{aligned}$$

(3.37): That $\mathrm{Sp}(A(A+B)^-B) \subset \mathrm{Sp}(A) \cap \mathrm{Sp}(B)$ is clear from $A(A+B)^-B = B(A+B)^-A$. On the other hand, let $\mathrm{Sp}(A) \cap \mathrm{Sp}(B) = \mathrm{Sp}(AX| AX = BY)$, where $X = (A+B)^-B$ and $Y = (A+B)^-A$. Then, $\mathrm{Sp}(A) \cap \mathrm{Sp}(B) \subset \mathrm{Sp}(AX) \cap \mathrm{Sp}(BY) = \mathrm{Sp}(A(A+B)^-B)$. Q.E.D.

Statement (3.35) is called the parallel sum of matrices A and B.

3.2.4 Generalized inverses of partitioned square matrices

In Section 1.4, we showed that the (regular) inverse of a symmetric nonsingular matrix

$$M = \begin{bmatrix} A & B \\ B' & C \end{bmatrix} \tag{3.38}$$

is given by (1.71) or (1.72). In this section, we consider a generalized inverse of M that may be singular.

Lemma 3.4 *Let* A *be symmetric and such that* $\mathrm{Sp}(A) \supset \mathrm{Sp}(B)$. *Then the following propositions hold:*

$$AA^-B = B, \tag{3.39}$$

$$B'A^-A = B', \tag{3.40}$$

and

$$(B'A^-B)' = B'A^-B \quad (B'A^-B \text{ is symmetric}). \tag{3.41}$$

Proof. Propositions (3.39) and (3.40) are clear from Theorem 3.11.

(3.41): Let $B = AW$. Then, $B'A^-B = W'A'A^-AW = W'AA^-AW$ $= W'AW$, which is symmetric. Q.E.D.

Theorem 3.13 *Let*

$$H = \begin{bmatrix} X & Y \\ Y' & Z \end{bmatrix} \tag{3.42}$$

represent a symmetric generalized inverse of M *defined in (3.38). If* Sp(A) $\supset$ Sp(B), X, Y, and Z *satisfy*

$$A = AXA + BY'A + AYB' + BZB', \tag{3.43}$$

$$(AY + BZ)D = O, \quad \text{where } D = C - B'A^-B, \tag{3.44}$$

and

$$Z = D^- = (C - B'A^-B)^-, \tag{3.45}$$

and if Sp(C) $\supset$ Sp(B'), *they satisfy*

$$C = (B'X + CY')B + (B'Y + CZ)C, \tag{3.46}$$

$$(AX + BY')E = O, \quad \text{where } E = A - BC^-B', \tag{3.47}$$

and

$$X = E^- = (A - BC^-B')^-. \tag{3.48}$$

Proof. From $MHM = M$, we obtain

$$(AX + BY')A + (AY + BZ)B' = A, \tag{3.49}$$

$$(AX + BY')B + (AY + BZ)C = B, \tag{3.50}$$

and

$$(B'X + CY')B + (B'Y + CZ)C = C. \tag{3.51}$$

Postmultiply (3.49) by A^-B and subtract it from (3.50). Then, by noting $AA^-B = B$, we obtain $(AY + BZ)(C - B'A^-B) = O$, which implies $(AY + BZ)D = O$, so that

$$AYD = -BZD. \tag{3.52}$$

Premultiply (3.50) by $\boldsymbol{B}'\boldsymbol{A}^-$ and subtract it from (3.51). We obtain

$$\boldsymbol{D}(\boldsymbol{Y}'\boldsymbol{B} + \boldsymbol{Z}\boldsymbol{C} - \boldsymbol{I}_p) = \boldsymbol{O} \tag{3.53}$$

by noting $\boldsymbol{B}'\boldsymbol{A}^-\boldsymbol{A} = \boldsymbol{B}'$, $\boldsymbol{D}' = \boldsymbol{D}$ ((3.40) in Lemma 3.4), $\boldsymbol{C} = \boldsymbol{C}'$, and $\boldsymbol{Z} = \boldsymbol{Z}'$. Hence, we have $\boldsymbol{D} = \boldsymbol{C}\boldsymbol{Z}\boldsymbol{D} + \boldsymbol{B}'\boldsymbol{Y}\boldsymbol{D} = \boldsymbol{C}\boldsymbol{Z}'\boldsymbol{D} + \boldsymbol{B}'\boldsymbol{A}^-\boldsymbol{A}\boldsymbol{Y}\boldsymbol{D}$. We substitute (3.52) into this to obtain $\boldsymbol{D} = \boldsymbol{C}\boldsymbol{Z}\boldsymbol{D} - \boldsymbol{B}'\boldsymbol{A}^-\boldsymbol{B}\boldsymbol{Z}\boldsymbol{D} = (\boldsymbol{C} - \boldsymbol{B}'\boldsymbol{A}^-\boldsymbol{B})\boldsymbol{Z}\boldsymbol{D} = \boldsymbol{D}\boldsymbol{Z}\boldsymbol{D}$, implying $\boldsymbol{Z} = \boldsymbol{D}^-$, from which (3.43), (3.44), and (3.45) follow. Equations (3.46), (3.47), and (3.48) follow similarly by deriving equations analogous to (3.52) and (3.53) by (3.50) – $\boldsymbol{B}\boldsymbol{C}^- \times$ (3.51), and (3.49) – (3.50) $\times \boldsymbol{C}^-\boldsymbol{B}'$. Q.E.D.

Corollary 1 *$\boldsymbol{H}$ defined in (3.42) can be expressed as*

$$\begin{bmatrix} \boldsymbol{A}^- + \boldsymbol{A}^-\boldsymbol{B}\boldsymbol{D}^-\boldsymbol{B}'\boldsymbol{A}^- & -\boldsymbol{A}^-\boldsymbol{B}\boldsymbol{D}^- \\ -\boldsymbol{D}^-\boldsymbol{B}'\boldsymbol{A}^- & \boldsymbol{D}^- \end{bmatrix}, \tag{3.54}$$

where $\boldsymbol{D} = \boldsymbol{C} - \boldsymbol{B}'\boldsymbol{A}^-\boldsymbol{B}$, or by

$$\begin{bmatrix} \boldsymbol{E}^- & -\boldsymbol{E}^-\boldsymbol{B}\boldsymbol{C}^- \\ -\boldsymbol{C}^-\boldsymbol{B}'\boldsymbol{E}^- & \boldsymbol{C}^- + \boldsymbol{C}^-\boldsymbol{B}'\boldsymbol{E}^-\boldsymbol{B}\boldsymbol{C}^- \end{bmatrix}, \tag{3.55}$$

where $\boldsymbol{E} = \boldsymbol{A} - \boldsymbol{B}\boldsymbol{C}^-\boldsymbol{B}'$.

Proof. It is clear from $\boldsymbol{A}\boldsymbol{Y}\boldsymbol{D} = -\boldsymbol{B}\boldsymbol{Z}\boldsymbol{D}$ and $\boldsymbol{A}\boldsymbol{A}^-\boldsymbol{B} = \boldsymbol{B}$ that $\boldsymbol{Y} = -\boldsymbol{A}^-\boldsymbol{B}\boldsymbol{Z}$ is a solution. Hence, $\boldsymbol{A}\boldsymbol{Y}\boldsymbol{B}' = -\boldsymbol{A}\boldsymbol{A}^-\boldsymbol{B}\boldsymbol{Z}\boldsymbol{B}' = -\boldsymbol{B}\boldsymbol{Z}\boldsymbol{B}'$, and $\boldsymbol{B}\boldsymbol{Y}'\boldsymbol{A} = \boldsymbol{B}(\boldsymbol{A}\boldsymbol{Y})' = \boldsymbol{B}(-\boldsymbol{A}\boldsymbol{A}^-\boldsymbol{B}\boldsymbol{Z})' = -\boldsymbol{B}\boldsymbol{Z}\boldsymbol{B}'$. Substituting these into (3.43) yields

$$\boldsymbol{A} = \boldsymbol{A}\boldsymbol{X}\boldsymbol{A} - \boldsymbol{B}\boldsymbol{Z}\boldsymbol{B}' = \boldsymbol{A}\boldsymbol{X}\boldsymbol{A} - \boldsymbol{B}\boldsymbol{D}^-\boldsymbol{B}'.$$

The equation above shows that $\boldsymbol{X} = \boldsymbol{A}^- + \boldsymbol{A}^-\boldsymbol{B}\boldsymbol{D}^-\boldsymbol{B}'\boldsymbol{A}^-$ satisfies (3.43), indicating that (3.54) gives an expression for $\boldsymbol{H}$. Equation (3.55) can be derived similarly using (3.46) through (3.48). Q.E.D.

Corollary 2 *Let*

$$\boldsymbol{F} = \begin{bmatrix} \boldsymbol{C}_1 & \boldsymbol{C}_2 \\ \boldsymbol{C}_2' & -\boldsymbol{C}_3 \end{bmatrix} \tag{3.56}$$

be a generalized inverse of

$$\boldsymbol{N} = \begin{bmatrix} \boldsymbol{A} & \boldsymbol{B} \\ \boldsymbol{B}' & \boldsymbol{O} \end{bmatrix}.$$

When Sp$(\boldsymbol{A}) \supset$ Sp$(\boldsymbol{B})$, *we have*

$$\begin{aligned} \boldsymbol{C}_1 &= \boldsymbol{A}^- - \boldsymbol{A}^-\boldsymbol{B}(\boldsymbol{B}'\boldsymbol{A}^-\boldsymbol{B})^-\boldsymbol{B}'\boldsymbol{A}^-, \\ \boldsymbol{C}_2 &= \boldsymbol{A}^-\boldsymbol{B}(\boldsymbol{B}'\boldsymbol{A}^-\boldsymbol{B})^-, \\ \boldsymbol{C}_3 &= (\boldsymbol{B}'\boldsymbol{A}^-\boldsymbol{B})^-. \end{aligned} \tag{3.57}$$

We omit the case in which Sp$(\boldsymbol{A}) \supset$ Sp$(\boldsymbol{B})$ does not necessarily hold in Theorem 3.13. (This is a little complicated but is left as an exercise for the reader.) Let

$$\tilde{\boldsymbol{F}} = \begin{bmatrix} \tilde{\boldsymbol{C}}_1 & \tilde{\boldsymbol{C}}_2 \\ \tilde{\boldsymbol{C}}_2' & -\tilde{\boldsymbol{C}}_3 \end{bmatrix}$$

be a generalized inverse of $\boldsymbol{N}$ defined above. Then,

$$\begin{aligned} \tilde{\boldsymbol{C}}_1 &= \boldsymbol{T}^- - \boldsymbol{T}^-\boldsymbol{B}(\boldsymbol{B}'\boldsymbol{T}^-\boldsymbol{B})^-\boldsymbol{B}'\boldsymbol{T}^-, \\ \tilde{\boldsymbol{C}}_2 &= \boldsymbol{T}^-\boldsymbol{B}(\boldsymbol{B}'\boldsymbol{T}^-\boldsymbol{B})^-, \\ \tilde{\boldsymbol{C}}_3 &= -\boldsymbol{U} + (\boldsymbol{B}'\boldsymbol{T}^-\boldsymbol{B})^-, \end{aligned} \tag{3.58}$$

where $\boldsymbol{T} = \boldsymbol{A} + \boldsymbol{B}\boldsymbol{U}\boldsymbol{B}'$, and $\boldsymbol{U}$ is an arbitrary matrix such that Sp$(\boldsymbol{T}) \supset$ Sp$(\boldsymbol{A})$ and Sp$(\boldsymbol{T}) \supset$ Sp$(\boldsymbol{B})$ (Rao, 1973).

3.3 A Variety of Generalized Inverse Matrices

As is clear from (3.46) in Theorem 3.13, a generalized inverse $\boldsymbol{A}^-$ of a given matrix $\boldsymbol{A}$ is not uniquely determined. The definition of the generalized inverse given in Theorem 3.2 allows arbitrariness in

(i) the choice of the complement space W of V,

(ii) the choice of the complement space $\tilde{V}$ of $\tilde{W}$, and

(iii) the choice of the subspace $\tilde{W}_r$ of $\tilde{W}$, including the choice of its dimensionality r,

despite the fact that $\tilde{W} =$ Ker$(\boldsymbol{A})$ is uniquely determined for $V =$ Sp$(\boldsymbol{A})$. Let W in (i) and $\tilde{V}$ in (ii) above be chosen so that $E^n = V \oplus W$ and $E^m = \tilde{V} \oplus \tilde{W}$, respectively. Then $\boldsymbol{A}\boldsymbol{A}^-$ is the projector onto V along W, and $\boldsymbol{A}^-\boldsymbol{A}$ is the projector onto $\tilde{V}$ along $\tilde{W}$. That is,

$$\boldsymbol{A}\boldsymbol{A}^- = \boldsymbol{P}_{V \cdot W} \tag{3.59}$$

and

$$\boldsymbol{A}^-\boldsymbol{A} = \boldsymbol{P}_{\tilde{V} \cdot \tilde{W}}. \tag{3.60}$$

3.3.1 Reflexive generalized inverse matrices

By the method presented in the previous section, we know $\boldsymbol{A}\boldsymbol{A}^-$ is the projector onto V along W (i.e., $\boldsymbol{P}_{V \cdot W}$), and $\boldsymbol{A}^-\boldsymbol{A}$ is the projector onto $\tilde{V}$ along $\tilde{W}$ (i.e., $\boldsymbol{P}_{\tilde{V}\cdot\tilde{W}}$). However, $\phi^-(\boldsymbol{y})$, an inverse transformation of an arbitrary n-component vector $\boldsymbol{y} \in E^n$, is not uniquely determined because there is some arbitrariness in the choice of $\phi_M^-(\boldsymbol{y}_2) = \boldsymbol{A}^-\boldsymbol{y}_2 \in \text{Ker}(\boldsymbol{A})$, where $\boldsymbol{y}_2$ is such that

$$\boldsymbol{y} = \boldsymbol{y}_1 + \boldsymbol{y}_2,$$

$\boldsymbol{y}_1 \in V$, and $\boldsymbol{y}_2 \in W$. Hence, an $\boldsymbol{A}^-$ that satisfies $\boldsymbol{P}_{V\cdot W} = \boldsymbol{A}\boldsymbol{A}^-$ and $\boldsymbol{P}_{W\cdot V} = \boldsymbol{A}^-\boldsymbol{A}$ is not uniquely determined. We therefore consider the condition under which $\boldsymbol{A}^-$ is uniquely determined for a given $\boldsymbol{A}$ and that satisfies the conditions above.

For an arbitrary $\boldsymbol{y} \in E^n$, we have $\boldsymbol{y}_1 = \boldsymbol{A}\boldsymbol{A}^-\boldsymbol{y} \in \text{Sp}(\boldsymbol{A})$ and $\boldsymbol{y}_2 = (\boldsymbol{I}_n - \boldsymbol{A}\boldsymbol{A}^-)\boldsymbol{y} \in \text{Sp}(\boldsymbol{A})^c$. Let $\boldsymbol{A}^-$ be an arbitrary generalized inverse of $\boldsymbol{A}$. From Theorem 3.2, we have

$$\begin{aligned} \boldsymbol{x} &= \boldsymbol{A}^-\boldsymbol{A}\boldsymbol{y} = \boldsymbol{A}^-\boldsymbol{y}_1 + \boldsymbol{A}^-\boldsymbol{y}_2 \\ &= \boldsymbol{A}^-(\boldsymbol{A}\boldsymbol{A}^-\boldsymbol{y}) + \boldsymbol{A}^-(\boldsymbol{I}_n - \boldsymbol{A}\boldsymbol{A}^-)\boldsymbol{y} \\ &= (\boldsymbol{A}^-\boldsymbol{A})\boldsymbol{A}^-\boldsymbol{y} + (\boldsymbol{I}_n - \boldsymbol{A}^-\boldsymbol{A})\boldsymbol{A}^-\boldsymbol{y} = \boldsymbol{x}_1 + \boldsymbol{x}_2, \end{aligned} \tag{3.61}$$

where $\boldsymbol{x}_1 \in \tilde{V} = \text{Sp}(\boldsymbol{A}^-\boldsymbol{A})$ and $\boldsymbol{x}_2 \in \tilde{W} = \text{Ker}(\boldsymbol{A}) = \text{Sp}(\boldsymbol{I}_n - \boldsymbol{A}\boldsymbol{A}^-)$. On the other hand,

$$\tilde{W}_r = \text{Sp}((\boldsymbol{I}_m - \boldsymbol{A}^-\boldsymbol{A})\boldsymbol{A}^-) \subset \text{Sp}(\boldsymbol{I}_m - \boldsymbol{A}^-\boldsymbol{A}) = \text{Ker}(\boldsymbol{A}). \tag{3.62}$$

Hence, $\boldsymbol{A}^-$ transforms $\boldsymbol{y}_1 \in \text{Sp}(\boldsymbol{A})$ into $\boldsymbol{x}_1 \in \text{Sp}(\boldsymbol{A}^-\boldsymbol{A})$, and $\boldsymbol{y}_2 \in \text{Sp}(\boldsymbol{I}_n - \boldsymbol{A}\boldsymbol{A}^-)$ into $\boldsymbol{x}_2 \in W = \text{Ker}(\boldsymbol{A})$. However, the latter mapping is not surjective. This allows an arbitrary choice of the dimensionality r in $\tilde{W}_r \subset \tilde{W} = \text{Ker}(\boldsymbol{A})$. Let $r = 0$, namely $\tilde{W}_r = \{\boldsymbol{0}\}$. Then, $(\boldsymbol{I}_m - \boldsymbol{A}^-\boldsymbol{A})\boldsymbol{A}^- = \boldsymbol{O}$, and it follows that

$$\boldsymbol{A}^-\boldsymbol{A}\boldsymbol{A}^- = \boldsymbol{A}^-. \tag{3.63}$$

Definition 3.2 *A generalized inverse $\boldsymbol{A}^-$ that satisfies both (3.1) and (3.63) is called a reflexive g-inverse matrix of $\boldsymbol{A}$ and is denoted as $\boldsymbol{A}_r^-$.*

As is clear from the proof of Theorem 3.3, $\boldsymbol{A}^-$ that satisfies

$$\boldsymbol{x}_2 = \boldsymbol{A}^-\boldsymbol{y}_2 = \boldsymbol{0} \tag{3.64}$$

is a reflexive g-inverse of $\boldsymbol{A}$, which transforms $\boldsymbol{y} \in V = \mathrm{Sp}(\boldsymbol{A})$ into $\boldsymbol{x}_1 \in \tilde{V} = \mathrm{Sp}(\boldsymbol{A}^-\boldsymbol{A})$ since $\boldsymbol{A}^-\boldsymbol{y} = \boldsymbol{A}^-\boldsymbol{y}_1 + \boldsymbol{A}^-\boldsymbol{y}_2 = \boldsymbol{A}^-\boldsymbol{y}_1 = \boldsymbol{x}_1$. Furthermore, $\boldsymbol{A}_r^-$ is uniquely determined only if W such that $\boldsymbol{E}^n = V \oplus W$ and $\tilde{V}$ such that $E^m = \tilde{V} \oplus \tilde{W}$ are simultaneously determined. In general, $\boldsymbol{A}_r^-$ is not uniquely determined because of the arbitrariness in the choice of W and $\tilde{V}$.

Note That $\boldsymbol{A}^-\boldsymbol{y} = \boldsymbol{0} \Leftrightarrow \boldsymbol{A}^-\boldsymbol{A}\boldsymbol{A}^- = \boldsymbol{A}^-$ can be shown as follows. From Theorem 3.2, we have $\boldsymbol{A}\boldsymbol{A}^-\boldsymbol{y}_1 = \boldsymbol{y}_1 \Rightarrow \boldsymbol{A}^-\boldsymbol{A}\boldsymbol{A}^-\boldsymbol{y}_1 = \boldsymbol{A}^-\boldsymbol{y}_1$. Furthermore, since $\boldsymbol{A}\boldsymbol{A}^-\boldsymbol{y}_2 = \boldsymbol{0} \Rightarrow \boldsymbol{A}^-\boldsymbol{A}\boldsymbol{A}^-\boldsymbol{y}_2 = \boldsymbol{0}$, we have $\boldsymbol{A}^-\boldsymbol{A}\boldsymbol{A}^-(\boldsymbol{y}_1 + \boldsymbol{y}_2) = \boldsymbol{A}^-\boldsymbol{y}_1$, the left-hand side of which is equal to $\boldsymbol{A}^-\boldsymbol{A}\boldsymbol{A}^-\boldsymbol{y}$. If we add $\boldsymbol{A}^-\boldsymbol{y}_2$ to the right-hand side, we obtain $\boldsymbol{A}^-\boldsymbol{y}_1 + \boldsymbol{A}^-\boldsymbol{y}_2 = \boldsymbol{A}^-\boldsymbol{y}$, and so $\boldsymbol{A}^-\boldsymbol{A}\boldsymbol{A}^-\boldsymbol{y} = \boldsymbol{A}^-\boldsymbol{y}$. Since this has to hold for any $\boldsymbol{y}$, it must hold that $\boldsymbol{A}^-\boldsymbol{A}\boldsymbol{A}^- = \boldsymbol{A}^-$.

Conversely, from Lemma 3.2, we have $\boldsymbol{y}_2 = (\boldsymbol{I}_n - \boldsymbol{A}\boldsymbol{A}^-)\boldsymbol{y}$. Thus, $\boldsymbol{A}^-\boldsymbol{A}\boldsymbol{A}^- = \boldsymbol{A}^- \Rightarrow \boldsymbol{A}^-\boldsymbol{y}_2 = \boldsymbol{A}^-(\boldsymbol{I}_n - \boldsymbol{A}\boldsymbol{A}^-)\boldsymbol{y} = \boldsymbol{0}$.

Theorem 3.14 *The following relation holds for a generalized inverse* $\boldsymbol{A}^-$ *that satisfies (3.1):*

$$\boldsymbol{A}^-\boldsymbol{A}\boldsymbol{A}^- = \boldsymbol{A}^- \Longleftrightarrow \mathrm{rank}(\boldsymbol{A}) = \mathrm{rank}(\boldsymbol{A}^-). \tag{3.65}$$

Proof. ($\Rightarrow$): Clear from (3.11).

($\Leftarrow$): Decompose $\boldsymbol{A}^-$ as $\boldsymbol{A}^- = (\boldsymbol{I}_m - \boldsymbol{A}^-\boldsymbol{A})\boldsymbol{A}^- + \boldsymbol{A}^-\boldsymbol{A}\boldsymbol{A}^-$. Since $\mathrm{Sp}(\boldsymbol{I}_m - \boldsymbol{A}^-\boldsymbol{A}) \cap \mathrm{Sp}(\boldsymbol{A}^-\boldsymbol{A}) = \{\boldsymbol{0}\}$, we have $\mathrm{rank}(\boldsymbol{A}^-) = \mathrm{rank}((\boldsymbol{I}_m - \boldsymbol{A}^-\boldsymbol{A})\boldsymbol{A}^-) + \mathrm{rank}(\boldsymbol{A}^-\boldsymbol{A}\boldsymbol{A}^-)$. From $\mathrm{rank}(\boldsymbol{A}^-\boldsymbol{A}\boldsymbol{A}^-) = \mathrm{rank}(\boldsymbol{A})$, we obtain $\mathrm{rank}((\boldsymbol{I}_m - \boldsymbol{A}^-\boldsymbol{A})\boldsymbol{A}^-) = 0 \Rightarrow (\boldsymbol{I}_m - \boldsymbol{A}^-\boldsymbol{A})\boldsymbol{A}^- = \boldsymbol{O}$, which implies $\boldsymbol{A}^-\boldsymbol{A}\boldsymbol{A}^- = \boldsymbol{A}^-$. Q.E.D.

Example 3.3 Let

$$\boldsymbol{A} = \begin{bmatrix} \boldsymbol{A}_{11} & \boldsymbol{A}_{12} \\ \boldsymbol{A}_{21} & \boldsymbol{A}_{22} \end{bmatrix},$$

where $\boldsymbol{A}_{11}$ is of order r and nonsingular. Let the rank of $\boldsymbol{A}$ be r. Then,

$$\boldsymbol{G} = \begin{bmatrix} \boldsymbol{A}_{11}^{-1} & \boldsymbol{O} \\ \boldsymbol{O} & \boldsymbol{O} \end{bmatrix}$$

is a reflexive g-inverse of $\boldsymbol{A}$ because $\mathrm{rank}(\boldsymbol{G}) = \mathrm{rank}(\boldsymbol{A}) = r$, and

$$\boldsymbol{A}\boldsymbol{G}\boldsymbol{A} = \begin{bmatrix} \boldsymbol{A}_{11} & \boldsymbol{A}_{12} \\ \boldsymbol{A}_{21} & \boldsymbol{A}_{21}\boldsymbol{A}_{11}^{-1}\boldsymbol{A}_{12}, \end{bmatrix},$$

where $A_{21}A_{11}^{-1}A_{12} = A_{22}$, and so $AGA = A$, since $\begin{bmatrix} A_{11} \\ A_{21} \end{bmatrix} W = \begin{bmatrix} A_{12} \\ A_{22} \end{bmatrix}$, and so $A_{11}W = A_{12}$ and $A_{21}W = A_{22}$. For example,

$$A = \begin{bmatrix} 3 & 2 & 1 \\ 2 & 2 & 2 \\ 1 & 2 & 3 \end{bmatrix}$$

is a symmetric matrix of rank 2. One expression of a reflexive g-inverse A_r^- of A is given by

$$\begin{bmatrix} \begin{bmatrix} 3 & 2 \\ 2 & 2 \end{bmatrix}^{-1} & \begin{matrix} 0 \\ 0 \end{matrix} \\ \begin{pmatrix} 0 & 0 \end{pmatrix} & 0 \end{bmatrix} = \begin{bmatrix} 1 & -1 & 0 \\ -1 & \frac{3}{2} & 0 \\ 0 & 0 & 0 \end{bmatrix}.$$

Example 3.4 Obtain a reflexive g-inverse A_r^- of $A = \begin{bmatrix} 1 & 1 \\ 1 & 1 \end{bmatrix}$.

$AA_r^-A = A$ implies $a + b + c + d = 1$. An additional condition may be derived from

$$\begin{bmatrix} a & b \\ c & d \end{bmatrix} \begin{bmatrix} 1 & 1 \\ 1 & 1 \end{bmatrix} \begin{bmatrix} a & b \\ c & d \end{bmatrix} = \begin{bmatrix} a & b \\ c & d \end{bmatrix}.$$

It may also be derived from $\text{rank}(A) = 1$, which implies $\text{rank}(A_r^-) = 1$. It follows that $\det(A_r^-) = ad - bc = 0$. A set of a, b, c, and d that satisfies both $a + b + c + d = 1$ and $ad - bc = 0$ defines a 2 by 2 square matrix A_r^-.

3.3.2 Minimum norm generalized inverse matrices

Let E^m be decomposed as $E^m = \tilde{V} \oplus \tilde{W}$, where $\tilde{W} = \text{Ker}(A)$, in Definition 3.3. If we choose $\tilde{V} = \tilde{W}^\perp$ (that is, when $\tilde{V}$ and $\tilde{W}$ are orthogonal), $A^-A = P_{\tilde{V}\cdot\tilde{W}}$ becomes an orthogonal projector, and it holds that

$$(A^-A)' = A^-A. \tag{3.66}$$

Since $\tilde{V} = \text{Sp}(A^-A)$ and $\tilde{W} = \text{Sp}(I_m - A^-A)$ from Lemmas 3.1 and 3.2, (3.66) can also be derived from

$$(A^-A)'(I_m - A^-A) = O \Longleftrightarrow (A^-A)' = A^-A. \tag{3.67}$$

Let $Ax = y$ be a linear equation, where $y \in \text{Sp}(A)$. Since $y_1 = Ax \in \text{Sp}(A)$ implies $y = y_1 + y_2 = y_1 + 0 = y_1$, we obtain

$$\tilde{x} = A^-y = A^-y_1 = A^-Ax. \tag{3.68}$$

Let $\boldsymbol{P} = \boldsymbol{A}^{-}\boldsymbol{A}$ be a projection matrix, and let $\boldsymbol{P}^*$ denote an orthogonal projector that satisfies $\boldsymbol{P}' = \boldsymbol{P}$. From Theorem 2.22, we have

$$\boldsymbol{P}' = \boldsymbol{P} \Longleftrightarrow ||\tilde{\boldsymbol{x}}|| = ||\boldsymbol{P}\boldsymbol{x}|| \leq ||\boldsymbol{x}||, \tag{3.69}$$

which indicates that the norm of $\boldsymbol{x}$ takes a minimum value $||\boldsymbol{x}|| = ||\boldsymbol{P}^*\boldsymbol{y}||$ when $\boldsymbol{P}' = \boldsymbol{P}$. That is, although infinitely many solutions exist for $\boldsymbol{x}$ in the linear equation $\boldsymbol{A}\boldsymbol{x} = \boldsymbol{y}$, where $\boldsymbol{y} \in \text{Sp}(\boldsymbol{A})$ and $\boldsymbol{A}$ is an n by m matrix of $\text{rank}(\boldsymbol{A}) < m$, $\boldsymbol{x} = \boldsymbol{A}^{-}\boldsymbol{y}$ gives a solution associated with the minimum sum of squares of elements when $\boldsymbol{A}^{-}$ satisfies (3.66).

Definition 3.3 *An $\boldsymbol{A}^{-}$ that satisfies both $\boldsymbol{A}\boldsymbol{A}^{-}\boldsymbol{A} = \boldsymbol{A}$ and $(\boldsymbol{A}^{-}\boldsymbol{A})' = \boldsymbol{A}^{-}\boldsymbol{A}$ is called a minimum norm g-inverse of $\boldsymbol{A}$, and is denoted by $\boldsymbol{A}_m^{-}$* (Rao and Mitra, 1971).

The following theorem holds for a minimum norm g-inverse $\boldsymbol{A}_m^{-}$.

Theorem 3.15 *The following three conditions are equivalent:*

$$\boldsymbol{A}_m^{-}\boldsymbol{A} = (\boldsymbol{A}_m^{-}\boldsymbol{A})' \text{ and } \boldsymbol{A}\boldsymbol{A}_m^{-}\boldsymbol{A} = \boldsymbol{A}, \tag{3.70}$$

$$\boldsymbol{A}_m^{-}\boldsymbol{A}\boldsymbol{A}' = \boldsymbol{A}', \tag{3.71}$$

$$\boldsymbol{A}_m^{-}\boldsymbol{A} = \boldsymbol{A}'(\boldsymbol{A}\boldsymbol{A}')^{-}\boldsymbol{A}. \tag{3.72}$$

Proof. (3.70) $\Rightarrow$ (3.71): $(\boldsymbol{A}\boldsymbol{A}_m^{-}\boldsymbol{A})' = \boldsymbol{A}' \Rightarrow (\boldsymbol{A}_m^{-}\boldsymbol{A})'\boldsymbol{A}' = \boldsymbol{A}' \Rightarrow \boldsymbol{A}_m^{-}\boldsymbol{A}\boldsymbol{A}' = \boldsymbol{A}'$.

(3.71) $\Rightarrow$ (3.72): Postmultiply both sides of $\boldsymbol{A}_m^{-}\boldsymbol{A}\boldsymbol{A}' = \boldsymbol{A}'$ by $(\boldsymbol{A}\boldsymbol{A}')^{-}\boldsymbol{A}$.

(3.72) $\Rightarrow$ (3.70): Use $\boldsymbol{A}'(\boldsymbol{A}\boldsymbol{A}')^{-}\boldsymbol{A}\boldsymbol{A}' = \boldsymbol{A}'$, and $(\boldsymbol{A}'(\boldsymbol{A}\boldsymbol{A}')^{-}\boldsymbol{A})' = \boldsymbol{A}'(\boldsymbol{A} \times \boldsymbol{A}')^{-}\boldsymbol{A}$ obtained by replacing $\boldsymbol{A}$ by $\boldsymbol{A}'$ in Theorem 3.5. Q.E.D.

Note Since $(\boldsymbol{A}_m^{-}\boldsymbol{A})'(\boldsymbol{I}_m - \boldsymbol{A}_m^{-}\boldsymbol{A}) = \boldsymbol{O}$, $\boldsymbol{A}_m^{-}\boldsymbol{A} = \boldsymbol{A}'(\boldsymbol{A}\boldsymbol{A}')^{-}\boldsymbol{A}$ is the orthogonal projector onto $\text{Sp}(\boldsymbol{A}')$.

When either one of the conditions in Theorem 3.15 holds, $\tilde{V}$ and $\tilde{W}$ are ortho-complementary subspaces of each other in the direct-sum decomposition $E^m = \tilde{V} \cap \tilde{W}$. In this case, $\tilde{V} = \text{Sp}(\boldsymbol{A}_m^{-}\boldsymbol{A}) = \text{Sp}(\boldsymbol{A}')$ holds from (3.72).

Note By Theorem 3.15, one expression for $\boldsymbol{A}_m^-$ is given by $\boldsymbol{A}'(\boldsymbol{A}\boldsymbol{A}')^-$. In this case, $\text{rank}(\boldsymbol{A}_m^-) = \text{rank}(\boldsymbol{A})$ holds. Let $\boldsymbol{Z}$ be an arbitrary m by n matrix. Then the following relation holds:

$$\boldsymbol{A}_m^- = \boldsymbol{A}'(\boldsymbol{A}\boldsymbol{A}')^- + \boldsymbol{Z}[\boldsymbol{I}_n - \boldsymbol{A}\boldsymbol{A}'(\boldsymbol{A}\boldsymbol{A}')^-]. \tag{3.73}$$

Let $\boldsymbol{x} = \boldsymbol{A}_m^-\boldsymbol{b}$ be a solution to $\boldsymbol{A}\boldsymbol{x} = \boldsymbol{b}$. Then, $\boldsymbol{A}\boldsymbol{A}'(\boldsymbol{A}\boldsymbol{A}')^-\boldsymbol{b} = \boldsymbol{A}\boldsymbol{A}'(\boldsymbol{A}\boldsymbol{A}')^-\boldsymbol{A}\boldsymbol{x} = \boldsymbol{A}\boldsymbol{x} = \boldsymbol{b}$. Hence, we obtain

$$\boldsymbol{x} = \boldsymbol{A}'(\boldsymbol{A}\boldsymbol{A}')^-\boldsymbol{b}. \tag{3.74}$$

The first term in (3.73) belongs to $\tilde{V} = \text{Sp}(\boldsymbol{A}')$ and the second term to $\tilde{W} = \tilde{V}^\perp$, and we have in general $\text{Sp}(\boldsymbol{A}_m^-) \supset \text{Sp}(\boldsymbol{A}')$, or $\text{rank}(\boldsymbol{A}_m^-) \geq \text{rank}(\boldsymbol{A}')$. A minimum norm g-inverse that satisfies $\text{rank}(\boldsymbol{A}_m^-) = \text{rank}(\boldsymbol{A})$ is called a minimum norm reflexive g-inverse and is denoted by

$$\boldsymbol{A}_{mr}^- = \boldsymbol{A}'(\boldsymbol{A}\boldsymbol{A}')^-. \tag{3.75}$$

Note Equation (3.74) can also be obtained directly by finding $\boldsymbol{x}$ that minimizes $\boldsymbol{x}'\boldsymbol{x}$ under $\boldsymbol{A}\boldsymbol{x} = \boldsymbol{b}$. Let $\boldsymbol{\lambda} = (\lambda_1, \lambda_2, \cdots, \lambda_p)'$ denote a vector of Lagrange multipliers, and define

$$f(\boldsymbol{x}, \boldsymbol{\lambda}) = \frac{1}{2}\boldsymbol{x}'\boldsymbol{x} - (\boldsymbol{A}\boldsymbol{x} - \boldsymbol{b})'\boldsymbol{\lambda}.$$

Differentiating f with respect to (the elements of) $\boldsymbol{x}$ and setting the results to zero, we obtain $\boldsymbol{x} = \boldsymbol{A}'\boldsymbol{\lambda}$. Substituting this into $\boldsymbol{A}\boldsymbol{x} = \boldsymbol{b}$, we obtain $\boldsymbol{b} = \boldsymbol{A}\boldsymbol{A}'\boldsymbol{\lambda}$, from which $\boldsymbol{\lambda} = (\boldsymbol{A}\boldsymbol{A}')^-\boldsymbol{b} + [\boldsymbol{I}_n - (\boldsymbol{A}\boldsymbol{A}')^-(\boldsymbol{A}\boldsymbol{A}')]\boldsymbol{z}$ is derived, where $\boldsymbol{z}$ is an arbitrary m-component vector. Hence, we obtain $\boldsymbol{x} = \boldsymbol{A}'(\boldsymbol{A}\boldsymbol{A}')^-\boldsymbol{b}$.

The solution above amounts to obtaining $\boldsymbol{x}$ that satisfies both $\boldsymbol{x} = \boldsymbol{A}'\boldsymbol{\lambda}$ and $\boldsymbol{A}\boldsymbol{x} = \boldsymbol{b}$, that is, to solving the simultaneous equation

$$\begin{bmatrix} \boldsymbol{I}_m & \boldsymbol{A}' \\ \boldsymbol{A} & \boldsymbol{O} \end{bmatrix} \begin{bmatrix} \boldsymbol{x} \\ -\boldsymbol{\lambda} \end{bmatrix} = \begin{bmatrix} \boldsymbol{0} \\ \boldsymbol{b} \end{bmatrix}$$

for the unknown vector $\begin{bmatrix} \boldsymbol{x} \\ -\boldsymbol{\lambda} \end{bmatrix}$.

Let

$$\begin{bmatrix} \boldsymbol{I}_m & \boldsymbol{A} \\ \boldsymbol{A}' & \boldsymbol{O} \end{bmatrix}^- = \begin{bmatrix} \boldsymbol{C}_1 & \boldsymbol{C}_2 \\ \boldsymbol{C}_2' & \boldsymbol{C}_3 \end{bmatrix}.$$

From $\text{Sp}(\boldsymbol{I}_m) \supset \text{Sp}(\boldsymbol{A})$ and the corollary of Theorem 3.13, we obtain (3.74) because $\boldsymbol{C}_2 = \boldsymbol{A}'(\boldsymbol{A}\boldsymbol{A}')^-$.

Example 3.5 Solving a simultaneous equation in three unknowns,

$$x + y - 2z = 2, \ \ x - 2y + z = -1, \ \ -2x + y + z = -1,$$

we obtain

$$x = k + 1, \ \ y = k + 1, \text{ and } z = k.$$

We therefore have

$$\begin{aligned} x^2 + y^2 + z^2 &= (k+1)^2 + (k+1)^2 + k^2 \\ &= 3k^2 + 4k + 2 = 3\left(k + \frac{2}{3}\right)^2 + \frac{2}{3} \geq \frac{2}{3}. \end{aligned}$$

Hence, the solution obtained by setting $k = -\frac{2}{3}$ (that is, $x = \frac{1}{3}$, $y = \frac{1}{3}$, and $z = -\frac{2}{3}$) minimizes $x^2 + y^2 + z^2$.

Let us derive the solution above via a minimum norm g-inverse. Let $\boldsymbol{Ax} = \boldsymbol{y}$ denote the simultaneous equation above in three unknowns. Then,

$$\boldsymbol{A} = \begin{bmatrix} 1 & 1 & -2 \\ 1 & -2 & 1 \\ -2 & 1 & 1 \end{bmatrix}, \ \boldsymbol{x} = \begin{bmatrix} x \\ y \\ z \end{bmatrix}, \text{ and } \boldsymbol{b} = \begin{bmatrix} 2 \\ -1 \\ -1 \end{bmatrix}.$$

A minimum norm reflexive g-inverse of $\boldsymbol{A}$, on the other hand, is, according to (3.75), given by

$$\boldsymbol{A}_{mr}^- = \boldsymbol{A}'(\boldsymbol{AA}')^- = \frac{1}{3}\begin{bmatrix} 1 & 1 & 0 \\ 0 & -1 & 0 \\ -1 & 0 & 0 \end{bmatrix}.$$

Hence,

$$\boldsymbol{x} = \boldsymbol{A}_{mr}^- \boldsymbol{b} = \left(\frac{1}{3}, \frac{1}{3}, -\frac{2}{3}\right)'.$$

(Verify that the $\boldsymbol{A}_{mr}^-$ above satisfies $\boldsymbol{AA}_{mr}^-\boldsymbol{A} = \boldsymbol{A}$, $(\boldsymbol{A}_{mr}^-\boldsymbol{A})' = \boldsymbol{A}_{mr}^-\boldsymbol{A}$, and $\boldsymbol{A}_{mr}^-\boldsymbol{AA}_{mr}^- = \boldsymbol{A}_{mr}^-$.)

3.3.3 Least squares generalized inverse matrices

As has already been mentioned, the necessary and sufficient condition for the simultaneous equation $\boldsymbol{Ax} = \boldsymbol{y}$ to have a solution is $\boldsymbol{y} \in \text{Sp}(\boldsymbol{A})$. When, on the other hand, $\boldsymbol{y} \notin \text{Sp}(\boldsymbol{A})$, no solution vector $\boldsymbol{x}$ exists. We therefore consider obtaining $\boldsymbol{x}^*$ that satisfies

$$||\boldsymbol{y} - \boldsymbol{Ax}^*||^2 = \min_{x \in E_m} ||\boldsymbol{y} - \boldsymbol{Ax}||^2. \tag{3.76}$$

Let $\boldsymbol{y} = \boldsymbol{y}_0 + \boldsymbol{y}_1$, where $\boldsymbol{y} \in E^n$, $\boldsymbol{y}_0 \in V = \text{Sp}(\boldsymbol{A})$, and $\boldsymbol{y}_1 \in W = \text{Sp}(\boldsymbol{I}_n - \boldsymbol{A}\boldsymbol{A}^-)$. Then a solution vector to $\boldsymbol{A}\boldsymbol{x} = \boldsymbol{y}_0$ can be expressed as $\boldsymbol{x} = \boldsymbol{A}^-\boldsymbol{y}_0$ using an arbitrary g-inverse $\boldsymbol{A}^-$. Since $\boldsymbol{y}_0 = \boldsymbol{y} - \boldsymbol{y}_1$, we have $\boldsymbol{x} = \boldsymbol{A}^-\boldsymbol{y}_0 = \boldsymbol{A}^-(\boldsymbol{y} - \boldsymbol{y}_1) = \boldsymbol{A}^-\boldsymbol{y} - \boldsymbol{A}^-\boldsymbol{y}_1$. Furthermore, since $\boldsymbol{y}_1 = (\boldsymbol{I}_n - \boldsymbol{A}\boldsymbol{A}^-)\boldsymbol{y}$, we have

$$\boldsymbol{A}\boldsymbol{x} = \boldsymbol{A}\boldsymbol{A}^-\boldsymbol{y} - \boldsymbol{A}\boldsymbol{A}^-(\boldsymbol{I}_n - \boldsymbol{A}\boldsymbol{A}^-)\boldsymbol{y} = \boldsymbol{A}\boldsymbol{A}^-\boldsymbol{y}.$$

Let $\boldsymbol{P}_A$ denote the orthogonal projector onto $\text{Sp}(\boldsymbol{A})$. From

$$||\boldsymbol{A}\boldsymbol{x} - \boldsymbol{y}||^2 = \\ ||(\boldsymbol{I}_n - \boldsymbol{A}\boldsymbol{A}^-)\boldsymbol{y}||^2 \geq ||(\boldsymbol{I}_n - \boldsymbol{P}_A)(\boldsymbol{I}_n - \boldsymbol{A}\boldsymbol{A}^-)\boldsymbol{y}||^2 = ||(\boldsymbol{I}_n - \boldsymbol{P}_A)\boldsymbol{y}||^2,$$

$\boldsymbol{A}^-$ that minimizes $||\boldsymbol{A}\boldsymbol{x} - \boldsymbol{y}||$ satisfies $\boldsymbol{A}\boldsymbol{A}^- = \boldsymbol{P}_A$. That is,

$$(\boldsymbol{A}\boldsymbol{A}^-)' = \boldsymbol{A}\boldsymbol{A}^-. \tag{3.77}$$

In this case, V and W are orthogonal, and the projector onto V along W, $\boldsymbol{P}_{V\cdot W} = \boldsymbol{P}_{V\cdot V^\perp} = \boldsymbol{A}\boldsymbol{A}^-$, becomes an orthogonal projector.

Definition 3.4 A generalized inverse $\boldsymbol{A}^-$ that satisfies both $\boldsymbol{A}\boldsymbol{A}^-\boldsymbol{A} = \boldsymbol{A}$ and $(\boldsymbol{A}\boldsymbol{A}')' = \boldsymbol{A}\boldsymbol{A}^-$ is called a least squares g-inverse matrix of $\boldsymbol{A}$ and is denoted as $\boldsymbol{A}_\ell^-$ (Rao and Mitra, 1971).

The following theorem holds for a least squares g-inverse.

Theorem 3.16 *The following three conditions are equivalent:*

$$\boldsymbol{A}\boldsymbol{A}_\ell^-\boldsymbol{A} = \boldsymbol{A} \textit{ and } (\boldsymbol{A}\boldsymbol{A}_\ell^-)' = \boldsymbol{A}\boldsymbol{A}_\ell^-, \tag{3.78}$$

$$\boldsymbol{A}'\boldsymbol{A}\boldsymbol{A}_\ell^- = \boldsymbol{A}', \tag{3.79}$$

$$\boldsymbol{A}\boldsymbol{A}_\ell^- = \boldsymbol{A}(\boldsymbol{A}'\boldsymbol{A})^-\boldsymbol{A}'. \tag{3.80}$$

Proof. (3.78) $\Rightarrow$ (3.79): $(\boldsymbol{A}\boldsymbol{A}_\ell^-\boldsymbol{A})' = \boldsymbol{A}' \Rightarrow \boldsymbol{A}'(\boldsymbol{A}\boldsymbol{A}_\ell^-)' = \boldsymbol{A}' \Rightarrow \boldsymbol{A}'\boldsymbol{A}\boldsymbol{A}_\ell^- = \boldsymbol{A}'$.

(3.79) $\Rightarrow$ (3.80): Premultiply both sides of $\boldsymbol{A}'\boldsymbol{A}\boldsymbol{A}_\ell^- = \boldsymbol{A}'$ by $\boldsymbol{A}(\boldsymbol{A}'\boldsymbol{A})^-$, and use the result in Theorem 3.5.

(3.80) $\Rightarrow$ (3.78): Similarly, clear from Theorem 3.5. Q.E.D.

Similarly to a minimum norm g-inverse A_m^-, a general form of a least squares g-inverse is given by

$$A_\ell^- = (A'A)^- A' + [I_m - (A'A)^- A'A]Z, \tag{3.81}$$

where Z is an arbitrary m by n matrix. In this case, we generally have $\text{rank}(A_\ell^-) \geq \text{rank}(A)$. A least squares reflexive g-inverse that satisfies $\text{rank}(A_\ell^-) = \text{rank}(A)$ is given by

$$A_{\ell r}^- = (A'A)^- A'. \tag{3.82}$$

We next prove a theorem that shows the relationship between a least squares g-inverse and a minimum norm g-inverse.

Theorem 3.17

$$\{(A')_m^-\} = \{(A_\ell^-)\}. \tag{3.83}$$

Proof. $AA_\ell^- A = A \Rightarrow A'(A_\ell^-)'A' = A'$. Furthermore, $(AA_\ell^-)' = AA_\ell^- \Rightarrow (A_\ell^-)'A' = ((A_\ell^-)'A')'$. Hence, from Theorem 3.15, $(A_\ell^-)' \in \{(A')_m^-\}$. On the other hand, from $A'(A')_m^- A' = A'$ and $((A')_m^- A')' = (A')_m^- A'$, we have

$$A((A')_m^-)' = (A((A')_m^-)')'.$$

Hence,

$$((A')_m^-)' \in \{A_\ell^-\} \Rightarrow (A')_m^- \in \{(A_\ell^-)'\},$$

resulting in (3.83). Q.E.D.

Example 3.6 The simultaneous equations $x + y = 2$, $x - 2y = 1$, and $-2x + y = 0$ obviously have no solution. Let

$$A = \begin{bmatrix} 1 & 1 \\ 1 & -2 \\ -2 & 1 \end{bmatrix}, \quad z = \begin{bmatrix} x \\ y \end{bmatrix}, \text{ and } b = \begin{bmatrix} 2 \\ 1 \\ 0 \end{bmatrix}.$$

The z that minimizes $||b - Ax||^2$ is given by

$$z = A_{\ell r}^- b = (A'A)^- A'b.$$

In this case, we have

$$A_{\ell r}^- = \frac{1}{3} \begin{bmatrix} 1 & 0 & -1 \\ 1 & -1 & 0 \end{bmatrix}.$$

Hence,

$$\boldsymbol{z} = \begin{bmatrix} x \\ y \end{bmatrix} = \frac{1}{3}\begin{bmatrix} 2 \\ 1 \end{bmatrix}, \quad \boldsymbol{Az} = \begin{bmatrix} 1 \\ 0 \\ -1 \end{bmatrix}.$$

The minimum is given by $||\boldsymbol{b} - \boldsymbol{Az}||^2 = (2-1)^2 + (1-0)^2 + (0-(-1))^2 = 3$.

3.3.4 The Moore-Penrose generalized inverse matrix

The kinds of generalized inverses discussed so far, reflexive g-inverses, minimum norm g-inverses, and least squares g-inverses, are not uniquely determined for a given matrix $\boldsymbol{A}$. However, $\boldsymbol{A}^-$ that satisfies (3.59) and (3.60) is determinable under the direct-sum decompositions $E^n = V \oplus W$ and $E^m = \tilde{V} \oplus \tilde{W}$, so that if $\boldsymbol{A}^-$ is a reflexive g-inverse (i.e., $\boldsymbol{A}^-\boldsymbol{A}\boldsymbol{A}^- = \boldsymbol{A}^-$), it can be uniquely determined. If in addition $W = V^\perp$ and $\tilde{V} = \tilde{W}^\perp$, then clearly (3.66) and (3.77) hold, and the following definition can be given.

Definition 3.5 *Matrix* $\boldsymbol{A}^+$ *that satisfies all of the following conditions is called the Moore-Penrose g-inverse matrix of* $\boldsymbol{A}$ (Moore, 1920; Penrose, 1955), *hereafter called merely the Moore-Penrose inverse*:

$$\boldsymbol{A}\boldsymbol{A}^+\boldsymbol{A} = \boldsymbol{A}, \tag{3.84}$$

$$\boldsymbol{A}^+\boldsymbol{A}\boldsymbol{A}^+ = \boldsymbol{A}^+, \tag{3.85}$$

$$(\boldsymbol{A}\boldsymbol{A}^+)' = \boldsymbol{A}\boldsymbol{A}^+, \tag{3.86}$$

$$(\boldsymbol{A}^+\boldsymbol{A})' = \boldsymbol{A}^+\boldsymbol{A}. \tag{3.87}$$

From the properties given in (3.86) and (3.87), we have $(\boldsymbol{A}\boldsymbol{A}^+)'(\boldsymbol{I}_n - \boldsymbol{A}\boldsymbol{A}^+) = \boldsymbol{O}$ and $(\boldsymbol{A}^+\boldsymbol{A})'(\boldsymbol{I}_m - \boldsymbol{A}^+\boldsymbol{A}) = \boldsymbol{O}$, and so

$$\boldsymbol{P}_A = \boldsymbol{A}\boldsymbol{A}^+ \text{ and } \boldsymbol{P}_{A^+} = \boldsymbol{A}^+\boldsymbol{A} \tag{3.88}$$

are the orthogonal projectors onto $\text{Sp}(\boldsymbol{A})$ and $\text{Sp}(\boldsymbol{A}^+)$, respectively. (Note that $(\boldsymbol{A}^+)^+ = \boldsymbol{A}$.) This means that the Moore-Penrose inverse can also be defined through (3.88). The definition using (3.84) through (3.87) was given by Penrose (1955), and the one using (3.88) was given by Moore (1920). If the reflexivity does not hold (i.e., $\boldsymbol{A}^+\boldsymbol{A}\boldsymbol{A}^+ \neq \boldsymbol{A}^+$), $\boldsymbol{P}_{A^+} = \boldsymbol{A}^+\boldsymbol{A}$ is the orthogonal projector onto $\text{Sp}(\boldsymbol{A}')$ but not necessarily onto $\text{Sp}(\boldsymbol{A}^+)$. This may be summarized in the following theorem.

Theorem 3.18 *Let $\boldsymbol{P}_A$, $\boldsymbol{P}_{A'}$, and $\boldsymbol{P}_G$ be the orthogonal projectors onto* $\mathrm{Sp}(\boldsymbol{A})$, $\mathrm{Sp}(\boldsymbol{A}')$, *and* $\mathrm{Sp}(\boldsymbol{G})$, *respectively. Then,*

(i) $\boldsymbol{AG} = \boldsymbol{P}_A$, $\boldsymbol{GA} = \boldsymbol{P}_G \Longleftrightarrow \boldsymbol{AGA} = \boldsymbol{A}$, $\boldsymbol{GAG} = \boldsymbol{G}$, $(\boldsymbol{AG})' = \boldsymbol{AG}$, $(\boldsymbol{GA})' = \boldsymbol{GA}$.

(ii) $\boldsymbol{AG} = \boldsymbol{P}_A$, $\boldsymbol{GA} = \boldsymbol{P}_{A'} \Longleftrightarrow \boldsymbol{AGA} = \boldsymbol{A}$, $(\boldsymbol{AG})' = \boldsymbol{AG}$, $(\boldsymbol{GA})' = \boldsymbol{GA}$.

(Proof omitted.)

Theorem 3.19 *The necessary and sufficient condition for $\boldsymbol{A}^-$ in $\boldsymbol{x} = \boldsymbol{A}^-\boldsymbol{b}$ to minimize $||\boldsymbol{Ax} - \boldsymbol{b}||$ is $\boldsymbol{A}^- = \boldsymbol{A}^+$.*

Proof. (Sufficiency) The $\boldsymbol{x}$ that minimizes $||\boldsymbol{Ax} - \boldsymbol{b}||$ can be expressed as

$$\boldsymbol{x} = \boldsymbol{A}^+\boldsymbol{b} + (\boldsymbol{I}_m - \boldsymbol{A}^+\boldsymbol{A})\boldsymbol{z}, \tag{3.89}$$

where $\boldsymbol{z}$ is an arbitrary m-component vector.

Furthermore, from (3.20) we have $\mathrm{Sp}(\boldsymbol{I}_m - \boldsymbol{A}^+\boldsymbol{A}) = \mathrm{Ker}(\boldsymbol{A})$, and from the fact that $\boldsymbol{A}^+$ is a reflexive g-inverse, we have $\mathrm{Sp}(\boldsymbol{A}^+) = \mathrm{Sp}(\boldsymbol{A}^+\boldsymbol{A})$. From the fact that $\boldsymbol{A}^+$ is also a minimum norm g-inverse, we have $E^m = \mathrm{Sp}(\boldsymbol{A}^+) \dot{\oplus} \mathrm{Sp}(\boldsymbol{I}_m - \boldsymbol{A}^+\boldsymbol{A})$, which together imply that the two vectors in (3.89), $\boldsymbol{A}^+\boldsymbol{b}$ and $(\boldsymbol{I}_m - \boldsymbol{A}^+\boldsymbol{A})\boldsymbol{b}$, are mutually orthogonal. We thus obtain

$$||\boldsymbol{x}||^2 = ||\boldsymbol{A}^+\boldsymbol{b}||^2 + ||(\boldsymbol{I}_m - \boldsymbol{A}^+\boldsymbol{A})\boldsymbol{z}||^2 \geq ||\boldsymbol{A}^+\boldsymbol{b}||^2, \tag{3.90}$$

indicating that $||\boldsymbol{A}^+\boldsymbol{b}||^2$ does not exceed $||\boldsymbol{x}||^2$.

(Necessity) Assume that $\boldsymbol{A}^+\boldsymbol{b}$ gives the minimum norm $||\boldsymbol{x}||$ among all possible $\boldsymbol{x}$'s. Then $\boldsymbol{A}^+$ that satisfies

$$||\boldsymbol{A}^+\boldsymbol{b}||^2 \leq ||\boldsymbol{x}||^2 = ||\boldsymbol{A}^+\boldsymbol{b} + (\boldsymbol{I}_m - \boldsymbol{A}^+\boldsymbol{A})\boldsymbol{z}||^2$$

also satisfies

$$(\boldsymbol{A}^+)'(\boldsymbol{I}_m - \boldsymbol{A}^+\boldsymbol{A}) = \boldsymbol{O} \Longleftrightarrow (\boldsymbol{A}^+)'\boldsymbol{A}^+\boldsymbol{A} = (\boldsymbol{A}^+)'.$$

Hence, by pre- and postmultiplying both sides of $(\boldsymbol{A}^+)'\boldsymbol{A}^+\boldsymbol{A} = (\boldsymbol{A}^+)'$ by $(\boldsymbol{AA}^+ - \boldsymbol{I}_n)'$ and $\boldsymbol{A}^+$, respectively, we obtain $(\boldsymbol{A}^+\boldsymbol{AA}^+ - \boldsymbol{A}^+)'(\boldsymbol{A}^+\boldsymbol{AA}^+ - \boldsymbol{A}^+) = \boldsymbol{O}$ after some manipulation. Furthermore, by premultiplying both sides of $(\boldsymbol{A}^+)'\boldsymbol{A}^+\boldsymbol{A} = (\boldsymbol{A}^+)'$ by $\boldsymbol{A}'$, we obtain $(\boldsymbol{A}^+\boldsymbol{A})' = \boldsymbol{A}^+\boldsymbol{A}$. The remaining two conditions, $\boldsymbol{AA}^+\boldsymbol{A} = \boldsymbol{A}$ and $(\boldsymbol{A}'\boldsymbol{A}^+)' = \boldsymbol{AA}^+$, can be derived from the fact that $\boldsymbol{A}^+$ is also a least squares g-inverse. Q.E.D.

We next introduce a theorem that shows the uniqueness of the Moore-Penrose inverse.

Theorem 3.20 *The Moore-Penrose inverse of* $\boldsymbol{A}$ *that satisfies the four conditions (3.84) through (3.87) in Definition 3.5 is uniquely determined.*

Proof. Let $\boldsymbol{X}$ and $\boldsymbol{Y}$ represent the Moore-Penrose inverses of $\boldsymbol{A}$. Then, $\boldsymbol{X} = \boldsymbol{XAX} = (\boldsymbol{XA})'\boldsymbol{X} = \boldsymbol{A}'\boldsymbol{X}'\boldsymbol{X} = \boldsymbol{A}'\boldsymbol{Y}'\boldsymbol{A}'\boldsymbol{X}'\boldsymbol{X} = \boldsymbol{A}'\boldsymbol{Y}'\boldsymbol{XAX} = \boldsymbol{A}'\boldsymbol{Y}'\boldsymbol{X} = \boldsymbol{YAX} = \boldsymbol{YAYAX} = \boldsymbol{YY}'\boldsymbol{A}'\boldsymbol{X}'\boldsymbol{A}' = \boldsymbol{YY}'\boldsymbol{A}' = \boldsymbol{YAY} = \boldsymbol{Y}$. (This proof is due to Kalman (1976).) Q.E.D.

We now consider expressions of the Moore-Penrose inverse.

Theorem 3.21 *The Moore-Penrose inverse of* $\boldsymbol{A}$ *can be expressed as*

$$\boldsymbol{A}^{+} = \boldsymbol{A}'\boldsymbol{A}(\boldsymbol{A}'\boldsymbol{A}\boldsymbol{A}'\boldsymbol{A})^{-}\boldsymbol{A}'. \tag{3.91}$$

Proof. Since $\boldsymbol{x} = \boldsymbol{A}^{+}\boldsymbol{b}$ minimizes $||\boldsymbol{b} - \boldsymbol{Ax}||$, it satisfies the normal equation $\boldsymbol{A}'\boldsymbol{Ax} = \boldsymbol{A}'\boldsymbol{b}$. To minimize $||\boldsymbol{x}||^2$ under this condition, we consider $f(\boldsymbol{x}, \boldsymbol{\lambda}) = \boldsymbol{x}'\boldsymbol{x} - 2\boldsymbol{\lambda}'(\boldsymbol{AA} - \boldsymbol{A}'\boldsymbol{b})$, where $\boldsymbol{\lambda} = (\lambda_1, \lambda_2, \cdots, \lambda_m)'$ is a vector of Lagrangean multipliers. We differentiate f with respect to $\boldsymbol{x}$, set the result to zero, and obtain $\boldsymbol{x} = \boldsymbol{A}'\boldsymbol{A}\boldsymbol{\lambda} \Rightarrow \boldsymbol{A}'\boldsymbol{A}\boldsymbol{\lambda} = \boldsymbol{A}^{+}\boldsymbol{b}$. Premultiplying both sides of this equation by $\boldsymbol{A}'\boldsymbol{A}(\boldsymbol{A}'\boldsymbol{A}\boldsymbol{A}'\boldsymbol{A})^{-}\boldsymbol{A}'\boldsymbol{A}$, we obtain $\boldsymbol{A}'\boldsymbol{A}\boldsymbol{A}^{+} = \boldsymbol{A}'$ and $\boldsymbol{A}'\boldsymbol{A}(\boldsymbol{A}'\boldsymbol{A}\boldsymbol{A}'\boldsymbol{A})^{-}\boldsymbol{A}'\boldsymbol{A}\boldsymbol{A}' = \boldsymbol{A}'$, leading to $\boldsymbol{A}'\boldsymbol{A}\boldsymbol{\lambda} = \boldsymbol{A}'\boldsymbol{A}(\boldsymbol{A}'\boldsymbol{A}\boldsymbol{A}'\boldsymbol{A})^{-}\boldsymbol{A}'\boldsymbol{b} = \boldsymbol{x}$, thereby establishing (3.91). Q.E.D.

Note Since $\boldsymbol{Ax} = \boldsymbol{AA}^{+}\boldsymbol{b}$ implies $\boldsymbol{A}'\boldsymbol{Ax} = \boldsymbol{A}'\boldsymbol{AA}^{+}\boldsymbol{b} = \boldsymbol{A}'\boldsymbol{b}$, it is also possible to minimize $\boldsymbol{x}'\boldsymbol{x}$ subject to the condition that $\boldsymbol{A}'\boldsymbol{Ax} = \boldsymbol{A}'\boldsymbol{b}$. Let $\tilde{\boldsymbol{\lambda}} = (\tilde{\lambda}_1, \tilde{\lambda}_2, \cdots, \tilde{\lambda}_m)'$, and define $f(\boldsymbol{x}, \boldsymbol{\lambda}) = \boldsymbol{x}'\boldsymbol{x} - 2\boldsymbol{\lambda}'(\boldsymbol{A}'\boldsymbol{Ax} - \boldsymbol{A}'\boldsymbol{b})$. Differentiating f with respect to $\boldsymbol{x}$ and $\boldsymbol{\lambda}$, and setting the results to zero, we obtain $\boldsymbol{x} = \boldsymbol{A}'\boldsymbol{A}\boldsymbol{\lambda}$ and $\boldsymbol{A}'\boldsymbol{Ax} = \boldsymbol{b}$.

Combining these two equations, we obtain $\begin{bmatrix} \boldsymbol{I}_m & \boldsymbol{A}'\boldsymbol{A} \\ \boldsymbol{A}'\boldsymbol{A} & \boldsymbol{O} \end{bmatrix} \begin{bmatrix} \boldsymbol{x} \\ \boldsymbol{\lambda} \end{bmatrix} = \begin{bmatrix} \boldsymbol{0} \\ \boldsymbol{A}'\boldsymbol{b} \end{bmatrix}$. Solving this equation using the corollary of Theorem 3.13, we also obtain (3.91).

Corollary

$$\boldsymbol{A}^{+} = \boldsymbol{A}'(\boldsymbol{AA}')^{-}\boldsymbol{A}(\boldsymbol{A}'\boldsymbol{A})^{-}\boldsymbol{A}'. \tag{3.92}$$

Proof. We use the fact that $(\boldsymbol{A}'\boldsymbol{A})^{-}\boldsymbol{A}'(\boldsymbol{AA}')^{-}\boldsymbol{A}(\boldsymbol{A}'\boldsymbol{A})^{-}$ is a g-inverse of $\boldsymbol{A}'\boldsymbol{AA}'\boldsymbol{A}$, which can be seen from

$$\boldsymbol{A}'\boldsymbol{AA}'\boldsymbol{A}(\boldsymbol{A}'\boldsymbol{A})^{-}\boldsymbol{A}'(\boldsymbol{AA}')^{-}\boldsymbol{A}(\boldsymbol{A}'\boldsymbol{A})^{-}\boldsymbol{A}'\boldsymbol{AA}'\boldsymbol{A}$$

$$= A'AA'(AA')^{-}A(A'A)^{-}A'AA'A$$
$$= A'A(A'A)^{-}A'AA'A = A'AA'A.$$

Q.E.D.

Example 3.7 Find A_ℓ^-, A_m^-, and A^+ for $A = \begin{bmatrix} 1 & 1 \\ 1 & 1 \end{bmatrix}$.

Let $A^- = \begin{bmatrix} a & b \\ c & d \end{bmatrix}$. From $AA^-A = A$, we obtain $a+b+c+d = 1$. A least squares g-inverse A_ℓ^- is given by

$$A_\ell^- = \begin{bmatrix} a & b \\ \frac{1}{2} - a & \frac{1}{2} - b \end{bmatrix}.$$

This is because

$$\begin{bmatrix} 1 & 1 \\ 1 & 1 \end{bmatrix} \begin{bmatrix} a & b \\ c & d \end{bmatrix} = \begin{bmatrix} a+c & b+d \\ a+c & b+d \end{bmatrix}$$

is symmetric, which implies $a+c = b+d$. This, combined with $a+b+c+d = 1$, yields $c = \frac{1}{2} - a$ and $d = \frac{1}{2} - b$.

Similarly, a minimum norm g-inverse A_m^- is given by

$$A_m^- = \begin{bmatrix} a & \frac{1}{2} - a \\ c & \frac{1}{2} - c \end{bmatrix}.$$

This derives from the fact that

$$\begin{bmatrix} a & b \\ c & d \end{bmatrix} \begin{bmatrix} 1 & 1 \\ 1 & 1 \end{bmatrix} = \begin{bmatrix} a+b & a+b \\ c+d & c+d \end{bmatrix}$$

is symmetric, which implies $a+b = c+d$. This, combined with $a+b+c+d = 1$, yields $b = \frac{1}{2} - a$ and $d = \frac{1}{2} - c$. A reflexive g-inverse has to satisfy $ad = bc$ from Example 3.4.

The Moore-Penrose inverse should satisfy all of the conditions above, and it is given by

$$A^+ = \begin{bmatrix} \frac{1}{4} & \frac{1}{4} \\ \frac{1}{4} & \frac{1}{4} \end{bmatrix}.$$

The Moore-Penrose inverse A^+ can also be calculated as follows instead of using (3.91) and (3.92). Let $x = A^+b$ for $\forall b \in E^n$. From (3.91), $x \in$

Sp($\boldsymbol{A}'$), and so there exists $\boldsymbol{x}$ such that $\boldsymbol{x} = \boldsymbol{A}'\boldsymbol{z}$ for some $\boldsymbol{z}$. Hence, $\boldsymbol{A}'\boldsymbol{b} = \boldsymbol{A}'\boldsymbol{z}$. Premultiplying both sides of this equation by $\boldsymbol{A}'\boldsymbol{A}$, we obtain $\boldsymbol{A}'\boldsymbol{b} = \boldsymbol{A}'\boldsymbol{A}\boldsymbol{x}$ from $\boldsymbol{A}'\boldsymbol{A}\boldsymbol{A}^+ = \boldsymbol{A}'$. Thus, by canceling out $\boldsymbol{z}$ from

$$\boldsymbol{A}'\boldsymbol{A}\boldsymbol{x} = \boldsymbol{A}'\boldsymbol{b} \text{ and } \boldsymbol{x} = \boldsymbol{A}'\boldsymbol{z},$$

we obtain $\boldsymbol{x} = \boldsymbol{A}^+\boldsymbol{b}$.

Example 3.8 Find $\boldsymbol{A}^+$ for $\boldsymbol{A} = \begin{bmatrix} 2 & 1 & 3 \\ 4 & 2 & 6 \end{bmatrix}$.

Let $\boldsymbol{x} = (x_1, x_2, x_3)'$ and $\boldsymbol{b} = (b_1, b_2)'$. Because $\boldsymbol{A}'\boldsymbol{A} = \begin{bmatrix} 20 & 10 & 30 \\ 10 & 5 & 15 \\ 30 & 15 & 45 \end{bmatrix}$, we obtain

$$10x_1 + 5x_2 + 15x_3 = b_1 + 2b_2 \tag{3.93}$$

from $\boldsymbol{A}'\boldsymbol{A}\boldsymbol{x} = \boldsymbol{A}'\boldsymbol{b}$. Furthermore, from $\boldsymbol{x} = \boldsymbol{A}'\boldsymbol{z}$, we have $x_1 = 2z_1 + 4z_2$, $x_2 = z_1 + 2z_2$, and $x_3 = 3z_1 + 6z_2$. Hence,

$$x_1 = 2x_2, \quad x_3 = 3x_2. \tag{3.94}$$

Substituting (3.94) into (3.93), we obtain

$$x_2 = \frac{1}{70}(b_1 + 2b_2). \tag{3.95}$$

Hence, we have

$$x_1 = \frac{2}{70}(b_1 + 2b_2), \quad x_3 = \frac{3}{70}(b_1 + 2b_2),$$

and so

$$\begin{pmatrix} x_1 \\ x_2 \\ x_3 \end{pmatrix} = \frac{1}{70}\begin{bmatrix} 2 & 4 \\ 1 & 2 \\ 3 & 6 \end{bmatrix}\begin{pmatrix} b_1 \\ b_2 \end{pmatrix},$$

leading to

$$\boldsymbol{A}^+ = \frac{1}{70}\begin{bmatrix} 2 & 4 \\ 1 & 2 \\ 3 & 6 \end{bmatrix}.$$

We now show how to obtain the Moore-Penrose inverse of $\boldsymbol{A}$ using (3.92) when an n by m matrix $\boldsymbol{A}$ admits a rank decomposition $\boldsymbol{A} = \boldsymbol{B}\boldsymbol{C}$, where

$\text{rank}(\boldsymbol{B}) = \text{rank}(\boldsymbol{C}) = r = \text{rank}(\boldsymbol{A})$. Substituting $\boldsymbol{A} = \boldsymbol{BC}$ into (3.92), we obtain

$$\boldsymbol{A}^+ = \boldsymbol{C}'\boldsymbol{B}'(\boldsymbol{BCC}'\boldsymbol{B}')^-\boldsymbol{BC}(\boldsymbol{C}'\boldsymbol{B}'\boldsymbol{BC})^-\boldsymbol{C}'\boldsymbol{B}'.$$

Note that $\boldsymbol{B}'\boldsymbol{B}$ and $\boldsymbol{CC}'$ are nonsingular matrices of order r and that $\boldsymbol{B}'(\boldsymbol{BB}')^-\boldsymbol{B}$ and $\boldsymbol{C}(\boldsymbol{C}'\boldsymbol{C})^-\boldsymbol{C}'$ are both identity matrices. We thus have

$$(\boldsymbol{BB}')^-\boldsymbol{B}(\boldsymbol{CC}')^-\boldsymbol{B}'(\boldsymbol{BB}')^- \in \{(\boldsymbol{BCC}'\boldsymbol{B}')^-\}$$

and

$$(\boldsymbol{C}'\boldsymbol{C})^-\boldsymbol{C}'(\boldsymbol{B}'\boldsymbol{B})^-\boldsymbol{C}(\boldsymbol{C}'\boldsymbol{C})^- \in \{(\boldsymbol{C}'\boldsymbol{B}'\boldsymbol{BC})^-\},$$

so that

$$\boldsymbol{A}^+ = \boldsymbol{C}'(\boldsymbol{CC}')^{-1}(\boldsymbol{B}'\boldsymbol{B})^{-1}\boldsymbol{B}', \tag{3.96}$$

where $\boldsymbol{A} = \boldsymbol{BC}$.

The following theorem is derived from the fact that $\boldsymbol{A}(\boldsymbol{A}'\boldsymbol{A})^-\boldsymbol{A}' = \boldsymbol{I}_n$ if $\text{rank}(\boldsymbol{A}) = n(\leq m)$ and $\boldsymbol{A}'(\boldsymbol{AA}')^-\boldsymbol{A} = \boldsymbol{I}_m$ if $\text{rank}(\boldsymbol{A}) = m(\leq n)$.

Theorem 3.22 If $\text{rank}(A) = n \leq m$,

$$\boldsymbol{A}^+ = \boldsymbol{A}'(\boldsymbol{AA}')^{-1} = \boldsymbol{A}^-_{mr}, \tag{3.97}$$

and if $\text{rank}(\boldsymbol{A}) = m \leq n$,

$$\boldsymbol{A}^+ = (\boldsymbol{A}'\boldsymbol{A})^{-1}\boldsymbol{A} = \boldsymbol{A}^-_{\ell r}. \tag{3.98}$$

(Proof omitted.)

Note Another expression of the Moore-Penrose inverse is given by

$$\boldsymbol{A}^+ = \boldsymbol{A}^-_{mr}\boldsymbol{A}\boldsymbol{A}^-_{\ell r} = \boldsymbol{A}^-_m\boldsymbol{A}\boldsymbol{A}^-_\ell. \tag{3.99}$$

This can be derived from the decomposition:

$$\begin{aligned}\boldsymbol{A}^- &= [\boldsymbol{A}^-_m\boldsymbol{A} + (\boldsymbol{I}_m - \boldsymbol{A}^-_m\boldsymbol{A})]\boldsymbol{A}^-[\boldsymbol{AA}^-_\ell + (\boldsymbol{I}_n - \boldsymbol{AA}^-_\ell)] \\ &= \boldsymbol{A}^-_m\boldsymbol{AA}^-_\ell + (\boldsymbol{I}_m - \boldsymbol{A}^-_m\boldsymbol{A})\boldsymbol{A}^-(\boldsymbol{I}_n - \boldsymbol{AA}^-_\ell).\end{aligned}$$

(It is left as an exercise for the reader to verify that the formula above satisfies the four conditions given in Definition 3.5.)

3.4 Exercises for Chapter 3

1. (a) Find $\boldsymbol{A}_{mr}^{-}$ when $\boldsymbol{A} = \begin{bmatrix} 1 & 2 & 3 \\ 2 & 3 & 1 \end{bmatrix}$.

(b) Find $\boldsymbol{A}_{\ell r}^{-}$ when $\boldsymbol{A} = \begin{bmatrix} 1 & 2 \\ 2 & 1 \\ 1 & 1 \end{bmatrix}$.

(c) Find $\boldsymbol{A}^{+}$ when $\boldsymbol{A} = \begin{bmatrix} 2 & -1 & -1 \\ -1 & 2 & -1 \\ -1 & -1 & 2 \end{bmatrix}$.

2. Show that the necessary and sufficient condition for $(\mathrm{Ker}(\boldsymbol{P}))^c = \mathrm{Ker}(\boldsymbol{I} - \boldsymbol{P})$ to hold is $\boldsymbol{P}^2 = \boldsymbol{P}$.

3. Let $\boldsymbol{A}$ be an n by m matrix. Show that $\boldsymbol{B}$ is an m by n g-inverse of $\boldsymbol{A}$ if any one of the following conditions holds:
(i) $\mathrm{rank}(\boldsymbol{I}_m - \boldsymbol{B}\boldsymbol{A}) = m - \mathrm{rank}(\boldsymbol{A})$.
(ii) $\mathrm{rank}(\boldsymbol{B}\boldsymbol{A}) = \mathrm{rank}(\boldsymbol{A})$ and $(\boldsymbol{B}\boldsymbol{A})^2 = \boldsymbol{B}\boldsymbol{A}$.
(iii) $\mathrm{rank}(\boldsymbol{A}\boldsymbol{B}) = \mathrm{rank}(\boldsymbol{A})$ and $(\boldsymbol{A}\boldsymbol{B})^2 = \boldsymbol{A}\boldsymbol{B}$.

4. Show the following:
(i) $\mathrm{rank}(\boldsymbol{A}\boldsymbol{B}) = \mathrm{rank}(\boldsymbol{A}) \Longleftrightarrow \boldsymbol{B}(\boldsymbol{A}\boldsymbol{B})^{-} \in \{\boldsymbol{A}^{-}\}$.
(ii) $\mathrm{rank}(\boldsymbol{C}\boldsymbol{A}\boldsymbol{D}) = \mathrm{rank}(\boldsymbol{A}) \Longleftrightarrow \boldsymbol{D}(\boldsymbol{C}\boldsymbol{A}\boldsymbol{D})^{-}\boldsymbol{C} \in \{\boldsymbol{A}^{-}\}$.

5. (i) Show that the necessary and sufficient condition for $\boldsymbol{B}^{-}\boldsymbol{A}^{-}$ to be a generalized inverse of $\boldsymbol{A}\boldsymbol{B}$ is $(\boldsymbol{A}^{-}\boldsymbol{A}\boldsymbol{B}\boldsymbol{B}^{-})^2 = \boldsymbol{A}^{-}\boldsymbol{A}\boldsymbol{B}\boldsymbol{B}^{-}$.
(ii) Show that $\{(\boldsymbol{A}\boldsymbol{B})_m^{-}\} = \{\boldsymbol{B}_m^{-}\boldsymbol{A}_m^{-}\}$ when $\boldsymbol{A}_m^{-}\boldsymbol{A}\boldsymbol{B}\boldsymbol{B}'$ is symmetric.
(iii) Show that $(\boldsymbol{Q}_A\boldsymbol{B})(\boldsymbol{Q}_A\boldsymbol{B})_\ell^{-} = \boldsymbol{P}_B - \boldsymbol{P}_A\boldsymbol{P}_B$ when $\boldsymbol{P}_A\boldsymbol{P}_B = \boldsymbol{P}_B\boldsymbol{P}_A$, where $\boldsymbol{P}_A = \boldsymbol{A}(\boldsymbol{A}'\boldsymbol{A})^{-}\boldsymbol{A}'$, $\boldsymbol{P}_B = \boldsymbol{B}(\boldsymbol{B}'\boldsymbol{B})^{-}\boldsymbol{B}'$, $\boldsymbol{Q}_A = \boldsymbol{I} - \boldsymbol{P}_A$, and $\boldsymbol{Q}_B = \boldsymbol{I} - \boldsymbol{P}_B$.

6. Show that the following three conditions are equivalent:
(i) $\boldsymbol{A} \in \{\boldsymbol{A}^{-}\}$.
(ii) $\boldsymbol{A}^2 = \boldsymbol{A}^4$ and $\mathrm{rank}(\boldsymbol{A}) = \mathrm{rank}(\boldsymbol{A}^2)$.
(iii) $\boldsymbol{A}^3 = \boldsymbol{A}$.

7. Show the following:
(i) $[\boldsymbol{A}, \boldsymbol{B}][\boldsymbol{A}, \boldsymbol{B}]^{-}\boldsymbol{A} = \boldsymbol{A}$.
(ii) $(\boldsymbol{A}\boldsymbol{A}' + \boldsymbol{B}\boldsymbol{B}')(\boldsymbol{A}\boldsymbol{A}' + \boldsymbol{B}\boldsymbol{B}')^{-}\boldsymbol{A} = \boldsymbol{A}$.

8. Show that $\boldsymbol{A}^{-} - \boldsymbol{A}^{-}\boldsymbol{U}(\boldsymbol{I} + \boldsymbol{V}\boldsymbol{A}^{-}\boldsymbol{U})^{-}\boldsymbol{V}\boldsymbol{A}^{-}$ is a generalized inverse of $\boldsymbol{A} + \boldsymbol{U}\boldsymbol{V}$ when $\boldsymbol{V} = \boldsymbol{W}_1\boldsymbol{A}$ and $\boldsymbol{U} = \boldsymbol{A}\boldsymbol{W}_2$ for some $\boldsymbol{W}_1$ and $\boldsymbol{W}_2$.

9. Let $\boldsymbol{A}$ be an n by m matrix of rank r, and let $\boldsymbol{B}$ and $\boldsymbol{C}$ be nonsingular ma-

trices of orders n and m, respectively, such that $\boldsymbol{BAC} = \begin{bmatrix} \boldsymbol{I}_r & \boldsymbol{O} \\ \boldsymbol{O} & \boldsymbol{O} \end{bmatrix}$. Show that $\boldsymbol{G} = \boldsymbol{C}\begin{bmatrix} \boldsymbol{I}_r & \boldsymbol{O} \\ \boldsymbol{O} & \boldsymbol{E} \end{bmatrix}\boldsymbol{B}$ is a generalized inverse of $\boldsymbol{A}$ with $\text{rank}(\boldsymbol{G}) = r + \text{rank}(\boldsymbol{E})$.

10. Let $\boldsymbol{A}$ be an n by m matrix. Show that the minimum of $||\boldsymbol{x} - \boldsymbol{Q}_{A'}\boldsymbol{\alpha}||^2$ with respect to $\boldsymbol{\alpha}$ is equal to $\boldsymbol{x}'\boldsymbol{P}_{A'}\boldsymbol{x}$, where $\boldsymbol{x} \in E^m$, $\boldsymbol{P}_{A'} = \boldsymbol{A}'(\boldsymbol{AA}')^-\boldsymbol{A}$, and $\boldsymbol{Q}_{A'} = \boldsymbol{I} - \boldsymbol{P}_{A'}$.

11. Show that $\boldsymbol{B} = \boldsymbol{A}^+$, where $\boldsymbol{B} = \boldsymbol{A}_m^-\boldsymbol{A}\boldsymbol{A}_\ell^-$.

12. Let $\boldsymbol{P}_1$ and $\boldsymbol{P}_2$ be the orthogonal projectors onto $V_1 \in E^n$ and $V_2 \in E^n$, respectively, and let $\boldsymbol{P}_{1\cap 2}$ be the orthogonal projectors onto $V_1 \cap V_2$. Show the following (Ben-Israel and Greville, 1974):

$$\begin{aligned} \boldsymbol{P}_{1\cap 2} &= 2\boldsymbol{P}_1(\boldsymbol{P}_1 + \boldsymbol{P}_2)^+\boldsymbol{P}_2 \\ &= 2\boldsymbol{P}_2(\boldsymbol{P}_1 + \boldsymbol{P}_2)^+\boldsymbol{P}_1. \end{aligned}$$

13. Let $\boldsymbol{G}$ (a transformation matrix from W to V) be a g-inverse of a transformation matrix $\boldsymbol{A}$ from V to W that satisfies the equation $\boldsymbol{AGA} = \boldsymbol{A}$. Define $\boldsymbol{N} = \boldsymbol{G} - \boldsymbol{GAG}$, $M = \text{Sp}(\boldsymbol{G} - \boldsymbol{N})$, and $L = \text{Ker}(\boldsymbol{G} - \boldsymbol{N})$. Show that the following propositions hold:
(i) $\boldsymbol{AN} = \boldsymbol{NA} = \boldsymbol{O}$.
(ii) $M \cap \text{Ker}(\boldsymbol{A}) = \{\boldsymbol{0}\}$ and $\boldsymbol{M} \oplus \text{Ker}(\boldsymbol{A}) = V$.
(iii) $L \cap \text{Sp}(\boldsymbol{A}) = \{\boldsymbol{0}\}$ and $L \oplus \text{Sp}(\boldsymbol{A}) = W$.

14. Let $\boldsymbol{A}$, $\boldsymbol{M}$, and $\boldsymbol{L}$ be matrices of orders $n \times m$, $n \times q$, and $m \times r$, respectively, such that $\text{rank}(\boldsymbol{M}'\boldsymbol{AL}) = \text{rank}(\boldsymbol{A})$. Show that the following three statements are equivalent:
(i) $\text{rank}(\boldsymbol{M}'\boldsymbol{A}) = \text{rank}(\boldsymbol{A})$.
(ii) $\boldsymbol{HA} = \boldsymbol{A}$, where $\boldsymbol{H} = \boldsymbol{A}(\boldsymbol{M}'\boldsymbol{A})^-\boldsymbol{M}'$.
(iii) $\text{Sp}(\boldsymbol{A}) \oplus \text{Ker}(\boldsymbol{H}) = E^n$.

Chapter 4

Explicit Representations

In this chapter, we present explicit representations of the projection matrix $\boldsymbol{P}_{V\cdot W}$ and generalized inverse (g-inverse) matrices given in Chapters 2 and 3, respectively, when basis vectors are given that generate $V = \mathrm{Sp}(\boldsymbol{A})$ and $W = \mathrm{Sp}(\boldsymbol{B})$, where $E^n = V \oplus W$.

4.1 Projection Matrices

We begin with the following lemma.

Lemma 4.1 *The following equalities hold if* $\mathrm{Sp}(\boldsymbol{A}) \cap \mathrm{Sp}(\boldsymbol{B}) = \{\boldsymbol{0}\}$, *where* $\mathrm{Sp}(\boldsymbol{A})$ *and* $\mathrm{Sp}(\boldsymbol{B})$ *are subspaces of* E^n:

$$\mathrm{rank}(\boldsymbol{A}) = \mathrm{rank}(\boldsymbol{Q}_B\boldsymbol{A}) = \mathrm{rank}(\boldsymbol{A}'\boldsymbol{Q}_B\boldsymbol{A}), \tag{4.1}$$

where $\boldsymbol{Q}_B = \boldsymbol{I}_n - \boldsymbol{P}_B$,

$$\mathrm{rank}(\boldsymbol{B}) = \mathrm{rank}(\boldsymbol{Q}_A\boldsymbol{B}) = \mathrm{rank}(\boldsymbol{B}'\boldsymbol{Q}_A\boldsymbol{B}), \tag{4.2}$$

where $\boldsymbol{Q}_A = \boldsymbol{I}_n - \boldsymbol{P}_A$, *and*

$$\boldsymbol{A}(\boldsymbol{A}'\boldsymbol{Q}_B\boldsymbol{A})^-\boldsymbol{A}'\boldsymbol{Q}_B\boldsymbol{A} = \boldsymbol{A} \text{ and } \boldsymbol{B}(\boldsymbol{B}'\boldsymbol{Q}_A\boldsymbol{B})^-\boldsymbol{B}'\boldsymbol{Q}_A\boldsymbol{B} = \boldsymbol{B}. \tag{4.3}$$

Proof. (4.1) and (4.2): Let $\boldsymbol{A}$ and $\boldsymbol{B}$ be n by p and n by q matrices, respectively, and let

$$\begin{aligned}[\boldsymbol{Q}_B\boldsymbol{A}, \boldsymbol{B}] &= [\boldsymbol{A} - \boldsymbol{B}(\boldsymbol{B}'\boldsymbol{B})^-\boldsymbol{B}'\boldsymbol{A}, \boldsymbol{B}] \\ &= [\boldsymbol{A}, \boldsymbol{B}]\begin{bmatrix} \boldsymbol{I}_p & \boldsymbol{O} \\ -(\boldsymbol{B}'\boldsymbol{B})^-\boldsymbol{B}'\boldsymbol{A} & \boldsymbol{I}_q \end{bmatrix} = [\boldsymbol{A}, \boldsymbol{B}]\boldsymbol{T}.\end{aligned}$$

Then $\boldsymbol{T}$ is a square matrix of order $p+q$, and $\det|\boldsymbol{T}| \neq 0$. Hence, $\mathrm{Sp}[\boldsymbol{Q}_B\boldsymbol{A}, \boldsymbol{B}] = \mathrm{Sp}[\boldsymbol{A}, \boldsymbol{B}]$. On the other hand, $\boldsymbol{Q}_B\boldsymbol{A}\boldsymbol{x} = \boldsymbol{B}\boldsymbol{y} \Rightarrow \boldsymbol{0} = \boldsymbol{P}_B\boldsymbol{Q}_B\boldsymbol{A}\boldsymbol{x} = \boldsymbol{P}_B\boldsymbol{B}\boldsymbol{y} \Rightarrow \boldsymbol{B}\boldsymbol{y} = \boldsymbol{0} \Rightarrow \boldsymbol{Q}_B\boldsymbol{A}\boldsymbol{x} = \boldsymbol{0}$, which implies that $\mathrm{Sp}(\boldsymbol{B})$ and $\mathrm{Sp}(\boldsymbol{Q}_B\boldsymbol{A})$ are disjoint. Since $\mathrm{Sp}(\boldsymbol{A})$ and $\mathrm{Sp}(\boldsymbol{B})$ are also disjoint, we obtain $\mathrm{rank}(\boldsymbol{A}) = \mathrm{rank}(\boldsymbol{Q}_B\boldsymbol{A})$. That $\mathrm{rank}(\boldsymbol{Q}_B\boldsymbol{A}) = \mathrm{rank}((\boldsymbol{Q}_B\boldsymbol{A})'\boldsymbol{Q}_B\boldsymbol{A})$ is clear from Theorem 1.8. Equality (4.2) can be proven similarly.

(4.3): From (4.1), $\mathrm{Sp}(\boldsymbol{A}') = \mathrm{Sp}(\boldsymbol{A}'\boldsymbol{Q}_B\boldsymbol{A})$ implies that there exists a $\boldsymbol{W}$ such that $\boldsymbol{A}' = \boldsymbol{A}'\boldsymbol{Q}_B\boldsymbol{A}\boldsymbol{W}$. Hence, we have

$$\boldsymbol{W}'\boldsymbol{A}'\boldsymbol{Q}_B\boldsymbol{A}(\boldsymbol{A}'\boldsymbol{Q}_B\boldsymbol{A})^-\boldsymbol{A}'\boldsymbol{Q}_B\boldsymbol{A} = \boldsymbol{W}'\boldsymbol{A}'\boldsymbol{Q}_B\boldsymbol{A} = \boldsymbol{A}.$$

The second half of (4.3) can be proven similarly. Q.E.D.

Corollary *Let $\boldsymbol{C}$ denote a matrix having the same number of columns m as $\boldsymbol{A}$, and let $\mathrm{Sp}(\boldsymbol{C}') \cap \mathrm{Sp}(\boldsymbol{A}') = \{\boldsymbol{0}\}$. Then the following relations hold:*

$$\mathrm{rank}(\boldsymbol{A}) = \mathrm{rank}(\boldsymbol{A}\boldsymbol{Q}_{C'}) = \mathrm{rank}(\boldsymbol{A}\boldsymbol{Q}_{C'}\boldsymbol{A}') \tag{4.4}$$

and

$$\boldsymbol{A}\boldsymbol{Q}_{C'}\boldsymbol{A}'(\boldsymbol{A}\boldsymbol{Q}_{C'}\boldsymbol{A}')^-\boldsymbol{A} = \boldsymbol{A}, \tag{4.5}$$

where $\boldsymbol{Q}_{C'} = \boldsymbol{I}_m - \boldsymbol{C}'(\boldsymbol{C}\boldsymbol{C}')^-\boldsymbol{C}$. (Proof omitted.)

Theorem 4.1 *Let $E^n \supset V \oplus W$, where $V = \mathrm{Sp}(\boldsymbol{A})$ and $W = \mathrm{Sp}(\boldsymbol{B})$. A general form of the projector $\boldsymbol{P}^*_{A\cdot B}$ onto V along W is given by*

$$\boldsymbol{P}^*_{A\cdot B} = \boldsymbol{A}(\boldsymbol{Q}^*_B\boldsymbol{A})^-\boldsymbol{Q}^*_B + \boldsymbol{Z}(\boldsymbol{I}_n - \boldsymbol{Q}^*_B\boldsymbol{A}(\boldsymbol{Q}^*_B\boldsymbol{A})^-)\boldsymbol{Q}^*_B, \tag{4.6}$$

where $\boldsymbol{Q}^*_B = \boldsymbol{I}_n - \boldsymbol{B}\boldsymbol{B}^-$ (with $\boldsymbol{B}^-$ being an arbitrary g-inverse of $\boldsymbol{B}$) and $\boldsymbol{Z}$ is an arbitrary square matrix of order n. Equation (4.6) can alternatively be expressed as

$$\boldsymbol{P}^*_{A\cdot B} = \boldsymbol{A}(\boldsymbol{A}'\boldsymbol{Q}_B\boldsymbol{A})^-\boldsymbol{A}'\boldsymbol{Q}_B + \boldsymbol{Z}(\boldsymbol{I}_n - \boldsymbol{Q}_B\boldsymbol{A}(\boldsymbol{A}'\boldsymbol{Q}_B\boldsymbol{A})^-\boldsymbol{A}')\boldsymbol{Q}_B, \tag{4.7}$$

where $\boldsymbol{Q}_B = \boldsymbol{I}_n - \boldsymbol{P}_B$ and $\boldsymbol{P}_B$ is the orthogonal projector onto $\mathrm{Sp}(\boldsymbol{B})$.

Proof. $\boldsymbol{P}^*_{A\cdot B}$ satisfies $\boldsymbol{P}^*_{A\cdot B}\boldsymbol{A} = \boldsymbol{A}$ and $\boldsymbol{P}^*_{A\cdot B}\boldsymbol{B} = \boldsymbol{O}$. The latter implies $\boldsymbol{P}^*_{A\cdot B}\boldsymbol{B} = \boldsymbol{K}\boldsymbol{Q}^*_B$ for some $\boldsymbol{K}$, a square matrix of order n. Substituting this into the former, we obtain $\boldsymbol{K}\boldsymbol{Q}^*_B\boldsymbol{A} = \boldsymbol{A}$. Hence,

$$\boldsymbol{K} = \boldsymbol{A}(\boldsymbol{Q}^*_B\boldsymbol{A})^- + \boldsymbol{Z}[\boldsymbol{I}_n - (\boldsymbol{Q}^*_B\boldsymbol{A})(\boldsymbol{Q}^*_B\boldsymbol{A})^-],$$

from which (4.6) follows. To derive (4.7) from (4.6), we use the fact that $(\boldsymbol{A}'\boldsymbol{Q}_B\boldsymbol{A})^-\boldsymbol{A}'$ is a g-inverse of $\boldsymbol{Q}_B^*\boldsymbol{A}$ when $\boldsymbol{Q}_B^* = \boldsymbol{Q}_B$. (This can be shown by the relation given in (4.3).) Q.E.D.

Corollary 1 *When* $E^n = \mathrm{Sp}(\boldsymbol{A}) \oplus \mathrm{Sp}(\boldsymbol{B})$, *the projector* $\boldsymbol{P}_{A\cdot B}$ *onto* $\mathrm{Sp}(\boldsymbol{A})$ *along* $\mathrm{Sp}(\boldsymbol{B})$ *can be expressed as*

$$\boldsymbol{P}_{A\cdot B} = \boldsymbol{A}(\boldsymbol{Q}_B^*\boldsymbol{A})^-\boldsymbol{Q}_B^*, \tag{4.8}$$

where $\boldsymbol{Q}_B^* = \boldsymbol{I}_n - \boldsymbol{B}\boldsymbol{B}^-$,

$$\boldsymbol{P}_{A\cdot B} = \boldsymbol{A}(\boldsymbol{A}'\boldsymbol{Q}_B\boldsymbol{A})^-\boldsymbol{A}'\boldsymbol{Q}_B, \tag{4.9}$$

where $\boldsymbol{Q}_B = \boldsymbol{I}_n - \boldsymbol{P}_B$, *or*

$$\boldsymbol{P}_{A\cdot B} = \boldsymbol{A}\boldsymbol{A}'(\boldsymbol{A}\boldsymbol{A}' + \boldsymbol{B}\boldsymbol{B}')^{-1}. \tag{4.10}$$

Proof. (4.8): Let the second term in (4.7) be denoted by $\boldsymbol{T}$. Then it is clear that $\boldsymbol{T}\boldsymbol{A} = \boldsymbol{O}$ and $\boldsymbol{T}\boldsymbol{B} = \boldsymbol{O}$ imply $\boldsymbol{T} = \boldsymbol{O}$.

(4.9): Let $\boldsymbol{T}$ denote the same as above. We have $\boldsymbol{T}\boldsymbol{B} = \boldsymbol{O}$, and

$$\begin{aligned} \boldsymbol{T}\boldsymbol{A} &= \boldsymbol{Z}(\boldsymbol{I}_n - \boldsymbol{Q}_B\boldsymbol{A}(\boldsymbol{A}'\boldsymbol{Q}_B\boldsymbol{A})^-\boldsymbol{A}')\boldsymbol{Q}_B\boldsymbol{A} \\ &= \boldsymbol{Z}(\boldsymbol{Q}_B\boldsymbol{A} - \boldsymbol{Q}_B\boldsymbol{A}(\boldsymbol{A}'\boldsymbol{Q}_B\boldsymbol{A})^-\boldsymbol{A}'\boldsymbol{Q}_B\boldsymbol{A}) \\ &= \boldsymbol{Z}(\boldsymbol{Q}_B\boldsymbol{A} - \boldsymbol{Q}_B\boldsymbol{A}) = \boldsymbol{O}. \end{aligned}$$

(Use (4.3).) We obtain (4.9) since $\boldsymbol{T}[\boldsymbol{A}, \boldsymbol{B}] = \boldsymbol{O}$ implies $\boldsymbol{T} = \boldsymbol{O}$.

(4.10): By the definition of a projection matrix (Theorem 2.2), $\boldsymbol{P}_{A\cdot B}\boldsymbol{A} = \boldsymbol{A}$ and $\boldsymbol{P}_{A\cdot B}\boldsymbol{B} = \boldsymbol{O}$, which imply $\boldsymbol{P}_{A\cdot B}\boldsymbol{A}\boldsymbol{A}' = \boldsymbol{A}\boldsymbol{A}'$ and $\boldsymbol{P}_{A\cdot B}\boldsymbol{B}\boldsymbol{B}' = \boldsymbol{O}$. Hence,

$$\boldsymbol{P}_{A\cdot B}(\boldsymbol{A}\boldsymbol{A}' + \boldsymbol{B}\boldsymbol{B}') = \boldsymbol{A}\boldsymbol{A}'.$$

On the other hand, we have

$$\mathrm{rank}(\boldsymbol{A}\boldsymbol{A}' + \boldsymbol{B}\boldsymbol{B}') = \mathrm{rank}\left([\boldsymbol{A}, \boldsymbol{B}]\begin{bmatrix} \boldsymbol{A}' \\ \boldsymbol{B}' \end{bmatrix}\right) = n$$

since $\mathrm{rank}[\boldsymbol{A}, \boldsymbol{B}] = \mathrm{rank}(\boldsymbol{A}) + \mathrm{rank}(\boldsymbol{B}) = n$. This means $\boldsymbol{A}\boldsymbol{A}' + \boldsymbol{B}\boldsymbol{B}'$ is nonsingular, so that its regular inverse exists, and (4.10) follows. Q.E.D.

Corollary 2 *Let* $E^m = \mathrm{Sp}(\boldsymbol{A}') \oplus \mathrm{Sp}(\boldsymbol{C}')$. *The projector* $\boldsymbol{P}_{A'\cdot C'}$ *onto* $\mathrm{Sp}(\boldsymbol{A}')$ *along* $\mathrm{Sp}(\boldsymbol{C}')$ *is given by*

$$\boldsymbol{P}_{A'\cdot C'} = \boldsymbol{A}'(\boldsymbol{A}\boldsymbol{Q}_{C'}\boldsymbol{A}')^-\boldsymbol{A}\boldsymbol{Q}_{C'}, \tag{4.11}$$

where $Q_{C'} = I_m - C'(CC')^- C$, *or*

$$P_{A' \cdot C'} = A'A(A'A + C'C)^{-1}. \tag{4.12}$$

Note Let $[A, B]$ be a square matrix. Then, it holds that $\text{rank}[A, B] = \text{rank}(A) + \text{rank}(B)$, which implies that the regular inverse exists for $[A, B]$. In this case, we have

$$P_{A \cdot B} = [A, O][A, B]^{-1} \text{ and } P_{B \cdot A} = [O.B][A, B]^{-1}. \tag{4.13}$$

Example 4.1 Let $A = \begin{bmatrix} 1 & 4 \\ 2 & 1 \\ 2 & 1 \end{bmatrix}$ and $B = \begin{pmatrix} 0 \\ 0 \\ 1 \end{pmatrix}$. Then, $[A, B]^{-1} = -\frac{1}{7} \begin{bmatrix} 1 & -4 & 0 \\ -2 & 1 & 0 \\ 0 & 7 & -7 \end{bmatrix}$. It follows from (4.13) that

$$P_{A \cdot B} = -\frac{1}{7} \begin{bmatrix} 1 & 4 & 0 \\ 2 & 1 & 0 \\ 2 & 1 & 0 \end{bmatrix} \begin{bmatrix} 1 & -4 & 0 \\ -2 & 1 & 0 \\ 0 & 7 & -7 \end{bmatrix} = \begin{bmatrix} 1 & 0 & 0 \\ 0 & 1 & 0 \\ 0 & 1 & 0 \end{bmatrix}$$

and

$$P_{B \cdot A} = -\frac{1}{7} \begin{bmatrix} 0 & 0 & 0 \\ 0 & 0 & 0 \\ 0 & 0 & 1 \end{bmatrix} \begin{bmatrix} 1 & -4 & 0 \\ -2 & 1 & 0 \\ 0 & 7 & -7 \end{bmatrix} = \begin{bmatrix} 0 & 0 & 0 \\ 0 & 0 & 0 \\ 0 & -1 & 1 \end{bmatrix}.$$

(Verify that $P_{A \cdot B}^2 = P_{A \cdot B}$, $P_{B \cdot A}^2 = P_{B \cdot A}$, $P_{A \cdot B} + P_{B \cdot A} = I_3$, and $P_{A \cdot B} \times P_{B \cdot A} = P_{B \cdot A} P_{A \cdot B} = O$.)

Let $\tilde{A} = \begin{bmatrix} 1 & 0 \\ 0 & 1 \\ 0 & 1 \end{bmatrix}$. From $\begin{bmatrix} 1 & 0 & 0 \\ 0 & 1 & 0 \\ 0 & 1 & 1 \end{bmatrix}^{-1} = \begin{bmatrix} 1 & 0 & 0 \\ 0 & 1 & 0 \\ 0 & -1 & 1 \end{bmatrix}$, we obtain

$$P_{\tilde{A} \cdot B} = \begin{bmatrix} 1 & 0 & 0 \\ 0 & 1 & 0 \\ 0 & 1 & 0 \end{bmatrix} \begin{bmatrix} 1 & 0 & 0 \\ 0 & 1 & 0 \\ 0 & -1 & 1 \end{bmatrix} = \begin{bmatrix} 1 & 0 & 0 \\ 0 & 1 & 0 \\ 0 & 1 & 0 \end{bmatrix}.$$

On the other hand, since

$$\begin{bmatrix} 1 & 4 \\ 2 & 1 \\ 2 & 1 \end{bmatrix} = \begin{bmatrix} 1 & 0 \\ 0 & 1 \\ 0 & 1 \end{bmatrix} \begin{bmatrix} 1 & 4 \\ 2 & 1 \end{bmatrix},$$

and so $\mathrm{Sp}(\boldsymbol{A}) = \mathrm{Sp}(\tilde{\boldsymbol{A}})$, we have

$$E^n = \mathrm{Sp}(\boldsymbol{A}) \oplus \mathrm{Sp}(\boldsymbol{B}) = \mathrm{Sp}(\tilde{\boldsymbol{A}}) \oplus \mathrm{Sp}(\boldsymbol{B}), \tag{4.14}$$

so that $\boldsymbol{P}_{A \cdot B} = \boldsymbol{P}_{\tilde{A} \cdot B}$. (See the note preceding Theorem 2.14.)

Corollary 2 *Let* $E^n = \mathrm{Sp}(\boldsymbol{A}) \oplus \mathrm{Sp}(\boldsymbol{B})$, *and let* $\mathrm{Sp}(\boldsymbol{A}) = \mathrm{Sp}(\tilde{\boldsymbol{A}})$ and $\mathrm{Sp}(\boldsymbol{B}) = \mathrm{Sp}(\tilde{\boldsymbol{B}})$. *Then,*

$$\boldsymbol{P}_{\tilde{A} \cdot \tilde{B}} = \boldsymbol{P}_{A \cdot B}. \tag{4.15}$$

It is clear that

$$\boldsymbol{P}_A = \boldsymbol{A}(\boldsymbol{A}'\boldsymbol{A})^- \boldsymbol{A}' = \tilde{\boldsymbol{A}}(\tilde{\boldsymbol{A}}'\tilde{\boldsymbol{A}})^- \tilde{\boldsymbol{A}}' = \boldsymbol{P}_{\tilde{A}}$$

follows as a special case of (4.15) when $\mathrm{Sp}(\boldsymbol{B}) = \mathrm{Sp}(\boldsymbol{A})^\perp$. *The* $\boldsymbol{P}_A$ *above can also be expressed as*

$$\boldsymbol{P}_A = \boldsymbol{P}_{AA'} = \boldsymbol{A}\boldsymbol{A}'(\boldsymbol{A}\boldsymbol{A}'\boldsymbol{A}\boldsymbol{A}')^- \boldsymbol{A}\boldsymbol{A}' \tag{4.16}$$

since $\mathrm{Sp}(\boldsymbol{A}) = \mathrm{Sp}(\boldsymbol{A}\boldsymbol{A}')$.

Note As is clear from (4.15), $\boldsymbol{P}_{A \cdot B}$ is not a function of the column vectors in $\boldsymbol{A}$ and $\boldsymbol{B}$ themselves but rather depends on the subspaces $\mathrm{Sp}(\boldsymbol{A})$ and $\mathrm{Sp}(\boldsymbol{B})$ spanned by the column vectors of $\boldsymbol{A}$ and $\boldsymbol{B}$. Hence, logically $\boldsymbol{P}_{A \cdot B}$ should be denoted as $\boldsymbol{P}_{Sp(A), Sp(B)}$. However, as for $\boldsymbol{P}_A$ and $\boldsymbol{P}_B$, we keep using the notation $\boldsymbol{P}_{A \cdot B}$ instead of $\boldsymbol{P}_{Sp(A), Sp(B)}$ for simplicity.

Note Since

$$[\boldsymbol{A}, \boldsymbol{B}] \begin{bmatrix} \boldsymbol{A}' \\ \boldsymbol{B}' \end{bmatrix} = \boldsymbol{A}\boldsymbol{A}' + \boldsymbol{B}\boldsymbol{B}',$$

we obtain, using (4.16),

$$\begin{aligned} \boldsymbol{P}_{A+B} &= (\boldsymbol{A}\boldsymbol{A}' + \boldsymbol{B}\boldsymbol{B}')(\boldsymbol{A}\boldsymbol{A}' + \boldsymbol{B}\boldsymbol{B}')^-_\ell \\ &= \boldsymbol{A}\boldsymbol{A}'(\boldsymbol{A}\boldsymbol{A}' + \boldsymbol{B}\boldsymbol{B}')^-_\ell + \boldsymbol{B}\boldsymbol{B}'(\boldsymbol{A}\boldsymbol{A}' + \boldsymbol{B}\boldsymbol{B}')^-_\ell, \end{aligned} \tag{4.17}$$

where $\boldsymbol{A}^-_\ell$ indicates a least squares g-inverse of $\boldsymbol{A}$.

If $\mathrm{Sp}(\boldsymbol{A})$ and $\mathrm{Sp}(\boldsymbol{B})$ are disjoint and cover the entire space of E^n, we have $(\boldsymbol{A}\boldsymbol{A}' + \boldsymbol{B}\boldsymbol{B}')^-_\ell = (\boldsymbol{A}\boldsymbol{A}' + \boldsymbol{B}\boldsymbol{B}')^{-1}$ and, from (4.17), we obtain

$$\boldsymbol{P}_{A \cdot B} = \boldsymbol{A}\boldsymbol{A}'(\boldsymbol{A}\boldsymbol{A}' + \boldsymbol{B}\boldsymbol{B}')^{-1} \text{ and } \boldsymbol{P}_{B \cdot A} = \boldsymbol{B}\boldsymbol{B}'(\boldsymbol{A}\boldsymbol{A}' + \boldsymbol{B}\boldsymbol{B}')^{-1}.$$

Theorem 4.2 *Let* $\boldsymbol{P}_{[A,B]}$ *denote the orthogonal projector onto* $\mathrm{Sp}[\boldsymbol{A},\boldsymbol{B}] = \mathrm{Sp}(\boldsymbol{A}) + \mathrm{Sp}(\boldsymbol{B})$, *namely*

$$\boldsymbol{P}_{[A,B]} = [\boldsymbol{A},\boldsymbol{B}]\begin{bmatrix} \boldsymbol{A}'\boldsymbol{A} & \boldsymbol{A}'\boldsymbol{B} \\ \boldsymbol{B}'\boldsymbol{A} & \boldsymbol{B}'\boldsymbol{B} \end{bmatrix}^{-}\begin{bmatrix} \boldsymbol{A}' \\ \boldsymbol{B}' \end{bmatrix}. \tag{4.18}$$

If $\mathrm{Sp}(\boldsymbol{A})$ *and* $\mathrm{Sp}(\boldsymbol{B})$ *are disjoint and cover the entire space* E^n, *the following decomposition holds:*

$$\boldsymbol{P}_{[A,B]} = \boldsymbol{P}_{A\cdot B}+\boldsymbol{P}_{B\cdot A} = \boldsymbol{A}(\boldsymbol{A}'\boldsymbol{Q}_B\boldsymbol{A})^{-}\boldsymbol{A}'\boldsymbol{Q}_B+\boldsymbol{B}(\boldsymbol{B}'\boldsymbol{Q}_A\boldsymbol{B})^{-}\boldsymbol{B}'\boldsymbol{Q}_A. \tag{4.19}$$

Proof. The decomposition of $\boldsymbol{P}_{[A,B]}$ follows from Theorem 2.13, while the representations of $\boldsymbol{P}_{A\cdot B}$ and $\boldsymbol{P}_{B\cdot A}$ follow from Corollary 1 of Theorem 4.1. Q.E.D.

Corollary 1 *Let* $E^n = \mathrm{Sp}(\boldsymbol{A}) \oplus \mathrm{Sp}(\boldsymbol{B})$. *Then,*

$$\boldsymbol{I}_n = \boldsymbol{A}(\boldsymbol{A}'\boldsymbol{Q}_B\boldsymbol{A})^{-}\boldsymbol{A}'\boldsymbol{Q}_B + \boldsymbol{B}(\boldsymbol{B}'\boldsymbol{Q}_A\boldsymbol{B})^{-}\boldsymbol{B}'\boldsymbol{Q}_A. \tag{4.20}$$

(Proof omitted.)

Corollary 2 *Let* $E^n = \mathrm{Sp}(\boldsymbol{A}) \oplus \mathrm{Sp}(\boldsymbol{B})$. *Then,*

$$\boldsymbol{Q}_A = \boldsymbol{Q}_A\boldsymbol{B}(\boldsymbol{B}'\boldsymbol{Q}_A\boldsymbol{B})^{-}\boldsymbol{B}'\boldsymbol{Q}_A \tag{4.21}$$

and

$$\boldsymbol{Q}_B = \boldsymbol{Q}_B\boldsymbol{A}(\boldsymbol{A}'\boldsymbol{Q}_B\boldsymbol{A})^{-}\boldsymbol{A}'\boldsymbol{Q}_B. \tag{4.22}$$

Proof. Formula (4.21) can be derived by premultiplying (4.20) by $\boldsymbol{Q}_A$, and (4.22) can be obtained by premultiplying it by $\boldsymbol{Q}_B$. Q.E.D.

Corollary 3 *Let* $E^m = \mathrm{Sp}(\boldsymbol{A}') \oplus \mathrm{Sp}(\boldsymbol{C}')$. *Then,*

$$\boldsymbol{Q}_{A'} = \boldsymbol{Q}_{A'}\boldsymbol{C}'(\boldsymbol{C}\boldsymbol{Q}_{A'}\boldsymbol{C}')^{-}\boldsymbol{C}\boldsymbol{Q}_{A'} \tag{4.23}$$

and

$$\boldsymbol{Q}_{C'} = \boldsymbol{Q}_{C'}\boldsymbol{A}'(\boldsymbol{A}\boldsymbol{Q}_{C'}\boldsymbol{A}')^{-}\boldsymbol{A}\boldsymbol{Q}_{C'}. \tag{4.24}$$

Proof. The proof is similar to that of Corollary 2. Q.E.D.

Theorem 4.1 can be generalized as follows:

Theorem 4.3 *Let $V \subset E^n$ and*

$$V = V_1 \oplus V_2 \oplus \cdots \oplus V_r, \tag{4.25}$$

where $V_j = \mathrm{Sp}(\boldsymbol{A}_j)$. Let $\boldsymbol{P}^*_{j\cdot(j)}$ denote a projector onto V_j along $V_{(j)} = V_1 \oplus \cdots \oplus V_{j-1} \oplus V_{j+1} \oplus \cdots \oplus V_r$. Then, the equation

$$\begin{aligned}\boldsymbol{P}^*_{j\cdot(j)} &= \boldsymbol{A}_j(\boldsymbol{A}_j'\boldsymbol{Q}_{(j)}\boldsymbol{A}_j)^-\boldsymbol{A}_j'\boldsymbol{Q}_{(j)} \\ &+\boldsymbol{Z}[\boldsymbol{I}_n - (\boldsymbol{Q}_{(j)}\boldsymbol{A}_j)(\boldsymbol{A}_j'\boldsymbol{Q}_{(j)}\boldsymbol{A}_j)^-\boldsymbol{A}_j']\boldsymbol{Q}_{(j)}\end{aligned} \tag{4.26}$$

holds, where $\boldsymbol{Q}_{(j)} = \boldsymbol{I}_n - \boldsymbol{P}_{(j)}$, $\boldsymbol{P}_{(j)}$ is the orthogonal projector onto $V_{(j)}$, and $\boldsymbol{Z}$ is an arbitrary square matrix of order n. (Proof omitted.)

Note If $V_1 \oplus V_2 \oplus \cdots \oplus V_r = E^n$, the second term in (4.26) will be null. Let $\boldsymbol{P}_{j\cdot(j)}$ denote the projector onto V_j along $V_{(j)}$. Then,

$$\boldsymbol{P}_{j\cdot(j)} = \boldsymbol{A}_j(\boldsymbol{A}_j'\boldsymbol{Q}_{(j)}\boldsymbol{A}_j)^-\boldsymbol{A}_j'\boldsymbol{Q}_{(j)}. \tag{4.27}$$

Let $\boldsymbol{A} = [\boldsymbol{A}_1, \boldsymbol{A}_2, \cdots, \boldsymbol{A}_r]$ be a nonsingular matrix of order n. Then,

$$\boldsymbol{P}_{j\cdot(j)} = \boldsymbol{A}_j\boldsymbol{A}_j'(\boldsymbol{A}_1\boldsymbol{A}_1' + \cdots + \boldsymbol{A}_r\boldsymbol{A}_r')^{-1} \tag{4.28}$$

can be derived in a manner similar to (4.10).

Let us again consider the case in which $V = V_1 \oplus V_2 \oplus \cdots \oplus V_r \subset E^n$. Let $\boldsymbol{P}_V$ denote the orthogonal projector onto $V = V_1 \oplus V_2 \oplus \cdots \oplus V_r = \mathrm{Sp}(\boldsymbol{A}_1) \oplus \mathrm{Sp}(\boldsymbol{A}_2) \oplus \cdots \oplus \mathrm{Sp}(\boldsymbol{A}_r)$. Then,

$$\boldsymbol{P}^*_{j\cdot(j)}\boldsymbol{P}_V = \boldsymbol{A}_j(\boldsymbol{A}_j'\boldsymbol{Q}_{(j)}\boldsymbol{A}_j)^-\boldsymbol{A}_j'\boldsymbol{Q}_{(j)} = \boldsymbol{P}_{j\cdot(j)}. \tag{4.29}$$

If (4.25) holds, $\boldsymbol{P}_V\boldsymbol{y} \in V$ for $\forall \boldsymbol{y} \in E^n$, so that

$$(\boldsymbol{P}^*_{1\cdot(1)} + \boldsymbol{P}^*_{2\cdot(2)} + \cdots + \boldsymbol{P}^*_{r\cdot(r)})\boldsymbol{P}_V\boldsymbol{y} = \boldsymbol{P}_V\boldsymbol{y}.$$

Since $\boldsymbol{y}$ is an arbitrary vector, the following theorem can be derived from (4.29).

Theorem 4.4 *Assume that (4.25) holds, and let $\boldsymbol{P}_{j\cdot(j)}$ denote the projector onto V_j along $V_{(j)} \dot{\oplus} V^\perp$. Then,*

$$\boldsymbol{P}_V = \boldsymbol{P}_{1\cdot(1)} + \boldsymbol{P}_{2\cdot(2)} + \cdots + \boldsymbol{P}_{r\cdot(r)}, \tag{4.30}$$

where $\boldsymbol{P}_{j\cdot(j)} = \boldsymbol{A}_j(\boldsymbol{A}_j'\boldsymbol{Q}_{(j)}\boldsymbol{A}_j)^-\boldsymbol{A}_j'\boldsymbol{Q}_{(j)}$. (Proof omitted.)

Note An alternative way of deriving (4.30 is as follows. Consider

$$E^n = V_1 \oplus V_2 \oplus \cdots \oplus V_r \oplus V^\perp, \tag{4.31}$$

where $V = V_1 \oplus \cdots \oplus V_r$. Let $V_j = \mathrm{Sp}(\boldsymbol{A}_j)$ and $V^\perp = \mathrm{Sp}(\boldsymbol{B})$. Then the projector onto V_j along $V_1 \oplus \cdots \oplus V_{j-1} \oplus V_{j+1} \oplus \cdots \oplus V_r \oplus V^\perp$ is given by

$$\boldsymbol{P}_{j\cdot(j)+B} = \boldsymbol{A}_j(\boldsymbol{A}_j'\boldsymbol{Q}_{(j)+B}\boldsymbol{A}_j)^-\boldsymbol{A}_j'\boldsymbol{Q}_{(j)+B}, \tag{4.32}$$

where $\boldsymbol{Q}_{(j)+B} = \boldsymbol{I}_n - \boldsymbol{P}_{(j)+B}$ and $\boldsymbol{P}_{(j)+B}$ is the orthogonal projector onto $V_{(j)} \dot{\oplus} V^\perp$. Since $V_j = \mathrm{Sp}(\boldsymbol{A}_j)$ $(j = 1, \cdots r)$ and $V^\perp = \mathrm{Sp}(\boldsymbol{B})$ are orthogonal, we have $\boldsymbol{A}_j'\boldsymbol{B} = \boldsymbol{O}$ and $\boldsymbol{A}_{(j)}'\boldsymbol{B} = \boldsymbol{O}$, so that

$$\begin{aligned}\boldsymbol{A}_j'\boldsymbol{Q}_{(j)+B} &= \boldsymbol{A}_j'(\boldsymbol{I}_n - \boldsymbol{P}_{(j)+B}) = \boldsymbol{A}_j'(\boldsymbol{I}_n - \boldsymbol{P}_{(j)} - \boldsymbol{P}_B)\\ &= \boldsymbol{A}_j'(\boldsymbol{I}_n - \boldsymbol{P}_{(j)}) = \boldsymbol{A}_j'\boldsymbol{Q}_{(j)}\end{aligned} \tag{4.33}$$

and

$$\boldsymbol{P}_{j\cdot(j)+B} = \boldsymbol{A}_j(\boldsymbol{A}_j'\boldsymbol{Q}_{(j)}\boldsymbol{A}_j)^-\boldsymbol{A}_j'\boldsymbol{Q}_{(j)} = \boldsymbol{P}_{j\cdot(j)}. \tag{4.34}$$

Hence, when $V_A = V_1 \oplus V_2 \oplus \cdots \oplus V_r$ and V_B are orthogonal, from now on we call the projector $\boldsymbol{P}_{j\cdot(j)+B}$ onto V_j along $V_{(j)} \dot{\oplus} V_B$ merely the projector onto V_j along $V_{(j)}$. However, when $V_A = \mathrm{Sp}(\boldsymbol{A}) = \mathrm{Sp}(\boldsymbol{A}_1) \oplus \cdots \oplus \mathrm{Sp}(\boldsymbol{A}_r)$ and $V_B = \mathrm{Sp}(B)$ are not orthogonal, we obtain the decomposition

$$\boldsymbol{P}_{A\cdot B} = \boldsymbol{P}_{1\cdot(1)+B} + \boldsymbol{P}_{2\cdot(2)+B} + \cdots + \boldsymbol{P}_{r\cdot(r)+B} \tag{4.35}$$

from $\boldsymbol{P}_{A\cdot B} + \boldsymbol{P}_{B\cdot A} = \boldsymbol{I}_n$, where $\boldsymbol{P}_{j\cdot(j)+B}$ is as given in (4.34).

Additionally, let $\boldsymbol{A}' = [\boldsymbol{A}_1', \boldsymbol{A}_2', \cdots, \boldsymbol{A}_r']$ and $\tilde{V}_j = \mathrm{Sp}(\boldsymbol{A}_j')$, and let

$$E^m = \tilde{V}_1 \oplus \tilde{V}_2 \oplus \cdots \oplus \tilde{V}_r.$$

Let $\tilde{\boldsymbol{P}}_{j\cdot(j)}$ denote the projector onto $\tilde{V}_j$ along $V_{(j)}$. Then,

$$\tilde{\boldsymbol{P}}_{j\cdot(j)} = \boldsymbol{A}_j'(\boldsymbol{A}_j\tilde{\boldsymbol{Q}}_{(j)}\boldsymbol{A}_j')^-\boldsymbol{A}_j\tilde{\boldsymbol{Q}}_{(j)}, \tag{4.36}$$

where $\tilde{\boldsymbol{Q}}_{(j)} = \boldsymbol{I}_m - \tilde{\boldsymbol{P}}_{(j)}$ and $\tilde{\boldsymbol{P}}_{(j)}$ is the orthogonal projector onto $\tilde{V}_{(j)} = \mathrm{Sp}(\boldsymbol{A}_1') \oplus \cdots \oplus \mathrm{Sp}(\boldsymbol{A}_{j-1}') \oplus \mathrm{Sp}(\boldsymbol{A}_{j+1}') \oplus \cdots \oplus \mathrm{Sp}(\boldsymbol{A}_r')$, and $\boldsymbol{A}_{(j)}' = [\boldsymbol{A}_1', \cdots, \boldsymbol{A}_{j-1}', \boldsymbol{A}_{j+1}', \cdots \boldsymbol{A}_r']$.

4.2 Decompositions of Projection Matrices

Let $V_A = \mathrm{Sp}(\boldsymbol{A})$ and $V_B = \mathrm{Sp}(\boldsymbol{B})$ be two nondisjoint subspaces, and let the corresponding projectors $\boldsymbol{P}_A$ and $\boldsymbol{P}_B$ be noncommutative. Then the space

$V = V_A + V_B$ can be decomposed in two ways, as shown in Lemma 2.4. Here we first consider a decomposition of the orthogonal projector $\boldsymbol{P}_{A\cup B}$ onto Sp$[\boldsymbol{A}, \boldsymbol{B}]$. Let $\boldsymbol{P}_A$ and $\boldsymbol{P}_B$ denote the orthogonal projectors onto V_A and V_B, and let $\boldsymbol{Q}_A = \boldsymbol{I}_n - \boldsymbol{P}_A$ and $\boldsymbol{Q}_B = \boldsymbol{I}_n - \boldsymbol{P}_B$ denote their orthogonal complements. From Lemma 2.4, the following theorem can be derived.

Theorem 4.5

$$\begin{aligned} \boldsymbol{P}_{[A,B]} &= \boldsymbol{P}_A + \boldsymbol{P}_{B[A]} &(4.37)\\ &= \boldsymbol{P}_B + \boldsymbol{P}_{A[B]}, &(4.38)\end{aligned}$$

where

$$\boldsymbol{P}_{A[B]} = \boldsymbol{Q}_B\boldsymbol{A}(\boldsymbol{Q}_B\boldsymbol{A})^-_\ell = \boldsymbol{Q}_B\boldsymbol{A}(\boldsymbol{A}'\boldsymbol{Q}_B\boldsymbol{A})^-\boldsymbol{A}'\boldsymbol{Q}_B$$

and

$$\boldsymbol{P}_{B[A]} = \boldsymbol{Q}_A\boldsymbol{B}(\boldsymbol{Q}_A\boldsymbol{B})^-_\ell = \boldsymbol{Q}_A\boldsymbol{B}(\boldsymbol{B}'\boldsymbol{Q}_A\boldsymbol{B})^-\boldsymbol{B}'\boldsymbol{Q}_A.$$

Proof. $(\boldsymbol{Q}_A\boldsymbol{B})'\boldsymbol{A} = \boldsymbol{B}'\boldsymbol{Q}_A\boldsymbol{A} = \boldsymbol{O}$ and $(\boldsymbol{Q}_B\boldsymbol{A})'\boldsymbol{B} = \boldsymbol{A}'\boldsymbol{Q}_B\boldsymbol{B} = \boldsymbol{O}$. Hence, $V_A = \text{Sp}(\boldsymbol{A})$ and $V_{B[A]} = \text{Sp}(\boldsymbol{Q}_B\boldsymbol{A})$ are orthogonal, $V_B = \text{Sp}(\boldsymbol{B})$ and $V_{A[B]} = \text{Sp}(\boldsymbol{Q}_A\boldsymbol{B})$ are orthogonal, and (4.37) and (4.38) follow. The expressions for $\boldsymbol{P}_{A[B]}$ and $\boldsymbol{P}_{B[A]}$ are clear from (3.78). Q.E.D.

Note $\boldsymbol{P}_{A[B]}$ and $\boldsymbol{P}_{B[A]}$ are often denoted as $\boldsymbol{P}_{Q_BA}$ and $\boldsymbol{P}_{Q_AB}$, respectively.

Note Decompositions (4.37) and (4.38) can also be derived by direct computation. Let

$$\boldsymbol{M} = \begin{bmatrix} \boldsymbol{A}'\boldsymbol{A} & \boldsymbol{A}'\boldsymbol{B} \\ \boldsymbol{B}'\boldsymbol{A} & \boldsymbol{B}'\boldsymbol{B} \end{bmatrix}.$$

A generalized inverse of $\boldsymbol{M}$ is then given by

$$\begin{bmatrix} (\boldsymbol{A}'\boldsymbol{A})^- + (\boldsymbol{A}'\boldsymbol{A})^-\boldsymbol{A}\boldsymbol{B}\boldsymbol{D}^-\boldsymbol{B}'\boldsymbol{A}(\boldsymbol{A}'\boldsymbol{A})^- & -(\boldsymbol{A}'\boldsymbol{A})^-\boldsymbol{A}'\boldsymbol{B}\boldsymbol{D}^- \\ -\boldsymbol{D}^-\boldsymbol{B}'\boldsymbol{A}(\boldsymbol{A}'\boldsymbol{A})^- & \boldsymbol{D}^- \end{bmatrix},$$

where $\boldsymbol{D} = \boldsymbol{B}'\boldsymbol{B} - \boldsymbol{B}'\boldsymbol{A}(\boldsymbol{A}'\boldsymbol{A})^-\boldsymbol{A}'\boldsymbol{B}$, using (3.44), since $\text{Sp}(\boldsymbol{A}'\boldsymbol{B}) \subset \text{Sp}(\boldsymbol{A}'\boldsymbol{A}) \subset \text{Sp}(\boldsymbol{A}')$. Let $\boldsymbol{P}_A = \boldsymbol{A}(\boldsymbol{A}'\boldsymbol{A})^-\boldsymbol{A}'$. Then,

$$\begin{aligned} \boldsymbol{P}_{[A,B]} &= \boldsymbol{P}_A + \boldsymbol{P}_A\boldsymbol{B}\boldsymbol{D}^-\boldsymbol{B}'\boldsymbol{P}_A - \boldsymbol{P}_A\boldsymbol{B}\boldsymbol{D}^-\boldsymbol{B}' - \boldsymbol{B}\boldsymbol{D}^-\boldsymbol{B}'\boldsymbol{P}_A + \boldsymbol{B}\boldsymbol{D}^-\boldsymbol{B}' \\ &= \boldsymbol{P}_A + (\boldsymbol{I}_n - \boldsymbol{P}_A)\boldsymbol{B}\boldsymbol{D}^-\boldsymbol{B}'(\boldsymbol{I}_n - \boldsymbol{P}_A) \\ &= \boldsymbol{P}_A + \boldsymbol{Q}_A\boldsymbol{B}(\boldsymbol{B}'\boldsymbol{Q}_A\boldsymbol{B})^-\boldsymbol{B}'\boldsymbol{Q}_A = \boldsymbol{P}_A + \boldsymbol{P}_{B[A]}. \end{aligned}$$

Corollary *Let $\boldsymbol{A}$ and $\boldsymbol{B}$ be matrices with m columns, and let $\tilde{V}_1 = \mathrm{Sp}(\boldsymbol{A}')$ and $\tilde{V}_2 = \mathrm{Sp}(\boldsymbol{B}')$. Then the orthogonal projector onto $\tilde{V}_1 + \tilde{V}_2$ is given by*

$$\boldsymbol{P}_{[A',B']} = [\boldsymbol{A}', \boldsymbol{B}'] \begin{bmatrix} \boldsymbol{A}\boldsymbol{A}' & \boldsymbol{A}\boldsymbol{B}' \\ \boldsymbol{B}\boldsymbol{A}' & \boldsymbol{B}\boldsymbol{B}' \end{bmatrix}^{-} \begin{bmatrix} \boldsymbol{A} \\ \boldsymbol{B} \end{bmatrix},$$

which is decomposed as

$$\begin{aligned} \boldsymbol{P}_{[A',B']} &= \boldsymbol{P}_{A'} + \boldsymbol{P}_{B'[A']} & (4.39) \\ &= \boldsymbol{P}_{B'} + \boldsymbol{P}_{A'[B']}, & (4.40) \end{aligned}$$

where

$$\boldsymbol{P}_{B'[A']} = (\boldsymbol{Q}_{A'}\boldsymbol{B}')(\boldsymbol{Q}_{A'}\boldsymbol{B}')^{-}_{\ell} = \boldsymbol{Q}_{A'}\boldsymbol{B}'(\boldsymbol{B}\boldsymbol{Q}_{A'}\boldsymbol{B}')^{-}\boldsymbol{B}\boldsymbol{Q}_{A'}$$

and

$$\boldsymbol{P}_{A'[B']} = (\boldsymbol{Q}_{B'}\boldsymbol{A}')(\boldsymbol{Q}_{B'}\boldsymbol{A}')^{-}_{\ell} = \boldsymbol{Q}_{B'}\boldsymbol{A}'(\boldsymbol{A}\boldsymbol{Q}_{B'}\boldsymbol{A}')^{-}\boldsymbol{A}\boldsymbol{Q}_{B'},$$

and $\boldsymbol{Q}_{A'} = \boldsymbol{I}_m - \boldsymbol{P}_{A'}$ and $\boldsymbol{Q}_{B'} = \boldsymbol{I}_m - \boldsymbol{P}_{B'}$, where $\boldsymbol{P}_{A'}$ and $\boldsymbol{P}_{B'}$ are orthogonal projectors onto $\mathrm{Sp}(\boldsymbol{A}')$ and $\mathrm{Sp}(\boldsymbol{B}')$, respectively.

(Proof omitted.)

Note The following equations can be derived from (3.72).

$$\boldsymbol{P}_{[A',B']} = \begin{bmatrix} \boldsymbol{A} \\ \boldsymbol{B} \end{bmatrix}^{-}_{m} \begin{bmatrix} \boldsymbol{A} \\ \boldsymbol{B} \end{bmatrix},$$

$$\boldsymbol{P}_{B'[A']} = (\boldsymbol{B}\boldsymbol{Q}_{A'})^{-}_{m}(\boldsymbol{B}\boldsymbol{Q}_{A'}),$$

and

$$\boldsymbol{P}_{A'[B']} = (\boldsymbol{A}\boldsymbol{Q}_{B'})^{-}_{m}(\boldsymbol{A}\boldsymbol{Q}_{B'}).$$

Theorem 4.6 *Let $E^n = (V_A + V_B) \oplus V_C$, where $V_C = \mathrm{Sp}(\boldsymbol{C})$, and let $\boldsymbol{P}_{[A,B]\cdot C}$ denote the projector onto $V_A + V_B$ along V_C. Then $\boldsymbol{P}_{[A,B]\cdot C}$ can be decomposed as follows:*

$$\begin{aligned} \boldsymbol{P}_{[A,B]\cdot C} &= \boldsymbol{P}_{A\cdot C} + \boldsymbol{P}_{B[A]\cdot C} & (4.41) \\ &= \boldsymbol{P}_{B\cdot C} + \boldsymbol{P}_{A[B]\cdot C}, & (4.42) \end{aligned}$$

where

$$\boldsymbol{P}_{A\cdot C} = \boldsymbol{A}(\boldsymbol{A}'\boldsymbol{Q}_C\boldsymbol{A})^{-}\boldsymbol{A}'\boldsymbol{Q}_C,$$

$$P_{B\cdot C} = B(B'Q_C B)^- B'Q_C,$$

$$P_{B[A]\cdot C} = P_{Q_A B\cdot C} = Q_A B(B'Q_A Q_C Q_A B)^- B'Q_A Q_C,$$

and

$$P_{A[B]\cdot C} = P_{Q_B A\cdot C} = Q_B A(A'Q_B Q_C Q_B A)^- A'Q_B Q_C.$$

Proof. From Lemma 2.4, we have

$$V_A + V_B = \mathrm{Sp}(A) \dot{\oplus} \mathrm{Sp}(Q_A B) = \mathrm{Sp}(B) \dot{\oplus} \mathrm{Sp}(Q_B A).$$

We then use Theorem 2.21. Q.E.D.

Note As has been stated in Theorem 2.18, when $P_A P_B = P_B P_A$, we have $Q_B P_A = P_A Q_B$, so that $Q_B A A_\ell^- Q_B A = Q_B P_A Q_B A = Q_B P_A A = Q_B A$ and $Q_B A A_\ell^- = P_A - P_A P_B = (Q_B A A_\ell^-)'$. Hence, $A_\ell^- \in \{(Q_B A)_\ell^-\}$, and so $Q_A B(Q_A B)_\ell^- = P_A - P_A P_B$, leading to

$$P_A P_B = P_B P_A \Longleftrightarrow P_{[A,B]} = P_A + P_B - P_A P_B. \tag{4.43}$$

Corollary 1 $P_{[A,B]} = P_A \Longleftrightarrow \mathrm{Sp}(B) \subset \mathrm{Sp}(A)$.

Proof. ($\Leftarrow$): From $\mathrm{Sp}(B) \subset \mathrm{Sp}(A)$, $B = AW$ for some W. In (4.37), $Q_A B = (I - P_A)B = (I - P_A)AW = O$. From $OO_\ell^- O = O$, we obtain $P_{[A,B]} = P_A$.

($\Rightarrow$): From (4.37), $(Q_A B)(Q_A B)_\ell^- = O$. Postmultiplying by $Q_A B$, we obtain $Q_A B = O$, which implies $Q_A P_B = O$, which in turn implies $P_A P_B = P_B$. By Theorem 2.11, we have $\mathrm{Sp}(B) \subset \mathrm{Sp}(A)$.

Q.E.D.

Corollary 2 *When* $\mathrm{Sp}(B) \subset \mathrm{Sp}(A)$,

$$P_{A[B]} = Q_B A(A'Q_B A)^- A'Q_B = P_A - P_B. \tag{4.44}$$

(Proof omitted.)

Let $V_1 = \mathrm{Sp}(A_1), \cdots, V_r = \mathrm{Sp}(A_r)$ be r subspaces that are not necessarily disjoint. Then Theorem 4.5 can be generalized as follows.

Theorem 4.7 *Let $\boldsymbol{P}$ denote the orthogonal projector onto $V = V_1 + V_2 + \cdots + V_r$. Then,*

$$\boldsymbol{P} = \boldsymbol{P}_1 + \boldsymbol{P}_{2[1]} + \boldsymbol{P}_{3[2]} + \cdots + \boldsymbol{P}_{r[r-1]}, \tag{4.45}$$

where $\boldsymbol{P}_{j[j-1]}$ indicates the orthogonal projector onto the space $V_{j[j-1]} = \{\boldsymbol{x}|\boldsymbol{x} = \boldsymbol{Q}_{[j-1]}\boldsymbol{y}, \boldsymbol{y} \in E^n\}$, $\boldsymbol{Q}_{[j-1]} = \boldsymbol{I}_n - \boldsymbol{P}_{[j-1]}$, and $\boldsymbol{P}_{[j-1]}$ is the orthogonal projector onto $\text{Sp}(\boldsymbol{A}_1) + \text{Sp}(\boldsymbol{A}_2) + \cdots + \text{Sp}(\boldsymbol{A}_{j-1})$.

(Proof omitted.)

Note The terms in the decomposition given in (4.45) correspond with $\text{Sp}(\boldsymbol{A}_1), \text{Sp}(\boldsymbol{A}_2), \cdots, \text{Sp}(\boldsymbol{A}_r)$ in that order. Rearranging these subspaces, we obtain $r!$ different decompositions of $\boldsymbol{P}$.

4.3 The Method of Least Squares

Explicit representations of projectors associated with subspaces given in Section 4.1 can also be derived by the method of least squares (LS).

Let $\boldsymbol{A}$ represent an n by m matrix, and let $\boldsymbol{b} \in E^n$ be a vector that does not necessarily belong to $\text{Sp}(\boldsymbol{A})$. Then $\boldsymbol{x}$ that minimizes $||\boldsymbol{b} - \boldsymbol{A}\boldsymbol{x}||^2$ should satisfy the normal equation $\boldsymbol{A}'\boldsymbol{A}\boldsymbol{x} = \boldsymbol{A}'\boldsymbol{b}$. Premultiplying both sides of this equation by $\boldsymbol{A}(\boldsymbol{A}'\boldsymbol{A})^-$, we obtain

$$\boldsymbol{A}\boldsymbol{x} = \boldsymbol{P}_A\boldsymbol{b},$$

where $\boldsymbol{P}_A = \boldsymbol{A}(\boldsymbol{A}'\boldsymbol{A})^-\boldsymbol{A}' = \boldsymbol{A}\boldsymbol{A}_\ell^-$. The following lemma can be immediately derived from the equation above.

Lemma 4.2

$$\min_x ||\boldsymbol{b} - \boldsymbol{A}\boldsymbol{x}||^2 = ||\boldsymbol{b} - \boldsymbol{P}_A\boldsymbol{b}||^2. \tag{4.46}$$

(Proof omitted.)

Let

$$||\boldsymbol{x}||_M^2 = \boldsymbol{x}'\boldsymbol{M}\boldsymbol{x} \tag{4.47}$$

denote a pseudo-norm, where $\boldsymbol{M}$ is an *nnd* matrix such that

$$\text{rank}(\boldsymbol{A}'\boldsymbol{M}\boldsymbol{A}) = \text{rank}(\boldsymbol{A}) = \text{rank}(\boldsymbol{A}'\boldsymbol{M}). \tag{4.48}$$

Then the following theorem holds.

Theorem 4.8 $\min_x ||\boldsymbol{b} - \boldsymbol{A}\boldsymbol{x}||^2_M = ||\boldsymbol{b} - \boldsymbol{P}_{A/M}\boldsymbol{b}||^2_M$, *where*

$$\boldsymbol{P}_{A/M} = \boldsymbol{A}(\boldsymbol{A}'\boldsymbol{M}\boldsymbol{A})^-\boldsymbol{A}'\boldsymbol{M}. \tag{4.49}$$

Proof. Since $\boldsymbol{M}$ is *nnd*, there exists an $\boldsymbol{N}$ such that $\boldsymbol{M} = \boldsymbol{N}\boldsymbol{N}'$. Hence,

$$||\boldsymbol{b} - \boldsymbol{P}_{A/M}\boldsymbol{b}||^2_M = (\boldsymbol{b} - \boldsymbol{A}\boldsymbol{x})'\boldsymbol{N}'\boldsymbol{N}(\boldsymbol{b} - \boldsymbol{A}\boldsymbol{x}) = ||\boldsymbol{N}\boldsymbol{b} - \boldsymbol{N}\boldsymbol{A}\boldsymbol{x}||^2.$$

By Lemma 4.2, $\boldsymbol{x}$ that minimizes the criterion above satisfies

$$\boldsymbol{N}'(\boldsymbol{N}\boldsymbol{A})\boldsymbol{x} = \boldsymbol{N}'\boldsymbol{N}\boldsymbol{A}(\boldsymbol{A}'\boldsymbol{N}'\boldsymbol{N}\boldsymbol{A})^-\boldsymbol{A}'\boldsymbol{N}'\boldsymbol{N}\boldsymbol{b},$$

that is, $\boldsymbol{M}\boldsymbol{A}\boldsymbol{x} = \boldsymbol{M}\boldsymbol{A}(\boldsymbol{A}'\boldsymbol{M}\boldsymbol{A})^-\boldsymbol{A}'\boldsymbol{M}\boldsymbol{b}$. Premultiplying both sides of this equation by $\boldsymbol{A}(\boldsymbol{A}'\boldsymbol{M}\boldsymbol{A})^-\boldsymbol{A}'$, we obtain

$$\boldsymbol{A}\boldsymbol{x} = \boldsymbol{P}_{A/M}\boldsymbol{b}$$

since $\boldsymbol{A}(\boldsymbol{A}'\boldsymbol{M}\boldsymbol{A})^-\boldsymbol{A}'\boldsymbol{M}\boldsymbol{A} = \boldsymbol{A}$ by (4.48).

An alternative proof. Differentiating $f(\boldsymbol{x}) = (\boldsymbol{b} - \boldsymbol{A}\boldsymbol{x})'\boldsymbol{M}(\boldsymbol{b} - \boldsymbol{A}\boldsymbol{x})$ with respect to $\boldsymbol{x}$ and setting the results equal to zero, we obtain

$$\frac{1}{2}\frac{\partial f}{\partial \boldsymbol{x}} = \boldsymbol{A}'\boldsymbol{M}\boldsymbol{A}\boldsymbol{x} - \boldsymbol{A}'\boldsymbol{M}\boldsymbol{b} = \boldsymbol{0}.$$

Premultiplying both sides by $\boldsymbol{A}(\boldsymbol{A}'\boldsymbol{M}\boldsymbol{A})^-$, we obtain the desired result.

Q.E.D.

Corollary *Let* Sp$(\boldsymbol{A})$ *and* Sp$(\boldsymbol{B})$ *be disjoint, and let* $\boldsymbol{Q}_B = \boldsymbol{I}_n - \boldsymbol{P}_B$. *Then*

$$\min_x ||\boldsymbol{b} - \boldsymbol{A}\boldsymbol{x}||^2_{Q_B} = ||\boldsymbol{b} - \boldsymbol{P}_{A\cdot B}\boldsymbol{b}||^2_{Q_B} \tag{4.50}$$

or

$$\min_x ||\boldsymbol{b} - \boldsymbol{A}\boldsymbol{x}||^2_{Q_B} = ||\boldsymbol{b} - \boldsymbol{P}_{A[B]}\boldsymbol{b}||^2_{Q_B}, \tag{4.51}$$

where $\boldsymbol{P}_{A\cdot B} = \boldsymbol{A}(\boldsymbol{A}'\boldsymbol{Q}_B\boldsymbol{A})^-\boldsymbol{A}'\boldsymbol{Q}_B$ *and* $\boldsymbol{P}_{A[B]} = \boldsymbol{Q}_B\boldsymbol{A}(\boldsymbol{A}'\boldsymbol{Q}_B\boldsymbol{A})^-\boldsymbol{A}'\boldsymbol{Q}_B$.

Proof. (4.50): Clear from rank$(\boldsymbol{A}'\boldsymbol{Q}_B\boldsymbol{A}) = $ rank$(\boldsymbol{A})$.
(4.51): Clear from $\boldsymbol{Q}_B\boldsymbol{P}_{A\cdot B} = \boldsymbol{P}_{A[B]}$. Q.E.D.

Hence, $\boldsymbol{P}_{A\cdot B}$, the projector onto Sp$(\boldsymbol{A})$ along Sp$(\boldsymbol{B})$, can be regarded as the orthogonal projector onto $\mathrm{Sp}(\boldsymbol{A})$ associated with the pseudo-norm $||\boldsymbol{x}||_{Q_B}$. (See Figure 4.1.) Furthermore, since $\boldsymbol{A}'\boldsymbol{Q}_A = \boldsymbol{O}$,

$$\boldsymbol{P}_{A\cdot B} = \boldsymbol{A}(\boldsymbol{A}'\boldsymbol{Q}_B\boldsymbol{A})^-\boldsymbol{A}'\boldsymbol{Q}_B = \boldsymbol{A}(\boldsymbol{A}'\boldsymbol{Q}^*\boldsymbol{A})^-\boldsymbol{A}'\boldsymbol{Q}^*,$$

where $\boldsymbol{Q}^* = \boldsymbol{Q}_A + \boldsymbol{Q}_B$, and so $\mathrm{rank}(\boldsymbol{Q}^*) = n$. Hence, $\boldsymbol{P}_{A\cdot B}$ is also considered as the orthogonal projector onto $\mathrm{Sp}(\boldsymbol{A})$ associated with the norm $||\boldsymbol{x}||_{Q^*}$ characterized by the *pd* matrix $\boldsymbol{Q}^*$. (See Figure 4.1.)

Theorem 4.9 *Consider $\boldsymbol{P}_{A/M}$ as defined in (4.49). Then (4.52) and (4.53) hold, or (4.54) holds:*

$$\boldsymbol{P}^2_{A/M} = \boldsymbol{P}_{A/M}, \tag{4.52}$$

$$(\boldsymbol{M}\boldsymbol{P}_{A/M})' = \boldsymbol{M}\boldsymbol{P}_{A/M}, \tag{4.53}$$

$$\boldsymbol{P}'_{A/M}\boldsymbol{M}\boldsymbol{P}_{A/M} = \boldsymbol{M}\boldsymbol{P}_{A/M} = \boldsymbol{P}'_{A/M}\boldsymbol{M}. \tag{4.54}$$

(Proof omitted.)

Definition 4.1 *When $\boldsymbol{M}$ satisfies (4.47), a square matrix $\boldsymbol{P}_{A/M}$ that satisfies (4.52) and (4.53), or (4.54) is called the orthogonal projector onto* $\mathrm{Sp}(\boldsymbol{A})$ *with respect to the pseudo-norm* $||\boldsymbol{x}||_M = (\boldsymbol{x}'\boldsymbol{M}\boldsymbol{x})^{1/2}$.

It is clear from the definition above that $\boldsymbol{I}_n - \boldsymbol{P}_{A\cdot B}$ is the orthogonal projector onto $\mathrm{Sp}(\boldsymbol{A})^{\perp}$ with respect to the pseudo-norm $||\boldsymbol{x}|||_M$.

Note When $\boldsymbol{M}$ does not satisfy (4.48), we generally have $\mathrm{Sp}(\boldsymbol{P}_{A/M}) \subset \mathrm{Sp}(\boldsymbol{A})$, and consequently $\boldsymbol{P}_{A/M}$ is not a mapping onto the entire space of $\boldsymbol{A}$. In this case, $\boldsymbol{P}_{A/M}$ is said to be a projector *into* $\mathrm{Sp}(\boldsymbol{A})$.

We next consider minimizing $||\boldsymbol{b} - \boldsymbol{A}\boldsymbol{x}||^2$ with respect to $\boldsymbol{x}$ under the constraint that $\boldsymbol{C}\boldsymbol{x} = \boldsymbol{d}$, where $\boldsymbol{C}$ and $\boldsymbol{d} \neq \boldsymbol{b}$ are a given matrix and a vector. The following lemma holds.

Lemma 4.3

$$\min_{Cx=d} ||\boldsymbol{b} - \boldsymbol{A}\boldsymbol{x}|| = \min_{x} ||\boldsymbol{b} - \boldsymbol{A}\boldsymbol{C}^-\boldsymbol{d} - \boldsymbol{A}\boldsymbol{Q}_{C'}\boldsymbol{z}||, \tag{4.55}$$

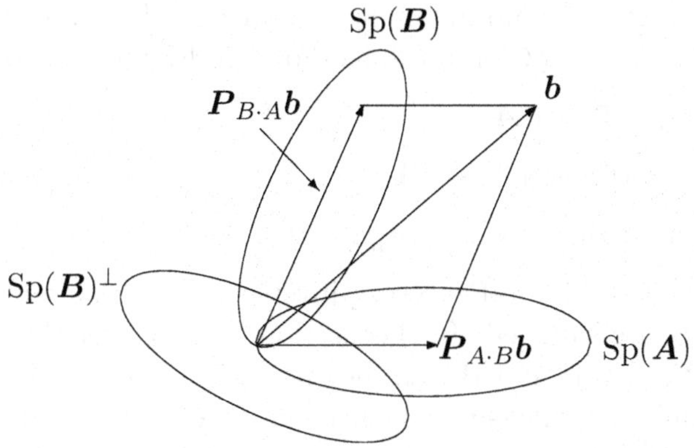

Figure 4.1: Geometric representation of the projection vector $\boldsymbol{P}_{A \cdot B}\boldsymbol{b}$.

where $\boldsymbol{Q}_{C'}$ is the orthogonal projector onto $\mathrm{Sp}(\boldsymbol{C}')^{\perp}$ *and $\boldsymbol{z}$ is an arbitrary m-component vector.*

Proof. Use the fact that $\boldsymbol{Cx} = \boldsymbol{d}$ implies $\boldsymbol{x} = \boldsymbol{C}^{-}\boldsymbol{d} + \boldsymbol{Q}_{C'}\boldsymbol{z}$. Q.E.D.

The following theorem can be derived from the lemma above and Theorem 2.25.

Theorem 4.10 *When*

$$\min_{Cx=d} ||\boldsymbol{b} - \boldsymbol{Ax}|| = ||(\boldsymbol{I}_n - \boldsymbol{P}_{AQ_{C'}})(\boldsymbol{b} - \boldsymbol{AC}^{-}\boldsymbol{d})||$$

holds,

$$\boldsymbol{x} = \boldsymbol{C}^{-}\boldsymbol{d} + \boldsymbol{Q}_{C'}(\boldsymbol{Q}_{C'}\boldsymbol{A}'\boldsymbol{A}\boldsymbol{Q}_{C'})^{-}\boldsymbol{Q}_{C'}\boldsymbol{A}'(\boldsymbol{b} - \boldsymbol{AC}^{-}\boldsymbol{d}), \tag{4.56}$$

where $\boldsymbol{P}_{AQ_{C'}}$ is the orthogonal projector onto $\mathrm{Sp}(\boldsymbol{AQ}_{C'})$.

(Proof omitted.)

4.4 Extended Definitions

Let

$$E^n = V \oplus W = \mathrm{Sp}(\boldsymbol{A}) \oplus (\boldsymbol{I}_n - \boldsymbol{AA}^{-})$$

and

$$E^m = \tilde{V} \oplus \tilde{W} = \mathrm{Sp}(\boldsymbol{A}^{-}\boldsymbol{A}) \oplus \mathrm{Sp}(\boldsymbol{I}_m - \boldsymbol{A}^{-}\boldsymbol{A}).$$

A reflexive g-inverse $\boldsymbol{A}_r^-$, a minimum norm g-inverse $\boldsymbol{A}_m^-$, and a least squares g-inverse $\boldsymbol{A}_\ell^-$ discussed in Chapter 3, as shown in Figure 4.2, correspond to:

(i) $\forall \boldsymbol{y} \in W$, $\boldsymbol{A}^- \boldsymbol{y} = \boldsymbol{0} \longrightarrow \boldsymbol{A}_r^-$,

(ii) V and W are orthogonal $\longrightarrow \boldsymbol{A}_\ell^-$,

(iii) $\tilde{V}$ and $\tilde{W}$ are orthogonal $\longrightarrow \boldsymbol{A}_m^-$,

and furthermore the Moore-Penrose g-inverse $\boldsymbol{A}^+$ follows when all of the conditions above are satisfied. In this section, we consider the situations in which V and W, and $\tilde{V}$ and $\tilde{W}$, are not necessarily orthogonal, and define generalized forms of g-inverses, which include $\boldsymbol{A}_m^-$, $\boldsymbol{A}_\ell^-$, and $\boldsymbol{A}^+$ as their special cases.

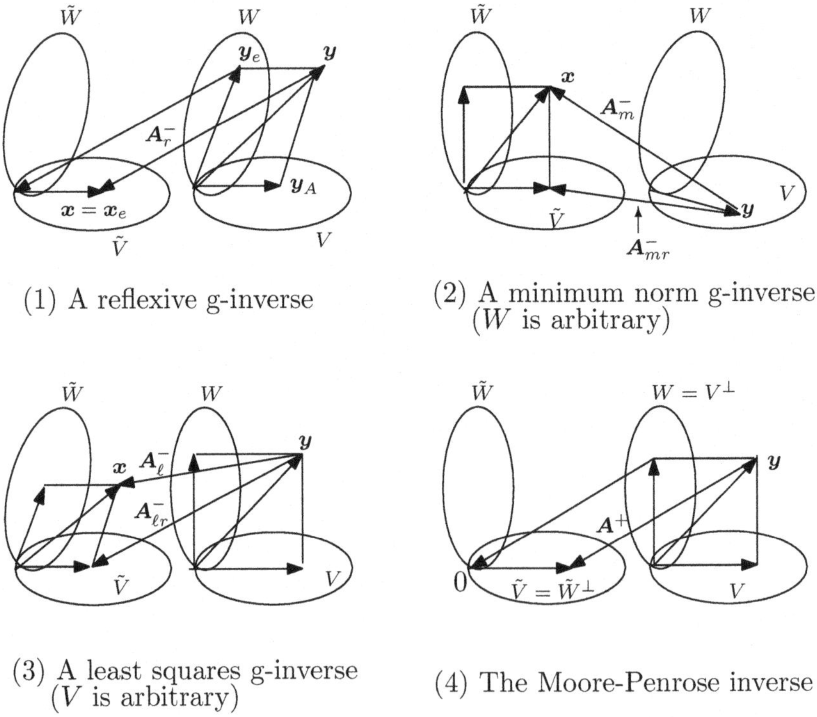
(1) A reflexive g-inverse
(2) A minimum norm g-inverse (W is arbitrary)
(3) A least squares g-inverse (V is arbitrary)
(4) The Moore-Penrose inverse

Figure 4.2: Geometric representation of the projection vector $\boldsymbol{P}_{A \cdot B}\boldsymbol{b}$.

For convenience, we start with a generalized form of least squares g-inverse, followed by minimum norm g-inverse and Moore-Penrose inverse.

4.4.1 A generalized form of least squares g-inverse

We consider the case in which a complement subspace of $V = \text{Sp}(\boldsymbol{A}) \in E^n$ is given as $W = \text{Sp}(\boldsymbol{B})$. Let us obtain $\boldsymbol{x}$ that minimizes $||\boldsymbol{b} - \boldsymbol{A}\boldsymbol{x}||^2_{Q_B}$ when $\boldsymbol{b} \notin \text{Sp}(\boldsymbol{A})$. According to Theorem 4.8 and its corollary, such an $\boldsymbol{x}$ should satisfy

$$\boldsymbol{A}\boldsymbol{x} = \boldsymbol{P}_{A \cdot B}\boldsymbol{b} = \boldsymbol{A}(\boldsymbol{A}'\boldsymbol{Q}_B\boldsymbol{A})^-\boldsymbol{A}'\boldsymbol{Q}_B\boldsymbol{b}. \tag{4.57}$$

Let $\boldsymbol{A}^-$ be an arbitrary g-inverse of $\boldsymbol{A}$, and substitute $\boldsymbol{x} = \boldsymbol{A}^-\boldsymbol{b}$ into (4.57). We obtain

$$\boldsymbol{A}\boldsymbol{A}^-\boldsymbol{b} = \boldsymbol{A}(\boldsymbol{A}'\boldsymbol{Q}_B\boldsymbol{A})^-\boldsymbol{A}'\boldsymbol{Q}_B\boldsymbol{b}.$$

This has to hold for any $\boldsymbol{b} \in E^n$, and so

$$\boldsymbol{A}\boldsymbol{A}^- = \boldsymbol{A}(\boldsymbol{A}'\boldsymbol{Q}_B\boldsymbol{A})^-\boldsymbol{A}'\boldsymbol{Q}_B \tag{4.58}$$

must hold. Premultiplying the equation above by $\boldsymbol{A}'\boldsymbol{Q}_B$, we further obtain, by (4.2),

$$\boldsymbol{A}'\boldsymbol{Q}_B\boldsymbol{A}\boldsymbol{A}^- = \boldsymbol{A}'\boldsymbol{Q}_B. \tag{4.59}$$

Let an $\boldsymbol{A}^-$ that satisfies (4.58) or (4.59) be written as $\boldsymbol{A}^-_{\ell(B)}$. Then the following theorem holds.

Theorem 4.11 *The following three conditions concerning $\boldsymbol{A}^-_{\ell(B)}$ are equivalent:*

$$\boldsymbol{A}\boldsymbol{A}^-_{\ell(B)}\boldsymbol{A} = \boldsymbol{A} \text{ and } (\boldsymbol{Q}_B\boldsymbol{A}\boldsymbol{A}^-_{\ell(B)})' = \boldsymbol{Q}_B\boldsymbol{A}\boldsymbol{A}^-_{\ell(B)}, \tag{4.60}$$

$$\boldsymbol{A}'\boldsymbol{Q}_B\boldsymbol{A}\boldsymbol{A}^-_{\ell(B)} = \boldsymbol{A}'\boldsymbol{Q}_B, \tag{4.61}$$

$$\boldsymbol{A}\boldsymbol{A}^-_{\ell(B)} = \boldsymbol{A}(\boldsymbol{A}'\boldsymbol{Q}_B\boldsymbol{A})^-\boldsymbol{A}'\boldsymbol{Q}_B. \tag{4.62}$$

Proof. (4.60) $\rightarrow$ (4.61): $\boldsymbol{A}\boldsymbol{A}^-_{\ell(B)}\boldsymbol{A} = \boldsymbol{A} \Rightarrow \boldsymbol{Q}_B\boldsymbol{A}\boldsymbol{A}^-_{\ell(B)}\boldsymbol{A} = \boldsymbol{Q}_B\boldsymbol{A}$. Transposing both sides, we obtain $\boldsymbol{A}'(\boldsymbol{Q}_B\boldsymbol{A}\boldsymbol{A}^-_{\ell(B)})' = \boldsymbol{A}'\boldsymbol{Q}_B$, the left-hand side of which is equal to $\boldsymbol{A}'\boldsymbol{Q}_B\boldsymbol{A}^-_{\ell(B)}$ due to the second equation in (4.60).

(4.61) $\rightarrow$ (4.62): Premultiply both sides by $\boldsymbol{A}(\boldsymbol{A}'\boldsymbol{Q}_B\boldsymbol{A})^-$ and use (4.3).

(4.62) $\rightarrow$ (4.60): Premultiplying both sides by $\boldsymbol{A}$, we obtain $\boldsymbol{A}\boldsymbol{A}^-_{\ell(B)}\boldsymbol{A} = \boldsymbol{A}$. That $\boldsymbol{Q}_B\boldsymbol{A}\boldsymbol{A}^-_{\ell(B)}$ is symmetric is clear from (4.21) and (4.22).

Q.E.D.

The three conditions in Theorem 4.11 indicate that $\boldsymbol{A}\boldsymbol{A}^-_{\ell(B)}$ is the projector onto $\text{Sp}(\boldsymbol{A})$ along $\text{Sp}(\boldsymbol{B})$ when $E^n = \text{Sp}(\boldsymbol{A}) \oplus \text{Sp}(\boldsymbol{B})$.

Definition 4.2 *A g-inverse* $\boldsymbol{A}^-_{\ell(B)}$ *that satisfies either one of the three conditions in Theorem 4.11 is called a B-constrained least squares g-inverse (a generalized form of the least squares g-inverse) of* $\boldsymbol{A}$.

A general expression of $\boldsymbol{A}^-_{\ell(B)}$ is, from Theorem 4.11, given by

$$\boldsymbol{A}^-_{\ell(B)} = (\boldsymbol{A}'\boldsymbol{Q}_B\boldsymbol{A})^-\boldsymbol{A}'\boldsymbol{Q}_B + [\boldsymbol{I}_m - (\boldsymbol{A}'\boldsymbol{Q}_B\boldsymbol{A})^-(\boldsymbol{A}'\boldsymbol{Q}_B\boldsymbol{A})]\boldsymbol{Z}, \tag{4.63}$$

where $\boldsymbol{Z}$ is an arbitrary m by n matrix. Let $\boldsymbol{A}^-_{\ell r(B)}$ denote an $\boldsymbol{A}^-_{\ell(B)}$ that satisfies the condition for reflexivity, namely $\boldsymbol{A}^-_{\ell r(B)}\boldsymbol{A}\boldsymbol{A}^-_{\ell r(B)} = \boldsymbol{A}^-_{\ell r(B)}$ or $\text{rank}(\boldsymbol{A}^-_{\ell r(B)}) = \text{rank}(\boldsymbol{A})$. Then,

$$\boldsymbol{A}^-_{\ell r(B)} = (\boldsymbol{A}'\boldsymbol{Q}_B\boldsymbol{A})^-\boldsymbol{A}'\boldsymbol{Q}_B. \tag{4.64}$$

Note When $\boldsymbol{B}$ is such that $\text{Sp}(\boldsymbol{B}) = \text{Sp}(\boldsymbol{A})^\perp$, $\boldsymbol{A}^-_{\ell(B)}$ reduces to $\boldsymbol{A}^-_\ell$ and $\boldsymbol{A}^-_{\ell r(B)}$ reduces to $\boldsymbol{A}^-_{\ell r}$.

Note When $\boldsymbol{M}$ is a *pd* matrix of order n,

$$\boldsymbol{A}^-_{\ell(M)} = (\boldsymbol{A}'\boldsymbol{M}\boldsymbol{A})^-\boldsymbol{A}'\boldsymbol{M} \tag{4.65}$$

is a g-inverse of $\boldsymbol{A}$ that satisfies $\boldsymbol{A}\boldsymbol{A}^-_{\ell(M)}\boldsymbol{A} = \boldsymbol{A}$, and $(\boldsymbol{M}\boldsymbol{A}\boldsymbol{A}^-_{\ell(M)})' = \boldsymbol{M}\boldsymbol{A}\boldsymbol{A}^-_{\ell(M)}$. This g-inverse is defined such that it minimizes $||\boldsymbol{A}\boldsymbol{x} - \boldsymbol{b}||^2_M$. If $\boldsymbol{M}$ is not *pd*, $\boldsymbol{A}^-_{\ell(M)}$ is not necessarily a g-inverse of $\boldsymbol{A}$.

Let $\boldsymbol{A} = [\boldsymbol{A}_1, \boldsymbol{A}_2, \cdots, \boldsymbol{A}_s]$ such that the $\boldsymbol{A}_j$'s are disjoint, namely

$$\text{Sp}(\boldsymbol{A}) = \text{Sp}(\boldsymbol{A}_1) \oplus \text{Sp}(\boldsymbol{A}_2) \oplus \cdots \oplus \text{Sp}(\boldsymbol{A}_s), \tag{4.66}$$

and let

$$\boldsymbol{A}_{(j)} = [\boldsymbol{A}_1, \cdots, \boldsymbol{A}_{j-1}, \boldsymbol{A}_{j+1}, \cdots, \boldsymbol{A}_s].$$

Then an $A_{(j)}$-constrained g-inverse of $\boldsymbol{A}$ is given by

$$\boldsymbol{A}^-_{j(j)} = (\boldsymbol{A}_j'\boldsymbol{Q}_{(j)}\boldsymbol{A}_j)^-\boldsymbol{A}_j'\boldsymbol{Q}_{(j)} + [\boldsymbol{I}_p - (\boldsymbol{A}_j'\boldsymbol{Q}_{(j)}\boldsymbol{A}_j)^-(\boldsymbol{A}_j'\boldsymbol{Q}_{(j)}\boldsymbol{A}_j)]\boldsymbol{Z}, \tag{4.67}$$

where $\boldsymbol{Q}_{(j)} = \boldsymbol{I}_n - \boldsymbol{P}_{(j)}$ and $\boldsymbol{P}_{(j)}$ is the orthogonal projector onto $\text{Sp}(\boldsymbol{A}_{(j)})$.

The existence of the $A^-_{j(j)}$ above is guaranteed by the following theorem.

Theorem 4.12 *A necessary and sufficient condition for* $A = [A_1, A_2, \cdots, A_s]$ *to satisfy (4.66) is that a g-inverse* Y *of* A *satisfies*

$$A_i Y_i A_i = A_i \text{ and } A_i Y_i A_j = O \ (i \neq j), \tag{4.68}$$

where $Y = [Y'_1, Y'_2, \cdots, Y'_s]'$.

Proof. (Necessity) Substituting $A = [A_1, A_2, \cdots, A_s]$ and $Y' = [Y'_1, Y'_2, \cdots, Y'_s]$ into $AYA = A$ and expanding, we obtain, for an arbitrary $i = 1, \cdots, s$,

$$A_1 Y_1 A_i + A_2 Y_2 A_i + \cdots + A_i Y_i A_i + \cdots + A_s Y_s A_i = A_i,$$

that is,

$$A_1 Y_1 A_i + A_2 Y_2 A_i + \cdots + A_i (Y_i A_i - I) + \cdots + A_s Y_s A_i = O.$$

Since $\mathrm{Sp}(A_i) \cap \mathrm{Sp}(A_j) = \{0\}$, (4.68) holds by Theorem 1.4.

(Sufficiency) Premultiplying $A_1 x_1 + A_2 x_2 + \cdots + A_s x_s = 0$ by $A_i Y_i$ that satisfies (4.68), we obtain $A_i x_i = 0$. Hence, $\mathrm{Sp}(A_1), \mathrm{Sp}(A_2), \cdots, \mathrm{Sp}(A_s)$ are disjoint, and $\mathrm{Sp}(A)$ is a direct-sum of these subspaces.

Q.E.D.

Let

$$A_{(j)} = [A_1, \cdots, A_{j-1}, A_{j+1}, \cdots, A_s]$$

as in Theorem 4.12. Then, $\mathrm{Sp}(A_{(j)}) \oplus \mathrm{Sp}(A_j) = \mathrm{Sp}(A)$, and so there exists A_j such that

$$A_j A^-_{j(j)} A_j = A_j \text{ and } A_j A^-_{j(j)} A_i = O \ (i \neq j). \tag{4.69}$$

$A^-_{j(j)}$ is an $A_{(j)}$-constrained g-inverse of A_j.

Let $E^n = \mathrm{Sp}(A) \oplus \mathrm{Sp}(B)$. There exist X and Y such that

$$AXA = A, \quad AXB = O,$$
$$BYB = B, \quad BYA = O.$$

However, X is identical to $A^-_{\ell(B)}$, and Y is identical to $B^-_{\ell(A)}$.

Corollary *A necessary and sufficient condition for* $A' = \begin{bmatrix} A_1' \\ A_2' \\ \vdots \\ A_s' \end{bmatrix}$ *to satisfy*

$$\mathrm{Sp}(A') = \mathrm{Sp}(A_1') \oplus \mathrm{Sp}(A_2') \oplus \cdots \oplus \mathrm{Sp}(A_s')$$

is that a g-inverse $Z = [Z_1, Z_2, \cdots, Z_s]$ *of* A *satisfy*

$$A_i Z_i A_i = A_i \text{ and } A_i Z_j A_j = O \ (i \neq j). \tag{4.70}$$

Proof. $AZA = A \Rightarrow A'Z'A' = A'$. By Theorem 4.12, $A_i'Z_i'A_i' = A_i'$ and $A_j'Z_j'A_i' = O$ $(j \neq i)$. Transposing these equations, we obtain (4.70).

Q.E.D.

4.4.2 A generalized form of minimum norm g-inverse

When $s = 2$ and $\mathrm{Sp}(A') = E^m$, namely $E^m = \tilde{V} \oplus \tilde{W}$ where $\tilde{V} = \mathrm{Sp}(A_1')$ and $\tilde{W} = \mathrm{Sp}(A_2')$, let a g-inverse of $A = [A_1', A_2']'$ be denoted by $Z = [Z_1, Z_2]$ as in the corollary to Theorem 4.12. The existence of Z_1 and Z_2 that satisfy

$$A_1Z_1A_1 = A_1, \ \ A_1Z_2A_2 = O, \ \ A_2Z_2A_2 = A_2, \text{ and } A_2Z_1A_1 = O \tag{4.71}$$

is assured. Let A and C denote m by n_1 and m by n_2 $(n_1+n_2 \geq n)$ matrices such that

$$AA^-A = A \text{ and } CA^-A = O. \tag{4.72}$$

Assume that $A'W_1 + C'W_2 = O$. Then, $(AA^-A)'W_1 + (CA^-A)'W_2 = O$, and so $A'W_1 = O$, which implies $C'W_2 = O$. That is, $\mathrm{Sp}(A')$ and $\mathrm{Sp}(C')$ are disjoint, and so we may assume $E^m = \mathrm{Sp}(A') \oplus \mathrm{Sp}(C')$. Taking the transpose of (4.72), we obtain

$$A'(A^-)'A' = A' \text{ and } A'(A^-)'C' = O. \tag{4.73}$$

Hence,

$$A'(A^-)' = P_{A' \cdot C'} = A'(AQ_{C'}A')^-AQ_{C'}, \tag{4.74}$$

where $Q_{C'} = I_m - C'(CC')^-C$, is the projector onto $\mathrm{Sp}(A')$ along $\mathrm{Sp}(C')$. Since $\{((AQ_{C'}A')^-)'\} = \{(AQ_{C'}A')^-\}$, this leads to

$$A^-A = Q_{C'}A'(AQ_{C'}A')^-A. \tag{4.75}$$

Let $A^-_{m(C)}$ denote an A^- that satisfies (4.74) or (4.75). Then,

$$A^-_{m(C)} = Q_{C'}A'(AQ_{C'}A')^- + \tilde{Z}[I_n - (AQ_{C'}A')(AQ_{C'}A')^-],$$

where $\tilde{Z}$ is an arbitrary m by n matrix. Furthermore, let $A^-_{mr(C)}$ denote an $A^-_{m(C)}$ that satisfies the reflexivity, namely $A^-_{mr(C)}AA^-_{mr(C)} = A^-_{mr(C)}$. Then,

$$A^-_{mr(C)} = Q_{C'}A'(AQ_{C'}A')^-. \tag{4.76}$$

By Corollary 2 of Theorem 4.1, the following theorem can be derived.

Theorem 4.13 *The following three conditions are equivalent:*

$$AA^-_{m(C)}A = A \text{ and } A^-_{m(C)}AA^-_{m(C)} = A^-_{m(C)}, \tag{4.77}$$

$$A^-_{m(C)}AQ_{C'}A' = Q_{C'}A', \tag{4.78}$$

$$A^-_{m(C)}A = Q_{C'}A'(AQ_{C'}A')^-A. \tag{4.79}$$

Proof. The proof is similar to that of Theorem 4.9. (Use Corollary 2 of Theorem 4.1 and Corollary 3 of Theorem 4.2.) Q.E.D.

Definition 4.3 *A g-inverse $A^-_{m(C)}$ that satisfies one of the conditions in Theorem 4.13 is called a C-constrained minimum norm g-inverse of A.*

Note $A^-_{m(C)}$ is a generalized form of A^-_m, and when $\mathrm{Sp}(C') = \mathrm{Sp}(A')^\perp$, it reduces to A^-_m.

Lemma 4.4 *Let $E^m = \mathrm{Sp}(A') \oplus \mathrm{Sp}(C')$. Then,*

$$E^m = \mathrm{Sp}(Q_{C'}) \oplus \mathrm{Sp}(Q_{A'}). \tag{4.80}$$

Proof. Let $Q_{C'}x + Q_{A'}y = 0$. Premultiplying both sides by $Q_{C'}A'(AQ_{C'} \times A')^-A$, we obtain $Q_{C'} = Q_{C'}A'(AQ_{C'}A')^-AQ_{C'}$ from (4.24), which implies $Q_{C'}x = 0$ and $Q_{A'}y = 0$. That is, $\mathrm{Sp}(Q_{C'})$ and $\mathrm{Sp}(Q_{A'})$ are disjoint. On the other hand, $\mathrm{rank}(Q_{C'}) + \mathrm{rank}(Q_{A'}) = (m - \mathrm{rank}(C)) + (m - \mathrm{rank}(A)) = 2m - m = m$, leading to (4.80). Q.E.D.

Theorem 4.14 *When (4.80) holds,* $\boldsymbol{A}^-_{m(C)}\boldsymbol{A}$ *is the projector onto* $\tilde{V} = \mathrm{Sp}(\boldsymbol{Q}_{C'}) = \mathrm{Ker}(\boldsymbol{C}')$ *along* $\tilde{W} = \mathrm{Sp}(\boldsymbol{Q}_{A'}) = \mathrm{Ker}(\boldsymbol{A}')$.

Proof. When $\boldsymbol{A}^-_{m(C)}\boldsymbol{A}$ is the projector onto $\mathrm{Sp}(\boldsymbol{Q}_{C'})$ along $\mathrm{Sp}(\boldsymbol{Q}_{A'})$, we have, from the definition of a projector in (4.9),

$$\boldsymbol{P}_{Q_{C'}\cdot Q_{A'}} = \boldsymbol{Q}_{C'}(\boldsymbol{Q}_{C'}\boldsymbol{P}_{A'}\boldsymbol{Q}_{C'})^-\boldsymbol{Q}_{C'}\boldsymbol{P}_{A'}. \tag{4.81}$$

From

$$\boldsymbol{P}_{A'}(\boldsymbol{P}_{A'}\boldsymbol{Q}_{C'}\boldsymbol{P}_{A'})^-\boldsymbol{P}_{A'}\boldsymbol{Q}_{C'}(\boldsymbol{Q}_{C'}\boldsymbol{P}_{A'}\boldsymbol{Q}_{C'})^- \in \{(\boldsymbol{Q}_{C'}\boldsymbol{P}_{A'}\boldsymbol{Q}_{C'})^-\}$$

and (4.20), we have

$$\boldsymbol{Q}_{C'}(\boldsymbol{Q}_{C'}\boldsymbol{P}_{A'}\boldsymbol{Q}_{C'})^-\boldsymbol{Q}_{C'}\boldsymbol{P}_{A'} + \boldsymbol{Q}_{A'}(\boldsymbol{Q}_{A'}\boldsymbol{P}_{C'}\boldsymbol{Q}_{A'})^-\boldsymbol{Q}_{A'}\boldsymbol{P}_{C'} = \boldsymbol{I}_m. \tag{4.82}$$

Premultiplying the equation above by $\boldsymbol{P}_{A'}$, we obtain

$$\boldsymbol{P}_{A'}\boldsymbol{Q}_{C'}(\boldsymbol{Q}_{C'}\boldsymbol{P}_{A'}\boldsymbol{Q}_{C'})^-\boldsymbol{Q}_{C'}\boldsymbol{P}_{A'} = \boldsymbol{P}_{A'},$$

which implies

$$\begin{aligned}\boldsymbol{P}_{Q_{C'}\cdot Q_{A'}} &= \boldsymbol{Q}_{C'}\boldsymbol{P}_{A'}(\boldsymbol{P}_{A'}\boldsymbol{Q}_{C'}\boldsymbol{P}_{A'})^-\boldsymbol{P}_{A'}\boldsymbol{Q}_{C'}(\boldsymbol{Q}_{C'}\boldsymbol{P}_{A'}\boldsymbol{Q}_{C'})^-\boldsymbol{Q}_{C'}\boldsymbol{P}_{A'}\\ &= \boldsymbol{Q}_{C'}\boldsymbol{P}_{A'}(\boldsymbol{P}_{A'}\boldsymbol{Q}_{C'}\boldsymbol{P}_{A'})^-\boldsymbol{P}_{A'} = \boldsymbol{Q}_{C'}\boldsymbol{A}'(\boldsymbol{A}\boldsymbol{Q}_{C'}\boldsymbol{A}')^-\boldsymbol{A}\\ &= \boldsymbol{A}^-_{m(C)}\boldsymbol{A},\end{aligned} \tag{4.83}$$

establishing Theorem 4.14. Q.E.D.

Corollary

$$(\boldsymbol{P}_{Q_{C'}\cdot Q_{A'}})' = \boldsymbol{P}_{A'\cdot C'}. \tag{4.84}$$

(Proof omitted.)

Note From Theorem 4.14, we have $\boldsymbol{A}^-_{m(C)}\boldsymbol{A} = \boldsymbol{P}_{\tilde{V}\cdot\tilde{W}}$ when (4.80) holds. This means that $\boldsymbol{A}^-_{m(C)}$ is constrained by $\mathrm{Sp}(\boldsymbol{C}')$ (not $\boldsymbol{C}'$ itself), so that it should have been written as $\boldsymbol{A}^-_{m(\tilde{V})}$. Hence, if $E^m = \tilde{V} \oplus \tilde{W}$, where $\tilde{V} = \mathrm{Sp}(\boldsymbol{A}^-\boldsymbol{A})$ and $\tilde{W} = \mathrm{Sp}(\boldsymbol{I}_m - \boldsymbol{A}^-\boldsymbol{A}) = \mathrm{Sp}(\boldsymbol{I}_m - \boldsymbol{P}_{A'}) = \mathrm{Sp}(\boldsymbol{Q}_{A'})$, we have

$$\tilde{V} = \mathrm{Sp}(\boldsymbol{Q}_{C'}) \tag{4.85}$$

by choosing $\boldsymbol{C}'$ such that $\mathrm{Sp}(\boldsymbol{A}') \oplus \mathrm{Sp}(\boldsymbol{C}') = E^m$.

Note One reason that $A^-_{m(C')}$ is a generalized form of a minimum norm g-inverse A^-_m is that $x = A^-_{m(C')}b$ is obtained as a solution that minimizes $||P_{Q_{C'}\cdot Q_{A'}}x||^2$ under the constraint $Ax = b$.

Note Let N be a *pd* matrix of order m. Then,

$$A^-_{m(N)} = NA'(ANA')^- \tag{4.86}$$

is a g-inverse that satisfies $AA^-_{m(N)}A = A$ and $(A^-_{m(N)}AN)' = A^-_{m(N)}AN$. This g-inverse can be derived as the one minimizing $||x||^2_N$ subject to the constraint that $b = Ax$.

We now give a generalization of Theorem 3.17.

Theorem 4.15

$$\{(A')^-_{m(B')}\} = \{(A^-_{\ell(B)})'\}. \tag{4.87}$$

Proof. From Theorem 4.11, $AA^-_{\ell(B)}A = A$ implies $A'(A^-_{\ell(B)})'A' = A'$. On the other hand, we have

$$(Q_BAA^-_{\ell(B)})' = Q_BAA^-_{\ell(B)} \Rightarrow (A^-_{\ell(B)})'A'Q_B = [(A^-_{\ell(B)})'A'Q_B]'.$$

Hence, from Theorem 4.13, $A^-_{\ell(B)} \in \{(A')^-_{m(B')}\}$. From Theorems 4.11 and 4.13, $(A')^-_{m(B')} \in \{A^-_{\ell(B)})'\}$, leading to (4.87). Q.E.D.

Example 4.2 (i) When $A = \begin{bmatrix} 1 & 1 \\ 1 & 1 \end{bmatrix}$ and $B = \begin{pmatrix} 1 \\ 2 \end{pmatrix}$, find $A^-_{\ell(B)}$ and $A^-_{\ell r(B)}$.

(ii) When $A = \begin{bmatrix} 1 & 1 \\ 1 & 1 \end{bmatrix}$ and $C = (1, 2)$, find $A^-_{m(C)}$ and $A^-_{mr(C)}$.

Solution. (i): Since $E^n = \mathrm{Sp}(A) \oplus \mathrm{Sp}(B)$, $AA^-_{\ell(B)}$ is the projector onto $\mathrm{Sp}(A)$ along $\mathrm{Sp}(B)$, so we obtain $P_{A\cdot B}$ by (4.10). We have

$$(AA' + BB')^{-1} = \begin{bmatrix} 3 & 4 \\ 4 & 6 \end{bmatrix}^{-1} = \frac{1}{2}\begin{bmatrix} 6 & -4 \\ -4 & 3 \end{bmatrix},$$

from which we obtain

$$P_{A\cdot B} = AA'(AA' + BB')^{-1} = \begin{bmatrix} 2 & -1 \\ 2 & -1 \end{bmatrix}.$$

Let

$$\boldsymbol{A}^-_{\ell(B)} = \begin{bmatrix} a & b \\ c & d \end{bmatrix}.$$

From $\begin{bmatrix} 1 & 1 \\ 1 & 1 \end{bmatrix}\begin{bmatrix} a & b \\ c & d \end{bmatrix} = \begin{bmatrix} 2 & -1 \\ 2 & -1 \end{bmatrix}$, we have $a + c = 2$ and $b + d = -1$. Hence,

$$\boldsymbol{A}^-_{\ell(B)} = \begin{bmatrix} a & b \\ 2-a & -1-b \end{bmatrix}.$$

Furthermore, from $\text{rank}(\boldsymbol{A}^-_{\ell r(B)}) = \text{rank}(\boldsymbol{A})$, we have $a(-1-b) = b(2-a)$, from which it follows that $b = -\frac{1}{2}a$ and

$$\boldsymbol{A}^-_{\ell r(B)} = \begin{bmatrix} a & -\frac{1}{2}a \\ 2-a & -1+\frac{1}{2}a \end{bmatrix}.$$

(ii): Note that $\text{Sp}(\boldsymbol{A}') \oplus \text{Sp}(\boldsymbol{C}') = E^2$. By (4.50), (4.51), and (4.10),

$$\boldsymbol{A}^-_{m(C)}\boldsymbol{A} = (\boldsymbol{P}_{A'\cdot C'})' = (\boldsymbol{A}'\boldsymbol{A} + \boldsymbol{C}'\boldsymbol{C})^{-1}\boldsymbol{A}'\boldsymbol{A}$$

and

$$\boldsymbol{A}'\boldsymbol{A}(\boldsymbol{A}'\boldsymbol{A} + \boldsymbol{C}'\boldsymbol{C})^{-1} = \frac{1}{3}\begin{bmatrix} 2 & 1 \\ 2 & 1 \end{bmatrix}.$$

Let

$$\boldsymbol{A}^-_{m(C)} = \begin{bmatrix} e & f \\ g & h \end{bmatrix}.$$

From

$$\begin{bmatrix} e & f \\ g & h \end{bmatrix}\begin{bmatrix} 1 & 1 \\ 1 & 1 \end{bmatrix} = \frac{1}{3}\begin{bmatrix} 2 & 2 \\ 1 & 1 \end{bmatrix},$$

we obtain $e + f = \frac{2}{3}$ and $g + h = \frac{1}{3}$. Hence,

$$\boldsymbol{A}^-_{m(C)} = \begin{bmatrix} e & \frac{2}{3}-e \\ g & \frac{1}{3}-g \end{bmatrix}.$$

Furthermore,

$$\boldsymbol{A}^-_{mr(C)} = \begin{bmatrix} e & \frac{2}{3}-e \\ \frac{1}{2}e & \frac{1}{3}-\frac{1}{2}e \end{bmatrix}.$$

4.4.3 A generalized form of the Moore-Penrose inverse

Let

$$E^n = V \oplus W = \mathrm{Sp}(\boldsymbol{A}) \oplus \mathrm{Sp}(\boldsymbol{B}) \tag{4.88}$$

and

$$E^m = \tilde{V} \oplus \tilde{W} = \mathrm{Sp}(\boldsymbol{Q}_{C'}) \oplus \mathrm{Sp}(\boldsymbol{Q}_{A'}), \tag{4.89}$$

where the complement subspace $W = \mathrm{Sp}(\boldsymbol{B})$ of $V = \mathrm{Sp}(\boldsymbol{A})$ and the complement subspace $\tilde{V} = \mathrm{Sp}(\boldsymbol{Q}_{C'})$ of $\tilde{W} = \mathrm{Ker}(\boldsymbol{A}) = \mathrm{Sp}(\boldsymbol{Q}_{A'})$ are prescribed. Let $\boldsymbol{A}^+_{B\cdot C}$ denote a transformation matrix from $\boldsymbol{y} \in E^n$ to $\boldsymbol{x} \in \tilde{V} = \mathrm{Sp}(\boldsymbol{Q}_{C'})$. (This matrix should ideally be written as $\boldsymbol{A}^+_{W\cdot\tilde{V}}$.) Since $\boldsymbol{A}^+_{B\cdot C}$ is a reflexive g-inverse of $\boldsymbol{A}$, it holds that

$$\boldsymbol{A}\boldsymbol{A}^+_{B\cdot C}\boldsymbol{A} = \boldsymbol{A} \tag{4.90}$$

and

$$\boldsymbol{A}^+_{B\cdot C}\boldsymbol{A}\boldsymbol{A}^+_{B\cdot C} = \boldsymbol{A}^+_{B\cdot C}. \tag{4.91}$$

Furthermore, from Theorem 3.3, $\boldsymbol{A}\boldsymbol{A}^+_{B\cdot C}$ is clearly the projector onto $V = \mathrm{Sp}(\boldsymbol{A})$ along $W = \mathrm{Sp}(\boldsymbol{B})$, and $\boldsymbol{A}^+_{B\cdot C}\boldsymbol{A}$ is the projector onto $\tilde{V} = \mathrm{Sp}(\boldsymbol{Q}_{C'})$ along $\tilde{W} = \mathrm{Ker}(\boldsymbol{A}) = \mathrm{Sp}(\boldsymbol{Q}_{A'})$. Hence, from Theorems 4.11 and 4.13, the following relations hold:

$$(\boldsymbol{Q}_B\boldsymbol{A}\boldsymbol{A}^+_{B\cdot C})' = \boldsymbol{Q}_B\boldsymbol{A}\boldsymbol{A}^+_{B\cdot C} \tag{4.92}$$

and

$$(\boldsymbol{A}^+_{B\cdot C}\boldsymbol{A}\boldsymbol{Q}_{C'})' = \boldsymbol{A}^+_{B\cdot C}\boldsymbol{A}\boldsymbol{Q}_{C'}. \tag{4.93}$$

Additionally, from the four equations above,

$$\boldsymbol{C}\boldsymbol{A}^+_{B\cdot C} = \boldsymbol{O} \text{ and } \boldsymbol{A}^+_{B\cdot C}\boldsymbol{B} = \boldsymbol{O} \tag{4.94}$$

hold.

When $W = V^\perp$ and $\tilde{V} = \tilde{W}^\perp$, the four equations (4.90) through (4.93) reduce to the four conditions for the Moore-Penrose inverse of $\boldsymbol{A}$.

Definition 4.4 *A g-inverse $\boldsymbol{A}^+_{B\cdot C}$ that satisfies the four equations (4.90) through (4.93) is called the B, C-constrained Moore-Penrose inverse of $\boldsymbol{A}$.* (See Figure 4.3.)

Theorem 4.16 *Let an m by n matrix $\boldsymbol{A}$ be given, and let the subspaces $W = \mathrm{Sp}(\boldsymbol{B})$ and $\tilde{W} = \mathrm{Sp}(\boldsymbol{Q}_{C'})$ be given such that $E^n = \mathrm{Sp}(\boldsymbol{A}) \oplus \mathrm{Sp}(\boldsymbol{B})$ and*

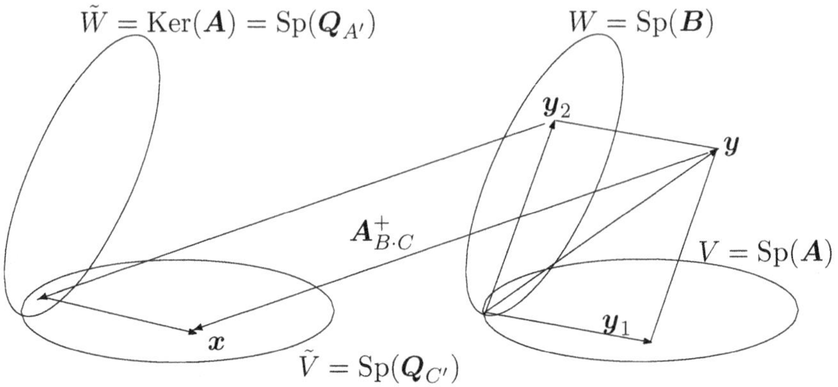

Figure 4.3: Spatial representation of the Moore-Penrose inverse.

$E^m = \mathrm{Sp}(\boldsymbol{Q}_{A'}) \oplus \mathrm{Sp}(\boldsymbol{Q}_{C'})$. *Then* $\boldsymbol{A}^+_{B\cdot C}$ *is uniquely determined by* $\boldsymbol{B}$ *and* $\boldsymbol{C}$ *that generate* W *and* $\tilde{W}$.

Proof. By (4.94), it holds that

$$\boldsymbol{Q}_{C'}\boldsymbol{A}^+_{B\cdot C} = \boldsymbol{A}^+_{B\cdot C} \text{ and } \boldsymbol{A}^+_{B\cdot C}\boldsymbol{Q}_B = \boldsymbol{A}^+_{B\cdot C}.$$

Hence, the four equations (4.90) through (4.93) can be rewritten as

$$(\boldsymbol{Q}_B\boldsymbol{A}\boldsymbol{Q}_{C'})\boldsymbol{A}^+_{B\cdot C}(\boldsymbol{Q}_B\boldsymbol{A}\boldsymbol{Q}_{C'}) = \boldsymbol{Q}_B\boldsymbol{A}\boldsymbol{Q}_{C'},$$

$$\boldsymbol{A}^+_{B\cdot C}(\boldsymbol{Q}_B\boldsymbol{A}\boldsymbol{Q}_{C'})\boldsymbol{A}^+_{B\cdot C} = \boldsymbol{A}^+_{B\cdot C}, \tag{4.95}$$

$$((\boldsymbol{Q}_B\boldsymbol{A}\boldsymbol{Q}_{C'})\boldsymbol{A}^+_{B\cdot C})' = (\boldsymbol{Q}_B\boldsymbol{A}\boldsymbol{Q}_{C'})\boldsymbol{A}^+_{B\cdot C},$$

and

$$(\boldsymbol{A}^+_{B\cdot C}(\boldsymbol{Q}_B\boldsymbol{A}\boldsymbol{Q}_{C'}))' = \boldsymbol{A}^+_{B\cdot C}(\boldsymbol{Q}_B\boldsymbol{A}\boldsymbol{Q}_{C'}).$$

This indicates that $\boldsymbol{A}^+_{B\cdot C}$ is the Moore-Penrose inverse of $\boldsymbol{A}_{B\cdot C} = \boldsymbol{Q}_B\boldsymbol{A}\boldsymbol{Q}_{C'}$. Since $\boldsymbol{Q}_B$ and $\boldsymbol{Q}_{C'}$ are the orthogonal projectors onto $\mathrm{Sp}(\boldsymbol{B})^\perp$ and $\mathrm{Sp}(\boldsymbol{C}')^\perp$, respectively, $\boldsymbol{A}^+_{B\cdot C}$ is uniquely determined by arbitrary $\tilde{\boldsymbol{B}}$ and $\tilde{\boldsymbol{C}}$ such that $\mathrm{Sp}(\boldsymbol{B}) = \mathrm{Sp}(\tilde{\boldsymbol{B}})$ and $\mathrm{Sp}(\boldsymbol{C}') = \mathrm{Sp}(\tilde{\boldsymbol{C}}')$. This indicates that $\boldsymbol{A}_{B\cdot C}$ is unique. $\boldsymbol{A}^+_{B\cdot C}$ is also unique, since the Moore-Penrose inverse is uniquely determined. Q.E.D.

Note It should be clear from the description above that $\boldsymbol{A}^+_{B\cdot C}$ that satisfies Theorem 4.16 generalizes the Moore-Penrose inverse given in Chapter 3. The Moore-Penrose inverse $\boldsymbol{A}^+$ corresponds with a linear transformation from E^n to $\tilde{V}$ when

$E^n = V \dot{\oplus} W$ and $E^m = \tilde{V} \dot{\oplus} \tilde{W}$. It is sort of an "orthogonalized" g-inverse, while $\boldsymbol{A}^+_{B\cdot C}$ is an "oblique" g-inverse in the sense that $W = \text{Sp}(\boldsymbol{B})$ and $\tilde{V} = \text{Sp}(\boldsymbol{Q}_{C'})$ are not orthogonal to V and $\tilde{W}$, respectively.

We now consider a representation of the generalized form of the Moore-Penrose inverse $\boldsymbol{A}^+_{B\cdot C}$.

Lemma 4.5

$$\boldsymbol{A}\boldsymbol{A}^+_{B\cdot C} = \boldsymbol{P}_{A\cdot B} \tag{4.96}$$

and

$$\boldsymbol{A}^+_{B\cdot C}\boldsymbol{A} = \boldsymbol{P}_{Q_{C'}\cdot Q_{A'}} = (\boldsymbol{P}_{A'\cdot C'})'. \tag{4.97}$$

Proof. (4.96): Clear from Theorem 4.1.
(4.97): Use Theorem 4.14 and (4.81). Q.E.D.

Theorem 4.17 $\boldsymbol{A}^+_{B\cdot C}$ *can be expressed as*

$$\boldsymbol{A}^+_{B\cdot C} = \boldsymbol{Q}^*_{C'}(\boldsymbol{A}\boldsymbol{Q}^*_{C'})^-\boldsymbol{A}(\boldsymbol{Q}^*_B\boldsymbol{A})^-\boldsymbol{Q}^*_B, \tag{4.98}$$

where $\boldsymbol{Q}^*_{C'} = \boldsymbol{I}_m - \boldsymbol{C}'(\boldsymbol{C}')^-$ and $\boldsymbol{Q}^*_B = \boldsymbol{I}_n - \boldsymbol{B}\boldsymbol{B}^-$,

$$\boldsymbol{A}^+_{B\cdot C} = \boldsymbol{Q}_{C'}\boldsymbol{A}'(\boldsymbol{A}\boldsymbol{Q}_{C'}\boldsymbol{A}')^-\boldsymbol{A}(\boldsymbol{A}'\boldsymbol{Q}_B\boldsymbol{A})^-\boldsymbol{A}'\boldsymbol{Q}_B, \tag{4.99}$$

and

$$\boldsymbol{A}^+_{B\cdot C} = (\boldsymbol{A}'\boldsymbol{A} + \boldsymbol{C}'\boldsymbol{C})^{-1}\boldsymbol{A}'\boldsymbol{A}\boldsymbol{A}'(\boldsymbol{A}\boldsymbol{A}' + \boldsymbol{B}\boldsymbol{B}')^{-1}. \tag{4.100}$$

Proof. From Lemma 4.5, it holds that $\boldsymbol{A}^+_{B\cdot C}\boldsymbol{A}\boldsymbol{A}^+_{B\cdot C} = \boldsymbol{A}^+_{B\cdot C}\boldsymbol{P}_{A\cdot B} = (\boldsymbol{P}_{A'\cdot C'})'\boldsymbol{A}^+_{B\cdot C} = \boldsymbol{A}^+_{B\cdot C}$. Apply Theorem 4.1 and its corollary.

Q.E.D.

Corollary (i) *When* $\text{Sp}(\boldsymbol{B}) = \text{Sp}(\boldsymbol{A})^\perp$,

$$\begin{aligned}\boldsymbol{A}^+_{B\cdot C} &= \boldsymbol{Q}_{C'}\boldsymbol{A}'(\boldsymbol{A}\boldsymbol{Q}_{C'}\boldsymbol{A}')^-\boldsymbol{A}(\boldsymbol{A}'\boldsymbol{A})^-\boldsymbol{A}' &(4.101)\\ &= (\boldsymbol{A}'\boldsymbol{A} + \boldsymbol{C}'\boldsymbol{C})^{-1}\boldsymbol{A}'. &(4.102)\end{aligned}$$

(The $\boldsymbol{A}^+_{B\cdot C}$ above is denoted as $\boldsymbol{A}^+_{m(C)}$.)

(ii) *When* $\text{Sp}(\boldsymbol{C}') = \text{Sp}(\boldsymbol{A}')^\perp$,

$$\begin{aligned}\boldsymbol{A}^+_{B\cdot C} &= \boldsymbol{A}'(\boldsymbol{A}\boldsymbol{A}')^-\boldsymbol{A}(\boldsymbol{A}'\boldsymbol{Q}_B\boldsymbol{A})^-\boldsymbol{A}'\boldsymbol{Q}_B &(4.103)\\ &= \boldsymbol{A}'(\boldsymbol{A}\boldsymbol{A}' + \boldsymbol{B}\boldsymbol{B}')^{-1}. &(4.104)\end{aligned}$$

(The $A^+_{B\cdot C}$ above is denoted as $A^+_{\ell(B)}$.)

(iii) *When* $\mathrm{Sp}(B) = \mathrm{Sp}(A)^\perp$ *and* $\mathrm{Sp}(C') = \mathrm{Sp}(A')^\perp$,

$$A^+_{B\cdot C} = A'(AA')^- A(A'A)^- A' = A^+. \tag{4.105}$$

(Proof omitted.)

Note When $\mathrm{rank}(A) = n$, $A^+_{m(C)} = A^+_{mr(C)}$, and when $\mathrm{rank}(A) = m$, $A^+_{\ell(B)} = A^+_{\ell r(B)}$, but they do not hold generally. However, A^+ in (4.105) always coincides with A^+ in (3.92).

Theorem 4.18 *The vector* x *that minimizes* $||P_{Q_{C'}\cdot Q_{A'}}x||^2$ *among those that minimize* $||Ax - b||^2_{Q_B}$ *is given by* $x = A^+_{B\cdot C}b$.

Proof. Since x minimizes $||Ax - b||^2_{Q_B}$, it satisfies the normal equation

$$A'Q_BAx = A'Q_Bb. \tag{4.106}$$

To minimize the norm $||P_{Q_{C'}\cdot Q_{A'}}x||^2$ subject to (4.106), we define

$$f(x, \lambda) = \frac{1}{2}x'\tilde{P}'\tilde{P}x - \lambda'(A'Q_BAx - A'Q_Bb),$$

where λ is a vector of Lagrangean multipliers and $\tilde{P} = P_{Q_{C'}\cdot Q_{A'}}$. Differentiating f with respect to x and setting the results to zero, we obtain

$$\tilde{P}'\tilde{P}x = A'Q_BA\lambda. \tag{4.107}$$

Putting together (4.106) and (4.107) in one equation, we obtain

$$\begin{bmatrix} \tilde{P}'\tilde{P} & A'Q_BA \\ A'Q_BA & O \end{bmatrix} \begin{pmatrix} x \\ \lambda \end{pmatrix} = \begin{pmatrix} 0 \\ A'Q_Bb \end{pmatrix}.$$

Hence,

$$\begin{pmatrix} x \\ \lambda \end{pmatrix} = \begin{bmatrix} \tilde{P}'\tilde{P} & A'Q_BA \\ A'Q_BA & O \end{bmatrix}^{-1} \begin{pmatrix} 0 \\ A'Q_Bb \end{pmatrix}$$
$$= \begin{bmatrix} C_1 & C_2 \\ C_2' & -C_3 \end{bmatrix} \begin{pmatrix} 0 \\ A'Q_Bb \end{pmatrix}.$$

Since $\tilde{\boldsymbol{P}}'\tilde{\boldsymbol{P}} = \boldsymbol{A}'(\boldsymbol{A}\boldsymbol{Q}_{C'}\boldsymbol{A}')^-\boldsymbol{A}$ and $\tilde{\boldsymbol{P}}\boldsymbol{Q}_{C'}$ is the projector onto $\text{Sp}(\boldsymbol{A}')$ along $\text{Sp}(\boldsymbol{C}')$, we have $\text{Sp}(\tilde{\boldsymbol{P}}'\tilde{\boldsymbol{P}}\boldsymbol{Q}_{C'}) = \text{Sp}(\boldsymbol{A})$, which implies $\text{Sp}(\tilde{\boldsymbol{P}}'\tilde{\boldsymbol{P}}) = \text{Sp}(\boldsymbol{A}') = \text{Sp}(\boldsymbol{A}'\boldsymbol{Q}_B\boldsymbol{A})$. Hence, by (3.57), we obtain

$$\begin{aligned} \boldsymbol{x} &= \boldsymbol{C}_2\boldsymbol{A}'\boldsymbol{Q}_B\boldsymbol{b} \\ &= (\tilde{\boldsymbol{P}}'\tilde{\boldsymbol{P}})^-\boldsymbol{A}'\boldsymbol{Q}_B\boldsymbol{A}(\boldsymbol{A}'\boldsymbol{Q}_B\boldsymbol{A}(\tilde{\boldsymbol{P}}'\tilde{\boldsymbol{P}})^-\boldsymbol{A}'\boldsymbol{Q}_B\boldsymbol{A})^-\boldsymbol{A}'\boldsymbol{Q}_B\boldsymbol{b}. \end{aligned}$$

We then use

$$\boldsymbol{Q}_{C'}\boldsymbol{A}'(\boldsymbol{A}\boldsymbol{Q}_{C'}\boldsymbol{A}')^-\boldsymbol{A}\boldsymbol{Q}_{C'} \in \{(\boldsymbol{A}'(\boldsymbol{A}\boldsymbol{Q}_{C'}\boldsymbol{A}')^-\boldsymbol{A})^-\} = \{(\tilde{\boldsymbol{P}}'\tilde{\boldsymbol{P}})^-\}$$

to establish

$$\boldsymbol{x} = \boldsymbol{Q}_{C'}\boldsymbol{A}'\boldsymbol{Q}_B\boldsymbol{A}(\boldsymbol{A}'\boldsymbol{Q}_B\boldsymbol{A}\boldsymbol{Q}_{C'}\boldsymbol{A}'\boldsymbol{Q}_B\boldsymbol{A})^-\boldsymbol{A}'\boldsymbol{Q}_B\boldsymbol{b}. \tag{4.108}$$

Furthermore, by noting that

$$(\boldsymbol{A}'\boldsymbol{Q}_B\boldsymbol{A})^-\boldsymbol{A}'(\boldsymbol{A}\boldsymbol{Q}_{C'}\boldsymbol{A}')^-\boldsymbol{A}(\boldsymbol{A}'\boldsymbol{Q}_B\boldsymbol{A})^- \in \{(\boldsymbol{A}'\boldsymbol{Q}_B\boldsymbol{A}\boldsymbol{Q}_{C'}\boldsymbol{A}'\boldsymbol{Q}_B\boldsymbol{A})^-\},$$

we obtain

$$\begin{aligned} \boldsymbol{x} &= \boldsymbol{Q}_{C'}\boldsymbol{A}'(\boldsymbol{A}\boldsymbol{Q}_{C'}\boldsymbol{A}')^-\boldsymbol{A}(\boldsymbol{A}'\boldsymbol{Q}_B\boldsymbol{A})^-\boldsymbol{A}'\boldsymbol{Q}_B\boldsymbol{b} \\ &= \boldsymbol{A}^+_{B\cdot C}\boldsymbol{b}. \end{aligned} \tag{4.109}$$

Q.E.D.

From the result above, Theorem 4.4 can be generalized as follows.

Theorem 4.19 *Let* $\text{Sp}(\boldsymbol{A}) = \text{Sp}(\boldsymbol{A}_1) \oplus \cdots \oplus \text{Sp}(\boldsymbol{A}_r)$. *If there exists a matrix* $\boldsymbol{C}_j$ *such that* $\text{Sp}(\boldsymbol{A}_j') \oplus \text{Sp}(\boldsymbol{C}_j') = E^{k_j}$, *where* k_j *is the number of columns in* $\boldsymbol{A}_j$, *then*

$$\boldsymbol{P}_A = \boldsymbol{A}_1(\boldsymbol{A}_1)^+_{A_{(1)}\cdot C_1} + \cdots + \boldsymbol{A}_r(\boldsymbol{A}_r)^+_{A_{(r)}\cdot C_r}, \tag{4.110}$$

where $\boldsymbol{A}_{(j)} = [\boldsymbol{A}_1, \cdots, \boldsymbol{A}_{j-1}, \boldsymbol{A}_{j+1}, \cdots, \boldsymbol{A}_r]$.

Proof. Clear from Theorem 4.4 and $\boldsymbol{A}_j(\boldsymbol{A}_j)^+_{A_{(j)}\cdot C_j} = \boldsymbol{P}_{j\cdot(j)}$. (See (4.27).)

Q.E.D.

Example 4.3 Find $\boldsymbol{A}^+_{B\cdot C}$ when $\boldsymbol{A} = \begin{bmatrix} 1 & 1 \\ 1 & 1 \end{bmatrix}$, $\boldsymbol{B} = \begin{pmatrix} 1 \\ 2 \end{pmatrix}$, and $\boldsymbol{C} = (1, 2)$.

Solution. Since $\text{Sp}(\boldsymbol{A}) \oplus \text{Sp}(\boldsymbol{B}) = E^2$ and $\text{Sp}(\boldsymbol{A}') \oplus \text{Sp}(\boldsymbol{C}') = E^2$, $\boldsymbol{A}^+_{B\cdot C}$

can be defined. To find $\boldsymbol{A}^+_{B\cdot C}$, we set e in $\boldsymbol{A}^-_{mr(C)}$ and a in $\boldsymbol{A}^-_{\ell r(B)}$ equal to each other in Example 4.2. Then $\boldsymbol{A}^-_{mr(C)} = \boldsymbol{A}^-_{\ell r(B)}$ and $a = e = \frac{4}{3}$, leading to

$$\boldsymbol{A}^+_{B\cdot C} = \frac{1}{3}\begin{bmatrix} 4 & -2 \\ 2 & -1 \end{bmatrix}.$$

An alternative solution. We calculate $\boldsymbol{A}^+_{B\cdot C}$ directly using (4.100).

$$\boldsymbol{A}'\boldsymbol{A} + \boldsymbol{C}'\boldsymbol{C} = \begin{bmatrix} 1 & 1 \\ 1 & 1 \end{bmatrix}^2 + \begin{pmatrix} 1 \\ -2 \end{pmatrix}(1, -2) = \begin{bmatrix} 3 & 0 \\ 0 & 6 \end{bmatrix},$$

and

$$\boldsymbol{A}\boldsymbol{A}' + \boldsymbol{B}\boldsymbol{B}' = \begin{bmatrix} 1 & 1 \\ 1 & 1 \end{bmatrix}^2 + \begin{pmatrix} 1 \\ 2 \end{pmatrix}(1, 2) = \begin{bmatrix} 3 & 4 \\ 4 & 6 \end{bmatrix}.$$

Hence, we obtain

$$\begin{bmatrix} 3 & 0 \\ 0 & 6 \end{bmatrix}^{-1}\begin{bmatrix} 1 & 1 \\ 1 & 1 \end{bmatrix}^3\begin{bmatrix} 3 & 4 \\ 4 & 6 \end{bmatrix}^{-1} = \frac{1}{3}\begin{bmatrix} 4 & -2 \\ 2 & -1 \end{bmatrix}.$$

(Verify that the $\boldsymbol{A}^+_{B\cdot C}$ above satisfies the four conditions (4.90) through (4.93).)

Note To be able to define $\boldsymbol{A}^+_{B\cdot C}$, $\boldsymbol{A}$ should be n by m of rank $r(< \min(n, m))$, $\boldsymbol{B}$ should be n by s of rank $n - r(\leq s)$, and $\boldsymbol{C}$ should be t by m of rank $m - r(\leq t)$.

Theorem 4.20 *Let* $\mathrm{Sp}(\boldsymbol{A}') \oplus \mathrm{Sp}(\boldsymbol{C}') = E^m$. *If* $\boldsymbol{d} = \boldsymbol{0}$, *(4.56) reduces to the equation*

$$\boldsymbol{x} = \boldsymbol{A}^+_{m(C)}\boldsymbol{b}, \tag{4.111}$$

where $\boldsymbol{A}^+_{m(C)}$ *is as given in (4.101) and (4.102).*

Proof. Since $\boldsymbol{A}'(\boldsymbol{A}\boldsymbol{Q}_{C'}\boldsymbol{A}')^-\boldsymbol{A}\boldsymbol{Q}_{C'}\boldsymbol{A}' = \boldsymbol{A}'$, we have

$$\begin{aligned}(\boldsymbol{Q}_{C'}\boldsymbol{A}'\boldsymbol{A}\boldsymbol{Q}_{C'})\boldsymbol{A}'(\boldsymbol{A}\boldsymbol{Q}_{C'}\boldsymbol{A}')^-\boldsymbol{A}(\boldsymbol{A}'\boldsymbol{A})^-\boldsymbol{A}'(\boldsymbol{A}'\boldsymbol{Q}_{C'}\boldsymbol{A})^-\boldsymbol{A}(\boldsymbol{Q}_{C'}\boldsymbol{A}'\boldsymbol{A}\boldsymbol{Q}_{C'}) \\ = \boldsymbol{Q}_{C'}\boldsymbol{A}'\boldsymbol{A}(\boldsymbol{A}'\boldsymbol{A})^-\boldsymbol{A}'(\boldsymbol{A}\boldsymbol{Q}_{C'}\boldsymbol{A}')^-\boldsymbol{A}\boldsymbol{Q}_{C'}\boldsymbol{A}'\boldsymbol{A}\boldsymbol{Q}_{C'} = \boldsymbol{Q}_{C'}\boldsymbol{A}'\boldsymbol{A}\boldsymbol{Q}_{C'},\end{aligned}$$

which indicates that

$$\boldsymbol{G} = \boldsymbol{A}'(\boldsymbol{A}\boldsymbol{Q}_{C'}\boldsymbol{A}')^-\boldsymbol{A}(\boldsymbol{A}'\boldsymbol{A})^-\boldsymbol{A}'(\boldsymbol{A}\boldsymbol{Q}_{C'}\boldsymbol{A}')^-\boldsymbol{A}$$

is a g-inverse of $\boldsymbol{Q}_{C'}\boldsymbol{A}'\boldsymbol{A}\boldsymbol{Q}_{C'}$. Hence, we have

$$\begin{aligned}\boldsymbol{x} &= \boldsymbol{Q}_{C'}\boldsymbol{G}\boldsymbol{Q}_{C'}\boldsymbol{A}'\boldsymbol{b}\\ &= \boldsymbol{Q}_{C'}\boldsymbol{A}'(\boldsymbol{A}\boldsymbol{Q}_{C'}\boldsymbol{A}')^-\boldsymbol{A}(\boldsymbol{A}'\boldsymbol{A})^-\boldsymbol{A}'(\boldsymbol{A}\boldsymbol{Q}_{C'}\boldsymbol{A}')^-\boldsymbol{A}\boldsymbol{Q}_{C'}\boldsymbol{A}'\boldsymbol{b}\\ &= \boldsymbol{Q}_{C'}\boldsymbol{A}'(\boldsymbol{A}\boldsymbol{Q}_{C'}\boldsymbol{A}')^-\boldsymbol{A}(\boldsymbol{A}'\boldsymbol{A})^-\boldsymbol{A}'\boldsymbol{b}.\end{aligned}$$

This leads to (4.111) by noting (4.101). Q.E.D.

Example 4.3 Let $\boldsymbol{b}$ and two items, each consisting of three categories, be given as follows:

$$\boldsymbol{b} = \begin{pmatrix} 72\\48\\40\\48\\28\\48\\40\\28 \end{pmatrix}, \quad \tilde{\boldsymbol{A}} = \left[\begin{array}{ccc|ccc} 0&1&0&1&0&0\\ 0&1&0&1&0&0\\ 1&0&0&0&0&1\\ 0&1&0&1&0&0\\ 0&0&1&0&1&0\\ 0&1&0&0&0&1\\ 1&0&0&1&0&0\\ 0&0&1&0&1&0 \end{array}\right].$$

Subtracting column means from the elements, we obtain

$$\boldsymbol{A} = \boldsymbol{Q}_M\tilde{\boldsymbol{A}} = \frac{1}{8}\begin{bmatrix} -2&-3&5&4&-2&-2\\ -2&5&-3&4&-2&-2\\ 6&-3&-3&-4&-2&6\\ -2&5&-3&4&-2&-2\\ -2&-3&5&-4&6&-2\\ -2&5&-3&-4&-2&6\\ 6&-3&-3&4&-2&-2\\ -2&-3&5&-4&6&-2 \end{bmatrix} = [\boldsymbol{a}_1, \boldsymbol{a}_2, \cdots, \boldsymbol{a}_6],$$

where $\boldsymbol{Q}_M = \boldsymbol{I}_8 - \frac{1}{8}\boldsymbol{1}\boldsymbol{1}'$. Note that $\text{rank}(\boldsymbol{A}) = \text{rank}(\tilde{\boldsymbol{A}}) - 2$. Since $\boldsymbol{\alpha} = (\alpha_1, \alpha_2, \alpha_3)'$ and $\boldsymbol{\beta} = (\beta_1, \beta_2, \beta_3)'$ that minimize

$$||\boldsymbol{b} - \alpha_1\boldsymbol{a}_1 - \alpha_2\boldsymbol{a}_2 - \alpha_3\boldsymbol{a}_3 - \beta_1\boldsymbol{a}_4 - \beta_2\boldsymbol{a}_5 - \beta_3\boldsymbol{a}_6||^2$$

cannot be determined uniquely, we add the condition that $\boldsymbol{C}\begin{pmatrix}\boldsymbol{\alpha}\\ \boldsymbol{\beta}\end{pmatrix} = \boldsymbol{0}$ and obtain

$$\begin{pmatrix}\hat{\boldsymbol{\alpha}}\\ \hat{\boldsymbol{\beta}}\end{pmatrix} = (\boldsymbol{A}'\boldsymbol{A} + \boldsymbol{C}'\boldsymbol{C})^{-1}\boldsymbol{A}'\boldsymbol{b}.$$

We vary the elements of $\boldsymbol{C}$ in three ways and obtain solutions:

$$\text{(a) } \boldsymbol{C} = \begin{bmatrix} 1 & 1 & 1 & 0 & 0 & 0 \\ 0 & 0 & 0 & 1 & 1 & 1 \end{bmatrix} \rightarrow \hat{\boldsymbol{\alpha}} = \begin{pmatrix} -1.67 \\ -0.67 \\ 2.33 \end{pmatrix}, \ \hat{\boldsymbol{\beta}} = \begin{pmatrix} 1.83 \\ -3.67 \\ 1.83 \end{pmatrix}.$$

$$\text{(b) } \boldsymbol{C} = \begin{bmatrix} 2 & 1 & 1 & 0 & 0 & 0 \\ 0 & 0 & 0 & 1 & 2 & 2 \end{bmatrix} \rightarrow \hat{\boldsymbol{\alpha}} = \begin{pmatrix} -1.24 \\ -0.24 \\ 2.74 \end{pmatrix}, \ \hat{\boldsymbol{\beta}} = \begin{pmatrix} 2.19 \\ -3.29 \\ 2.19 \end{pmatrix}.$$

$$\text{(c) } \boldsymbol{C} = \begin{bmatrix} 1 & 1 & 1 & 1 & 1 & 1 \\ 1 & -1 & 1 & -1 & 1 & -1 \end{bmatrix} \rightarrow \hat{\boldsymbol{\alpha}} = \begin{pmatrix} 1.33 \\ 2.33 \\ 5.33 \end{pmatrix}, \ \hat{\boldsymbol{\beta}} = \begin{pmatrix} -1.16 \\ -6.67 \\ -1.16 \end{pmatrix}.$$

Note The method above is equivalent to the method of obtaining weight coefficients called Quantification Method I (Hayashi, 1952). Note that different solutions are obtained depending on the constraints imposed on $\boldsymbol{\alpha}$ and $\boldsymbol{\beta}$.

Theorem 4.21 *Let* $\mathrm{Sp}(\boldsymbol{A}) \oplus \mathrm{Sp}(\boldsymbol{B}) = E^n$ *and* $\mathrm{Sp}(\boldsymbol{A}') \oplus \mathrm{Sp}(\boldsymbol{B}') = E^m$. *The vector* $\boldsymbol{x}$ *that minimizes* $||\boldsymbol{y} - \boldsymbol{A}\boldsymbol{x}||^2_{Q_B}$ *subject to the constraint that* $\boldsymbol{C}\boldsymbol{x} = \boldsymbol{0}$ *is given by*

$$\boldsymbol{x} = \boldsymbol{A}^+_{B \cdot C}\boldsymbol{y}, \tag{4.112}$$

where $\boldsymbol{A}^+_{B \cdot C}$ *is given by (4.98) through (4.100).*

Proof. From the corollary of Theorem 4.8, we have $\min_x ||\boldsymbol{y} - \boldsymbol{A}\boldsymbol{x}||^2_{Q_B} = ||\boldsymbol{P}_{A \cdot B}\boldsymbol{y}||^2_{Q_B}$. Using the fact that $\boldsymbol{P}_{A \cdot B} = \boldsymbol{A}\boldsymbol{A}^+_{B \cdot C}$, we obtain $\boldsymbol{A}\boldsymbol{x} = \boldsymbol{A}\boldsymbol{A}^+_{B \cdot C}\boldsymbol{y}$. Premultiplying both sides of this by $\boldsymbol{A}^+_{B \cdot C}$, we obtain $(\boldsymbol{A}^+_{B \cdot C}\boldsymbol{A})\boldsymbol{Q}_{C'} = \boldsymbol{Q}_{C'}$, leading to $\boldsymbol{x} = \boldsymbol{A}^+_{B \cdot C}\boldsymbol{y}$. Q.E.D.

4.4.4 Optimal g-inverses

The generalized form of the Moore-Penrose inverse $\boldsymbol{A}^+_{B \cdot C}$ discussed in the previous subsection minimizes $||\boldsymbol{x}||^2_{Q_{C'}}$ among all $\boldsymbol{x}$'s that minimize $||\boldsymbol{A}\boldsymbol{x} - \boldsymbol{b}||^2_{Q_B}$. In this subsection, we obtain $\boldsymbol{x}$ that minimizes

$$\begin{aligned} & ||\boldsymbol{A}\boldsymbol{x} - \boldsymbol{b}||^2_{Q_B} + ||\boldsymbol{x}||^2_{Q_{C'}} \\ & \quad = (\boldsymbol{A}\boldsymbol{x} - \boldsymbol{b})'\boldsymbol{Q}_B(\boldsymbol{A}\boldsymbol{x} - \boldsymbol{b}) + \boldsymbol{x}'\boldsymbol{Q}_{C'}\boldsymbol{x} \\ & \quad = \boldsymbol{x}'(\boldsymbol{A}'\boldsymbol{Q}_B\boldsymbol{A} + \boldsymbol{Q}_{C'})\boldsymbol{x} - \boldsymbol{x}'\boldsymbol{A}'\boldsymbol{Q}_B\boldsymbol{b} - \boldsymbol{b}'\boldsymbol{Q}_B\boldsymbol{A}\boldsymbol{x} + \boldsymbol{b}'\boldsymbol{Q}_B\boldsymbol{b}. \end{aligned} \tag{4.113}$$

Differentiating the criterion above with respect to $\boldsymbol{x}$ and setting the results to zero gives

$$(\boldsymbol{A}'\boldsymbol{Q}_B\boldsymbol{A} + \boldsymbol{Q}_{C'})\boldsymbol{x} = \boldsymbol{A}'\boldsymbol{Q}_B\boldsymbol{b}. \tag{4.114}$$

Assuming that the regular inverse exists for $\boldsymbol{A}'\boldsymbol{Q}_B\boldsymbol{A} + \boldsymbol{Q}_{C'}$, we obtain

$$\boldsymbol{x} = \boldsymbol{A}^+_{Q(B)\oplus Q(C)}\boldsymbol{b}, \tag{4.115}$$

where

$$\boldsymbol{A}^+_{Q(B)\oplus Q(C)} = (\boldsymbol{A}'\boldsymbol{Q}_B\boldsymbol{A} + \boldsymbol{Q}_{C'})^{-1}\boldsymbol{A}'\boldsymbol{Q}_B. \tag{4.116}$$

Let $\boldsymbol{G}$ denote $\boldsymbol{A}^+_{Q(B)\oplus Q(C)}$ above. Then the following theorem holds.

Theorem 4.22

$$\text{rank}(\boldsymbol{G}) = \text{rank}(\boldsymbol{A}), \tag{4.117}$$

$$(\boldsymbol{Q}_{C'}\boldsymbol{G}\boldsymbol{A})' = \boldsymbol{Q}_{C'}\boldsymbol{G}\boldsymbol{A}, \tag{4.118}$$

and

$$(\boldsymbol{Q}_B\boldsymbol{A}\boldsymbol{G})' = \boldsymbol{Q}_B\boldsymbol{A}\boldsymbol{G}. \tag{4.119}$$

Proof. (4.117): Since Sp($\boldsymbol{A}$) and Sp($\boldsymbol{B}$) are disjoint, we have rank($\boldsymbol{G}$) = rank($\boldsymbol{A}\boldsymbol{Q}_B$) = rank($\boldsymbol{A}'$) = rank($\boldsymbol{A}$).

4.118): We have

$$\begin{aligned}\boldsymbol{Q}_{C'}\boldsymbol{G}\boldsymbol{A} &= \boldsymbol{Q}_{C'}(\boldsymbol{A}'\boldsymbol{Q}_B\boldsymbol{A} + \boldsymbol{Q}_{C'})^{-1}\boldsymbol{A}'\boldsymbol{Q}_B\boldsymbol{A} \\ &= (\boldsymbol{Q}_{C'} + \boldsymbol{A}'\boldsymbol{Q}_B\boldsymbol{A} - \boldsymbol{A}'\boldsymbol{Q}_B\boldsymbol{A}) \\ &\qquad \times(\boldsymbol{A}'\boldsymbol{Q}_B\boldsymbol{A} + \boldsymbol{Q}_{C'})^{-1}\boldsymbol{A}'\boldsymbol{Q}_B\boldsymbol{A} \\ &= \boldsymbol{A}'\boldsymbol{Q}_B\boldsymbol{A} - \boldsymbol{A}'\boldsymbol{Q}_B\boldsymbol{A}(\boldsymbol{A}'\boldsymbol{Q}_B\boldsymbol{A} + \boldsymbol{Q}_{C'})^{-1}\boldsymbol{A}'\boldsymbol{Q}_B\boldsymbol{A}.\end{aligned}$$

Since $\boldsymbol{Q}_B$ and $\boldsymbol{Q}_{C'}$ are symmetric, the equation above is also symmetric.

(4.119): $\boldsymbol{Q}_B\boldsymbol{A}\boldsymbol{G} = \boldsymbol{Q}_B\boldsymbol{A}(\boldsymbol{A}'\boldsymbol{Q}_B\boldsymbol{A}) + \boldsymbol{Q}_{C'})^{-1}\boldsymbol{A}'\boldsymbol{Q}_B$ is clearly symmetric.

Q.E.D.

Corollary Sp($\boldsymbol{Q}_{C'}\boldsymbol{G}\boldsymbol{A}$) = Sp($\boldsymbol{Q}_{C'}$) $\cap$ Sp($\boldsymbol{A}'\boldsymbol{Q}_B\boldsymbol{A}$).

Proof. This is clear from (3.37) and the fact that $\boldsymbol{Q}_{C'}(\boldsymbol{A}'\boldsymbol{Q}_B\boldsymbol{A}+\boldsymbol{Q}_{C'})^{-1}\boldsymbol{A}'$ $\times\boldsymbol{Q}_B\boldsymbol{A}$ is a parallel sum of $\boldsymbol{Q}_{C'}$ and $\boldsymbol{A}'\boldsymbol{Q}_B\boldsymbol{A}$. Q.E.D.

Note Since $\boldsymbol{A} - \boldsymbol{A}\boldsymbol{G}\boldsymbol{A} = \boldsymbol{A}(\boldsymbol{A}'\boldsymbol{Q}_B\boldsymbol{A}+\boldsymbol{Q}_{C'})^{-1}\boldsymbol{Q}_{C'}$, $\boldsymbol{G}$ is not a g-inverse of $\boldsymbol{A}$. The three properties in Theorem 3.22 are, however, very similar to those for the general form of the Moore-Penrose inverse $\boldsymbol{A}^+_{B\cdot C}$. Mitra (1975) called

$$\boldsymbol{A}^+_{M\oplus N} = (\boldsymbol{A}'\boldsymbol{M}\boldsymbol{A} + \boldsymbol{N})^{-1}\boldsymbol{A}'\boldsymbol{M} \tag{4.120}$$

an optimal inverse (instead of (4.116)), where $\boldsymbol{M}$ and $\boldsymbol{N}$ are *pd* matrices of orders n and p, respectively. Note that $\boldsymbol{x} = \boldsymbol{A}^{+}_{M \oplus N}\boldsymbol{b}$ minimizes

$$||\boldsymbol{A}\boldsymbol{x} - \boldsymbol{b}||^2_M + ||\boldsymbol{x}||^2_N. \tag{4.121}$$

If (4.120) is denoted by $\boldsymbol{G}$, (4.118) becomes $(\boldsymbol{NGA})' = \boldsymbol{NGA}$ and (4.119) becomes $(\boldsymbol{MAG})' = \boldsymbol{MAG}$. Additionally, it holds that

$$(\boldsymbol{A}')^{+}_{N \oplus M} = \boldsymbol{A}^{+}_{M^{-1} \oplus N^{-1}}. \tag{4.122}$$

Note If we set $\boldsymbol{M} = \boldsymbol{I}_n$ and $\boldsymbol{N} = \lambda \boldsymbol{I}_p$ in (4.120), where λ is a small positive scalar called a ridge parameter, we obtain

$$\boldsymbol{A}^{+}_{I_n \oplus I_p} = (\boldsymbol{A}'\boldsymbol{A} + \lambda \boldsymbol{I}_p)^{-1}\boldsymbol{A}', \tag{4.123}$$

which is often called the Tikhonov regularized inverse (Tikhonov and Arsenin, 1977). Using (4.123), Takane and Yanai (2008) defined a ridge operator $\boldsymbol{R}_X(\lambda)$ by

$$\boldsymbol{R}_X(\lambda) = \boldsymbol{A}\boldsymbol{A}^{+}_{I_n \oplus I_p} = \boldsymbol{A}(\boldsymbol{A}'\boldsymbol{A} + \lambda \boldsymbol{I}_p)^{-1}\boldsymbol{A}', \tag{4.124}$$

which has many properties similar to an orthogonal projector. Let

$$\boldsymbol{M}_X(\lambda) = \boldsymbol{I}_n + \lambda(\boldsymbol{X}\boldsymbol{X}')^{+}. \tag{4.125}$$

(This is called a ridge metric matrix.) Then $\boldsymbol{A}'\boldsymbol{A} + \lambda \boldsymbol{I}_p$ can be rewritten as $\boldsymbol{A}'\boldsymbol{A} + \lambda \boldsymbol{I}_p = \boldsymbol{A}'\boldsymbol{M}_X(\lambda)\boldsymbol{A}$, so that the ridge operator defined above can be rewritten as

$$\boldsymbol{R}_X(\lambda) = \boldsymbol{A}(\boldsymbol{A}'\boldsymbol{M}_X(\lambda)\boldsymbol{A})^{-1}\boldsymbol{A}'. \tag{4.126}$$

Takane and Yanai (2008) considered a variety of decompositions of ridge operators analogous to those for orthogonal projectors such as those given in Theorems 2.10, 2.16, 4.2, and 4.5.

4.5 Exercises for Chapter 4

1. Find $\boldsymbol{A}^{-}_{mr(C)}$ when $\boldsymbol{A} = \begin{bmatrix} 1 & 2 & 3 \\ 2 & 3 & 1 \end{bmatrix}$ and $\boldsymbol{C} = (1, 1, 1)$.

2. Let $\boldsymbol{A} = \begin{bmatrix} 1 & 2 \\ 2 & 1 \\ 1 & 1 \end{bmatrix}$.

(i) Find $\boldsymbol{A}^{-}_{\ell r(B)}$ when $\boldsymbol{B} = \begin{bmatrix} 1 \\ 1 \\ 1 \end{bmatrix}$.

(ii) Find $A^-_{\ell r(\tilde{B})}$ when $\tilde{B} = \begin{bmatrix} 1 \\ a \\ b \end{bmatrix}$, and verify that $A^-_{\ell r(\tilde{B})} = A^-\ell r$ when $a = -3$ and $b = 1$.

3. Let $A = \begin{bmatrix} 2 & -1 & -1 \\ -1 & 2 & -1 \\ -1 & -1 & 2 \end{bmatrix}$, $B = (1, 2, 1)'$, and $C = (2, 1, 1)$. Then, $\mathrm{Sp}(A) \oplus \mathrm{Sp}(B) = E^3$ and $\mathrm{Sp}(A') \oplus \mathrm{Sp}(C') = E^3$. Obtain $A^+_{B \cdot C}$.

4. Let $\mathrm{Sp}(A) \oplus \mathrm{Sp}(B)$, and let P_A and P_B denote the orthogonal projectors onto $\mathrm{Sp}(A)$ and $\mathrm{Sp}(B)$.
(i) Show that $I_n - P_A P_B$ is nonsingular.
(ii) Show that $(I_n - P_A P_B)^{-1} P_A = P_A (I_n - P_B P_A)^{-1}$.
(iii) Show that $(I_n - P_A P_B)^{-1} P_A (I_n - P_A P_B)^{-1}$ is the projector onto $\mathrm{Sp}(A)$ along $\mathrm{Sp}(B)$.

5. Let $\mathrm{Sp}(A') \oplus \mathrm{Sp}(C') \subset E^m$. Show that x that minimizes $||Ax - b||^2$ under the constraint that $Cx = 0$ is given by

$$x = (A'A + C'C + D'D)^{-1} A'b,$$

where D is an arbitrary matrix that satisfies $\mathrm{Sp}(D') = (\mathrm{Sp}(A') \oplus \mathrm{Sp}(C'))^c$.

6. Let A be an n by m matrix, and let G be an *nnd* matrix of order n such that $E^n = \mathrm{Sp}(A) \oplus \mathrm{Sp}(GZ)$, where $\mathrm{Sp}(Z) = \mathrm{Sp}(A)^\perp$. Show that the relation

$$P_{A \cdot TZ} = P_{A/T^{-1}}$$

holds, where the right-hand side is the projector defined by the pseudo-norm $||x||^2 = x'T^{-1}x$ given in (4.49). Furthermore, T is given by $T = G + AUA'$, where U is an arbitrary matrix of order m satisfying $\mathrm{Sp}(T) = \mathrm{Sp}(G) + \mathrm{Sp}(A)$.

7. Let A be an n by m matrix, and let M be an *nnd* matrix of order n such that $\mathrm{rank}(A'MA) = \mathrm{rank}(A)$. Show the following:
(i) $E^n = \mathrm{Sp}(A) \oplus \mathrm{Sp}(A'M)$.
(ii) $P_{A/M} = A(A'MA)^- A'M$ is the projector onto $\mathrm{Sp}(A)$ along $\mathrm{Ker}(A'M)$.
(iii) Let $M = Q_B$. Show that $\mathrm{Ker}(A'M) = \mathrm{Sp}(B)$ and $P_{A/Q_B} = P_{A \cdot B} = A(A'Q_B A)^- A'Q_B$, when $E^n = \mathrm{Sp}(A) \oplus \mathrm{Sp}(B)$.

8. Let $E^n = \mathrm{Sp}(A) \oplus \mathrm{Sp}(B) = \mathrm{Sp}(A) \oplus \mathrm{Sp}(\tilde{B})$ and $E^m = \mathrm{Sp}(A') \oplus \mathrm{Sp}(C')$. Show that

$$A^+_{\tilde{B} \cdot C} A A^+_{B \cdot C} = A^+_{B \cdot C}.$$

9. Let M be a symmetric *pd* matrix of order n, and let A and B be n by r and n by $n - r$ matrices having full column rank such that $\mathrm{Ker}(A') = \mathrm{Sp}(B)$. Show that

$$M^{-1} = M^{-1}A(A'M^{-1}A)^{-1}A'M^{-1} + B(B'MB)^{-1}B'. \tag{4.127}$$

(The formula above is often called Khatri's (1966) lemma. See also Khatri (1990).)

10. Let $\boldsymbol{A}$ be an n by m matrix, and let $V \subset E^m$ and $W \subset E^n$ be two subspaces. Consider the following four conditions:
(a) $\boldsymbol{G}$ maps an arbitrary vector in E^n to V.
(b) $\boldsymbol{G}'$ maps an arbitrary vector in E^m to W.
(c) $\boldsymbol{GA}$ is an identity transformation when its domain is restricted to V.
(d) $(\boldsymbol{AG})'$ is an identity transformation when its domain is restricted to W.
(i) Let $V = \text{Sp}(\boldsymbol{H})$ and

$$\text{rank}(\boldsymbol{AH}) = \text{rank}(\boldsymbol{H}) = \text{rank}(\boldsymbol{A}), \tag{4.128}$$

and let $\boldsymbol{G}$ satisfy conditions (a) and (c) above. Show that

$$\boldsymbol{G} = \boldsymbol{H}(\boldsymbol{AH})^- \tag{4.129}$$

is a g-inverse of $\boldsymbol{A}$.
(ii) Let $W = \text{Sp}(\boldsymbol{F}')$ and

$$\text{rank}(\boldsymbol{FA}) = \text{rank}(\boldsymbol{F}) = \text{rank}(\boldsymbol{A}), \tag{4.130}$$

and let $\boldsymbol{G}$ satisfy conditions (b) and (d) above. Show that

$$\boldsymbol{G} = (\boldsymbol{FA})^-\boldsymbol{F} \tag{4.131}$$

is a g-inverse of $\boldsymbol{A}$.
(iii) Let $V = \text{Sp}(\boldsymbol{H})$ and $W = \text{Sp}(\boldsymbol{F}')$, and

$$\text{rank}(\boldsymbol{FAH}) = \text{rank}(\boldsymbol{H}) = \text{rank}(\boldsymbol{F}) = \text{rank}(\boldsymbol{A}), \tag{4.132}$$

and let $\boldsymbol{G}$ satisfy all of the conditions (a) through (d). Show that

$$\boldsymbol{G} = \boldsymbol{H}(\boldsymbol{FAH})^-\boldsymbol{F} \tag{4.133}$$

is a g-inverse of $\boldsymbol{A}$.
(The g-inverses defined this way are called constrained g-inverses (Rao and Mitra, 1971).)
(iv) Show the following:

In (i), let $E^m = \text{Sp}(\boldsymbol{A}') \oplus \text{Sp}(\boldsymbol{C}')$ and $\boldsymbol{H} = \boldsymbol{I}_p - \boldsymbol{C}'(\boldsymbol{CC}')^-\boldsymbol{C}$. Then (4.128) and

$$\boldsymbol{G} = \boldsymbol{A}^-_{mr(C)} \tag{4.134}$$

hold.

In (ii), let $E^n = \text{Sp}(\boldsymbol{A}) \oplus \text{Sp}(\boldsymbol{B})$ and $\boldsymbol{F} = \boldsymbol{I}_n - \boldsymbol{B}(\boldsymbol{B}'\boldsymbol{B})^-\boldsymbol{B}'$. Then (4.130) and

$$\boldsymbol{G} = \boldsymbol{A}^-_{\ell r(B)} \tag{4.135}$$

hold.

In (iii), let $E^m = \text{Sp}(\boldsymbol{A}') \oplus \text{Sp}(\boldsymbol{C}')$, $E^n = \text{Sp}(\boldsymbol{A}) \oplus \text{Sp}(\boldsymbol{B})$, $\boldsymbol{H} = \boldsymbol{I}_p - \boldsymbol{C}'(\boldsymbol{C}\boldsymbol{C}')^- \boldsymbol{C}$, and $\boldsymbol{F} = I_n - \boldsymbol{B}(\boldsymbol{B}'\boldsymbol{B})^- \boldsymbol{B}'$. Then (4.132) and

$$\boldsymbol{G} = \boldsymbol{A}^+_{B \cdot C} \tag{4.136}$$

hold.
(v) Assume that $\boldsymbol{FAH}$ is square and nonsingular. Show that

$$\begin{aligned} &\text{rank}(\boldsymbol{A} - \boldsymbol{AH}(\boldsymbol{FAH})^{-1}\boldsymbol{FA}) \\ &\quad = \text{rank}(\boldsymbol{A}) - \text{rank}(\boldsymbol{AH}(\boldsymbol{FAH})^{-1}\boldsymbol{FA}) \qquad (4.137) \\ &\quad = \text{rank}(\boldsymbol{A}) - \text{rank}(\boldsymbol{FAH}). \qquad (4.138) \end{aligned}$$

This rank formula is often called the Wedderburn-Guttman theorem (Guttman, 1944, 1952, 1957; see also Takane and Yanai, 2005).

11. Show the following:
(i) $\boldsymbol{P}^+_{A/M} = \boldsymbol{P}_{MA}\boldsymbol{P}_A$, where $\boldsymbol{P}_{A/M} = \boldsymbol{A}(\boldsymbol{A}'\boldsymbol{M}\boldsymbol{A})^-\boldsymbol{A}'\boldsymbol{M}$, $\boldsymbol{P}_{MA} = \boldsymbol{M}\boldsymbol{A}(\boldsymbol{A}'\boldsymbol{M}^2\boldsymbol{A})^- \boldsymbol{A}'\boldsymbol{M}$, and $\boldsymbol{P}_A = \boldsymbol{A}(\boldsymbol{A}'\boldsymbol{A})^-\boldsymbol{A}'$.
(ii) $(\boldsymbol{M}\boldsymbol{P}_{A/M})^+ = \boldsymbol{P}_{MA}\boldsymbol{M}^-\boldsymbol{P}_{MA}$, where $\text{Sp}(\boldsymbol{A}) \subset \text{Sp}(\boldsymbol{M})$, which may be assumed without loss of generality.
(iii) $\boldsymbol{Q}^+_{A/M} = \boldsymbol{Q}_A\boldsymbol{Q}_{MA}$, where $\boldsymbol{Q}_{A/M} = \boldsymbol{I} - \boldsymbol{P}_{A/M}$, $\boldsymbol{Q}_A = \boldsymbol{I} - \boldsymbol{P}_A$, and $\boldsymbol{Q}_{MA} = \boldsymbol{I} - \boldsymbol{P}_{MA}$.
(iv) $(\boldsymbol{M}\boldsymbol{Q}_{A/M})^+ = \boldsymbol{Q}_A\boldsymbol{M}^+\boldsymbol{Q}_A$, where $\text{Sp}(\boldsymbol{A}) \subset \text{Sp}(\boldsymbol{M}) = \text{Sp}(\boldsymbol{M}^+)$, which may be assumed without loss of generality.

12. Show that minimizing

$$\phi(\boldsymbol{B}) = ||\boldsymbol{Y} - \boldsymbol{X}\boldsymbol{B}||^2 + \lambda||\boldsymbol{B}||^2$$

with respect to $\boldsymbol{B}$ leads to

$$\hat{\boldsymbol{B}} = (\boldsymbol{X}'\boldsymbol{X} + \lambda\boldsymbol{I})^{-1}\boldsymbol{X}'\boldsymbol{Y},$$

where $(\boldsymbol{X}'\boldsymbol{X} + \lambda\boldsymbol{I})^{-1}\boldsymbol{X}'$ is the Tikhonov regularized inverse defined in (4.123). (Regression analysis that involves a minimization of the criterion above is called ridge regression (Hoerl and Kennard, 1970).)
13. Show that:
(i) $\boldsymbol{R}_X(\lambda)\boldsymbol{M}_X(\lambda)\boldsymbol{R}_X(\lambda) = \boldsymbol{R}_X(\lambda)$ (i.e., $\boldsymbol{M}_X(\lambda) \in \{\boldsymbol{R}_X(\lambda)^-\}$), where $\boldsymbol{R}_X(\lambda)$ and $\boldsymbol{M}_X(\lambda)$ are as defined in (4.124) (and rewritten as in (4.126) and (4.125), respectively.
(ii) $\boldsymbol{R}_X(\lambda)^+ = \boldsymbol{M}_X(\lambda)$.

Chapter 5

Singular Value Decomposition (SVD)

5.1 Definition through Linear Transformations

In the previous section, we utilized the orthogonal direct-sum decompositions

$$E^n = V_1 \dot{\oplus} W_1 \text{ and } E^m = V_2 \dot{\oplus} W_2, \tag{5.1}$$

where $V_1 = \text{Sp}(\boldsymbol{A})$, $W_1 = V_1^{\perp}$, $W_2 = \text{Ker}(\boldsymbol{A})$, and $V_2 = W_2^{\perp}$, to define the Moore-Penrose inverse $\boldsymbol{A}^+$ of the n by m matrix $\boldsymbol{A}$ in $\boldsymbol{y} = \boldsymbol{A}\boldsymbol{x}$, a linear transformation from E^m to E^n. Let $\boldsymbol{A}'$ be a matrix that represents a linear transformation $\boldsymbol{x} = \boldsymbol{A}'\boldsymbol{y}$ from E^n to E^m. Then the following theorem holds.

Theorem 5.1

(i) $V_2 = \text{Sp}(\boldsymbol{A}') = \text{Sp}(\boldsymbol{A}'\boldsymbol{A})$.

(ii) *The transformation* $\boldsymbol{y} = \boldsymbol{A}\boldsymbol{x}$ *from* V_2 *to* V_1 *and the transformation* $\boldsymbol{x} = \boldsymbol{A}'\boldsymbol{y}$ *from* V_1 *to* V_2 *are one-to-one.*

(iii) *Let* $f(\boldsymbol{x}) = \boldsymbol{A}'\boldsymbol{A}\boldsymbol{x}$ *be a transformation from* V_2 *to* V_2, *and let*

$$\text{Sp}_{V_2}(\boldsymbol{A}'\boldsymbol{A}) = \{f(\boldsymbol{x}) = \boldsymbol{A}'\boldsymbol{A}\boldsymbol{x} | \boldsymbol{x} \in V_2\} \tag{5.2}$$

denote the image space of $f(\boldsymbol{x})$ *when* $\boldsymbol{x}$ *moves around within* V_2. *Then,*

$$\text{Sp}_{V_2}(\boldsymbol{A}'\boldsymbol{A}) = V_2, \tag{5.3}$$

and the transformation from V_2 *to* V_2 *is one-to-one.*

Note Since $V_2 = \mathrm{Sp}(\boldsymbol{A}')$, $\mathrm{Sp}_{V_2}(\boldsymbol{A}'\boldsymbol{A})$ is often written as $\mathrm{Sp}_{A'}(\boldsymbol{A}'\boldsymbol{A})$. We may also use the matrix and the subspace interchangeably as in $\mathrm{Sp}_{V_1}(V_2)$ or $\mathrm{Sp}_A(V_2)$, and so on.

Proof of Theorem 5.1 (i): Clear from the corollary of Theorem 1.9 and Lemma 3.1.

(ii): From $\mathrm{rank}(\boldsymbol{A}'\boldsymbol{A}) = \mathrm{rank}(\boldsymbol{A})$, we have $\dim(V_1) = \dim(V_2)$, from which it follows that the transformations $\boldsymbol{y} = \boldsymbol{A}\boldsymbol{x}$ from V_2 to V_1 and $\boldsymbol{x} = \boldsymbol{A}'\boldsymbol{y}$ from V_1 to V_2 are both one-to-one.

(iii): For an arbitrary $\boldsymbol{x} \in E^m$, let $\boldsymbol{x} = \boldsymbol{x}_1 + \boldsymbol{x}_2$, where $\boldsymbol{x}_1 \in V_2$ and $\boldsymbol{x}_2 \in W_2$. Then, $\boldsymbol{z} = \boldsymbol{A}'\boldsymbol{A}\boldsymbol{x} = \boldsymbol{A}'\boldsymbol{A}\boldsymbol{x}_1 \in \mathrm{Sp}_{V_2}(\boldsymbol{A}'\boldsymbol{A})$. Hence, $\mathrm{Sp}_{V_2}(\boldsymbol{A}'\boldsymbol{A}) = \mathrm{Sp}(\boldsymbol{A}'\boldsymbol{A}) = \mathrm{Sp}(\boldsymbol{A}') = V_2$. Also, $\boldsymbol{A}'\boldsymbol{A}\boldsymbol{x}_1 = \boldsymbol{A}\boldsymbol{A}\boldsymbol{x}_2 \Rightarrow \boldsymbol{A}'\boldsymbol{A}(\boldsymbol{x}_2 - \boldsymbol{x}_1) = \boldsymbol{0} \Rightarrow \boldsymbol{x}_2 - \boldsymbol{x}_1 \in \mathrm{Ker}(\boldsymbol{A}'\boldsymbol{A}) = \mathrm{Ker}(\boldsymbol{A}) = W_r$. Hence, $\boldsymbol{x}_1 = \boldsymbol{x}_2$ if $\boldsymbol{x}_1, \boldsymbol{x}_2 \in V_2$. Q.E.D.

Let $\boldsymbol{y} = \boldsymbol{T}\boldsymbol{x}$ be an arbitrary linear transformation from E^n to E^n (i.e., $\boldsymbol{T}$ is a square matrix of order n), and let $V = \{\boldsymbol{T}\boldsymbol{x} | \boldsymbol{x} \in V\}$ be a subspace of E^n ($V \subset E^n$). Then V is said to be invariant over $\boldsymbol{T}$. Hence, $V_2 = \mathrm{Sp}(\boldsymbol{A}')$ is invariant over $\boldsymbol{A}'\boldsymbol{A}$. Let $\boldsymbol{y} = \boldsymbol{T}\boldsymbol{x}$ be a linear transformation from E^m to E^n, and let its conjugate transpose $\boldsymbol{x} = \boldsymbol{T}'\boldsymbol{y}$ be a linear transformation from E^n to E^m. When the two subspaces $V_1 \subset E^n$ and $V_2 \subset E^m$ satisfy

$$V_1 = \{\boldsymbol{y} | \boldsymbol{y} = \boldsymbol{T}\boldsymbol{x}, \boldsymbol{x} \in V_2\} \tag{5.4}$$

and

$$V_2 = \{\boldsymbol{x} | \boldsymbol{x} = \boldsymbol{T}'\boldsymbol{y}, \boldsymbol{y} \in V_1\}, \tag{5.5}$$

V_1 and V_2 are said to be bi-invariant. (Clearly, V_1 and V_2 defined above are bi-invariant with respect to $\boldsymbol{A}$ and $\boldsymbol{A}'$, where $\boldsymbol{A}$ is an n by m matrix.)

Let us now consider making V_{11} and V_{21}, which are subspaces of V_1 and V_2, respectively, bi-invariant. That is,

$$\mathrm{Sp}_{V_1}(V_{21}) = V_{11} \text{ and } \mathrm{Sp}_{V_2}(V_{11}) = V_{21}. \tag{5.6}$$

Since $\dim(V_{11}) = \dim(V_{21})$, let us consider the case of minimum dimensionality, namely $\dim(V_{11}) = \dim(V_{21}) = 1$. This means that we are looking for

$$\boldsymbol{A}\boldsymbol{x} = c_1\boldsymbol{y} \text{ and } \boldsymbol{A}'\boldsymbol{y} = c_2\boldsymbol{x}, \tag{5.7}$$

where $\boldsymbol{x} \in E^m$, $\boldsymbol{y} \in E^n$, and c_1 and c_2 are nonzero constants. One possible pair of such vectors, $\boldsymbol{x}$ and $\boldsymbol{y}$, can be obtained as follows.

Lemma 5.1

$$\max_{x} \phi(\boldsymbol{x}) = \max_{x} \frac{||\boldsymbol{A}\boldsymbol{x}||^2}{||\boldsymbol{x}||^2} = \lambda_1(\boldsymbol{A}'\boldsymbol{A}), \tag{5.8}$$

where $\lambda_1(\boldsymbol{A}'\boldsymbol{A})$ *is the largest eigenvalue of* $\boldsymbol{A}'\boldsymbol{A}$.

Proof. Since $\phi(\boldsymbol{x})$ is continuous with respect to (each element of) $\boldsymbol{x}$ and is bounded, it takes its maximum and minimum values on the surface of the sphere $c = \{\boldsymbol{x} | ||\boldsymbol{x}|| = 1\}$. Maximizing $\phi(\boldsymbol{x})$ with respect to $\boldsymbol{x}$ is equivalent to maximizing its numerator $\boldsymbol{x}'\boldsymbol{A}'\boldsymbol{A}\boldsymbol{x}$ subject to the constraint that $||\boldsymbol{x}||^2 = \boldsymbol{x}'\boldsymbol{x} = 1$, which may be done via the Lagrange multiplier method. Define

$$f(\boldsymbol{x}, \lambda) = \boldsymbol{x}'\boldsymbol{A}'\boldsymbol{A}\boldsymbol{x} - \lambda(\boldsymbol{x}'\boldsymbol{x} - 1),$$

where λ is a Lagrange multiplier. Differentiating f with respect to (each element of) $\boldsymbol{x}$ and setting the result to zero, we obtain

$$\frac{1}{2}\frac{\partial f}{\partial \boldsymbol{x}} = \boldsymbol{A}'\boldsymbol{A}\boldsymbol{x} - \lambda\boldsymbol{x} = \boldsymbol{0}.$$

Premultiplying the equation above by $\boldsymbol{x}'$, we obtain

$$\boldsymbol{x}'\boldsymbol{A}'\boldsymbol{A}\boldsymbol{x} = \lambda\boldsymbol{x}'\boldsymbol{x} = \lambda.$$

This shows that the maximum of $\phi(\boldsymbol{x})$ corresponds with the largest eigenvalue λ_1 of $\boldsymbol{A}'\boldsymbol{A}$ (often denoted as $\lambda_1(\boldsymbol{A}'\boldsymbol{A})$). Q.E.D.

Let $\boldsymbol{x}_1$ denote a vector that maximizes $||\boldsymbol{A}\boldsymbol{x}||^2/||\boldsymbol{x}||^2$, and let $\boldsymbol{y}_1 = \boldsymbol{A}\boldsymbol{x}$. Then,

$$\boldsymbol{A}'\boldsymbol{y}_1 = \boldsymbol{A}'\boldsymbol{A}\boldsymbol{x}_1 = \lambda_1\boldsymbol{x}_1, \tag{5.9}$$

which indicates that $\boldsymbol{x}_1$ and $\boldsymbol{y}_1$ constitute a solution that satisfies (5.7). Let $V_{11} = \{c\boldsymbol{y}_1\}$ and $V_{21} = \{d\boldsymbol{x}_1\}$, where c and d are arbitrary real numbers. Let V_{11}^* and V_{21}^* denote the sets of vectors orthogonal to $\boldsymbol{y}_i$ and $\boldsymbol{x}_i$ in V_1 and V_2, respectively. Then, $\boldsymbol{A}\boldsymbol{x}^* \in V_{11}^*$ if $\boldsymbol{x}^* \in V_{21}^*$ since $\boldsymbol{y}_1'\boldsymbol{A}\boldsymbol{x}^* = \lambda_1\boldsymbol{x}_1'\boldsymbol{x}^* = 0$. Also, $\boldsymbol{A}'\boldsymbol{y}^* \in V_{21}^*$ if $\boldsymbol{y}^* \in V_{11}^*$, since $\boldsymbol{x}_1'\boldsymbol{A}'\boldsymbol{y}^* = \boldsymbol{y}'\boldsymbol{y}^* = 0$. Hence, $\text{Sp}_A(V_{21}^*) \subset V_{11}^*$ and $\text{Sp}_{A'}(V_{11}^*) \subset V_{21}^*$, which implies $V_{11} \dot{\oplus} V_{11}^* = V_1$ and $V_{21} \dot{\oplus} V_{21}^* = V_2$. Hence, we have $\text{Sp}_A(V_2) = V_1$ and $\text{Sp}_{A'}(V_1) = V_2$, and so $\text{Sp}_A(V_{21}) = V_{11}$ and $\text{Sp}_{A'}(V_{11}) = V_{21}$. We now let

$$\boldsymbol{A}_1 = \boldsymbol{A} - \boldsymbol{y}_1\boldsymbol{x}_1'. \tag{5.10}$$

Then, if $\boldsymbol{x}^* \in V_{21}^*$,

$$\boldsymbol{A}_1\boldsymbol{x}^* = \boldsymbol{A}\boldsymbol{x}^* - \boldsymbol{y}_1\boldsymbol{x}_1'\boldsymbol{x}^* = \boldsymbol{A}\boldsymbol{x}^*$$

and

$$\boldsymbol{A}_1\boldsymbol{x}_1 = \boldsymbol{A}\boldsymbol{x}_1 - \boldsymbol{y}_1\boldsymbol{x}_1'\boldsymbol{x}_1 = \boldsymbol{y}_1 - \boldsymbol{y}_1 = \boldsymbol{0},$$

which indicate that $\boldsymbol{A}_1$ defines the same transformation as $\boldsymbol{A}$ from V_{21}^* to V_{11}^* and that V_{21} is the subspace of the null space of $\boldsymbol{A}_1$ (i.e., $\text{Ker}(\boldsymbol{A}_1)$). Similarly, since

$$\boldsymbol{y}^* \in V_{11}^* \Longrightarrow \boldsymbol{A}_1'\boldsymbol{y}^* = \boldsymbol{A}'\boldsymbol{y}^* - \boldsymbol{x}_1\boldsymbol{y}_1'\boldsymbol{y}^* = \boldsymbol{A}'\boldsymbol{y}^*$$

and

$$\boldsymbol{y}_1 \in V_{11} \Longrightarrow \boldsymbol{A}_1'\boldsymbol{y}_1 = \boldsymbol{A}'\boldsymbol{y}_1 - \boldsymbol{x}_1\boldsymbol{y}_1'\boldsymbol{y}_1 = \lambda\boldsymbol{x}_1 - \lambda\boldsymbol{x}_1 = \boldsymbol{0},$$

$\boldsymbol{A}_1'$ defines the same transformation as $\boldsymbol{A}'$ from V_{11}^* to V_{21}^*. The null space of $\boldsymbol{A}_1$ is given by $V_{11} \oplus W_1$, whose dimensionality is equal to $\dim(W_1) + 1$. Hence $\text{rank}(\boldsymbol{A}_1) = \text{rank}(\boldsymbol{A}) - 1$.

Similarly, let $\boldsymbol{x}_2$ denote a vector that maximizes $||\boldsymbol{A}_1\boldsymbol{x}||^2/||\boldsymbol{x}||^2$, and let $\boldsymbol{A}_1\boldsymbol{x}_2 = \boldsymbol{A}\boldsymbol{x}_2 = \boldsymbol{y}_2$. Then, $\boldsymbol{A}'\boldsymbol{y}_2 = \lambda_2\boldsymbol{y}_2$, where λ_2 is the second largest eigenvalue of $\boldsymbol{A}'\boldsymbol{A}$. Define

$$V_{22} = \{c\boldsymbol{x}_2\} \text{ and } V_{12} = \{d\boldsymbol{y}_2\},$$

where c and d are arbitrary real numbers. Then, $\text{Sp}_A(V_{22}) = V_{12}$ and $\text{Sp}_{A'}(V_{12}) = V_{22}$, implying that V_{22} and V_{12} are bi-invariant with respect to $\boldsymbol{A}$ as well. We also have $\boldsymbol{x}_2 \in V_{21}^*$ and $\boldsymbol{y}_2 \in V_{11}^*$, so that $\boldsymbol{x}_1'\boldsymbol{x}_2 = 0$ and $\boldsymbol{y}_1'\boldsymbol{y}_2 = 0$. Let us next define

$$\boldsymbol{A}_2 = \boldsymbol{A}_1 - \boldsymbol{y}_2\boldsymbol{x}_2' = \boldsymbol{A} - \boldsymbol{y}_1\boldsymbol{x}_1' - \boldsymbol{y}_2\boldsymbol{x}_2'. \tag{5.11}$$

Then, $\text{rank}(\boldsymbol{A}_2) = \text{rank}(\boldsymbol{A}) - 2$.

Applying the same operation repeatedly, we obtain a matrix with all elements being zero, namely a zero matrix, $\boldsymbol{O}$. That is,

$$\boldsymbol{A} - \boldsymbol{y}_1\boldsymbol{x}_1' - \cdots - \boldsymbol{y}_r\boldsymbol{x}_r' = \boldsymbol{O}$$

or

$$\boldsymbol{A} = \boldsymbol{y}_1\boldsymbol{x}_1' + \cdots + \boldsymbol{y}_r\boldsymbol{x}_r'. \tag{5.12}$$

Here, $\boldsymbol{x}_1, \boldsymbol{x}_2, \cdots, \boldsymbol{x}_r$ and $\boldsymbol{y}_1, \boldsymbol{y}_2, \cdots \boldsymbol{y}_r$ constitute orthogonal basis vectors for $V_2 = \text{Sp}(\boldsymbol{A}')$ and $V_1 = \text{Sp}(\boldsymbol{A})$, respectively, and it holds that

$$\boldsymbol{A}\boldsymbol{x}_j = \boldsymbol{y}_j \text{ and } \boldsymbol{A}'\boldsymbol{y}_j = \lambda\boldsymbol{x}_j \ (j = 1, \cdots, r), \tag{5.13}$$

where $\lambda_1 > \lambda_2 > \cdots > \lambda_r > 0$ are nonzero eigenvalues of $\boldsymbol{A}'\boldsymbol{A}$ (or of $\boldsymbol{A}\boldsymbol{A}'$). Since

$$||\boldsymbol{y}_j||^2 = \boldsymbol{y}_j'\boldsymbol{y}_j = \boldsymbol{y}_j'\boldsymbol{A}\boldsymbol{x}_j = \lambda_j\boldsymbol{x}_j'\boldsymbol{x}_j = \lambda_j > 0,$$

there exists $\mu_j = \sqrt{\lambda_j}$ such that $\lambda_j^2 = \mu_j$ ($\mu_j > 0$). Let $\boldsymbol{y}_j^* = \boldsymbol{y}_j/\mu_j$. Then,

$$\boldsymbol{A}\boldsymbol{x}_j = \boldsymbol{y}_j = \mu_j \boldsymbol{y}_j^* \tag{5.14}$$

and

$$\boldsymbol{A}'\boldsymbol{y}_j^* = \lambda_j \boldsymbol{x}_j/\mu_j = \mu_j \boldsymbol{x}_j. \tag{5.15}$$

Hence, from (5.12), we obtain

$$\boldsymbol{A} = \mu_1 \boldsymbol{y}_1^* \boldsymbol{x}_1' + \cdots, +\mu_r \boldsymbol{y}_r^* \boldsymbol{x}_r'.$$

Let $\boldsymbol{u}_j = \boldsymbol{y}_j^*$ ($j = 1, \cdots, r$) and $\boldsymbol{v}_j = \boldsymbol{x}_j$ ($j = 1, \cdots, r$), meaning

$$\boldsymbol{V}_{[r]} = [\boldsymbol{v}_1, \boldsymbol{v}_2, \cdots, \boldsymbol{v}_r] \text{ and } \boldsymbol{U}_{[r]} = [\boldsymbol{u}_1, \boldsymbol{u}_2, \cdots, \boldsymbol{u}_r], \tag{5.16}$$

and let

$$\boldsymbol{\Delta}_r = \begin{bmatrix} \mu_1 & 0 & \cdots & 0 \\ 0 & \mu_2 & \cdots & 0 \\ \vdots & \vdots & \ddots & \vdots \\ 0 & 0 & \cdots & \mu_r \end{bmatrix}. \tag{5.17}$$

Then the following theorem can be derived.

Theorem 5.2 *An n by m matrix $\boldsymbol{A}$ of rank r can be decomposed as*

$$\begin{aligned} \boldsymbol{A} &= \mu_1 \boldsymbol{u}_1 \boldsymbol{v}_1' + \mu_2 \boldsymbol{u}_2 \boldsymbol{v}_2' + \cdots + \mu_r \boldsymbol{u}_r \boldsymbol{v}_r' && (5.18) \\ &= \boldsymbol{U}_{[r]} \boldsymbol{\Delta}_r \boldsymbol{V}_{[r]}', && (5.19) \end{aligned}$$

where $\lambda_j = \mu_j^2$ ($j = 1, \cdots, r$) are nonzero eigenvalues of $\boldsymbol{A}'\boldsymbol{A}$. (It is assumed that there are no identical eigenvalues.)

Corollary 1 *Vectors $\boldsymbol{v}_j$ and $\boldsymbol{u}_j$ ($j = 1, \cdots, r$) that satisfy (5.18) also satisfy the equations*

$$\boldsymbol{A}\boldsymbol{v}_j = \mu_j \boldsymbol{u}_j \text{ and } \boldsymbol{A}'\boldsymbol{u}_j = \mu_j \boldsymbol{v}_j, \tag{5.20}$$

$$\boldsymbol{A}'\boldsymbol{A}\boldsymbol{v}_j = \lambda_j \boldsymbol{v}_j \text{ and } \boldsymbol{A}\boldsymbol{v}_j = \mu_j \boldsymbol{u}_j, \tag{5.21}$$

and

$$\boldsymbol{A}\boldsymbol{A}'\boldsymbol{u}_j = \lambda_j \boldsymbol{u}_j \text{ and } \boldsymbol{A}'\boldsymbol{u}_j = \mu_j \boldsymbol{v}_j. \tag{5.22}$$

Proof. (5.20): Postmultiplying (5.18) by $\boldsymbol{v}_j$, we obtain $\boldsymbol{A}\boldsymbol{v}_j = \mu_j \boldsymbol{u}_j$, and by postmultiplying the transpose $\boldsymbol{A}'$ of (5.18) by $\boldsymbol{v}_j$, we obtain $\boldsymbol{A}'\boldsymbol{u}_j = \mu_j \boldsymbol{v}_j$. Q.E.D.

Corollary 2 *When* $\boldsymbol{A}'\boldsymbol{A} = \boldsymbol{A}\boldsymbol{A}'$, *matrix* $\boldsymbol{A}$ *is called a normal matrix. A normal matrix can be decomposed as*

$$\boldsymbol{A} = \mu_1 \boldsymbol{u}_1 \boldsymbol{u}_1' + \mu_2 \boldsymbol{u}_2 \boldsymbol{u}_2' + \cdots + \mu_r \boldsymbol{u}_r \boldsymbol{u}_r'.$$

Proof. It is clear from (5.21) and (5.22) that $\boldsymbol{u}_j = \boldsymbol{v}_j$ when $\boldsymbol{A}'\boldsymbol{A} = \boldsymbol{A}\boldsymbol{A}'$. Q.E.D.

Definition 5.1 *Decomposition (5.18) (and (5.19)) is called the singular value decomposition (SVD) of the matrix* $\boldsymbol{A}$, *where* μ_j *indicates the* j*th largest singular value of* $\boldsymbol{A}$ *and is often denoted as* $\mu_j = \mu_j(\boldsymbol{A})$.

Note that $\boldsymbol{U}_{[r]}$ and $\boldsymbol{V}_{[r]}$ are columnwise orthogonal, that is,

$$\boldsymbol{U}_{[r]}'\boldsymbol{U}_{[r]} = \boldsymbol{V}_{[r]}'\boldsymbol{V}_{[r]} = \boldsymbol{I}_r. \tag{5.23}$$

Furthermore, we can add $\boldsymbol{U}_{[0]} = [\boldsymbol{u}_{r+1}, \cdots, \boldsymbol{u}_n]$ to $\boldsymbol{U}_{[r]}$, where $\boldsymbol{U}_{[0]}$ is an n by $n-r$ columnwise orthogonal matrix ($\boldsymbol{U}_{[0]}'\boldsymbol{U}_{[0]} = \boldsymbol{I}_{n-r}$) that is also orthogonal to $\boldsymbol{U}_{[r]}$ ($\boldsymbol{U}_{[r]}'\boldsymbol{U}_{[0]} = \boldsymbol{O}$). The resultant matrix $\boldsymbol{U} = [\boldsymbol{U}_{[r]}, \boldsymbol{U}_{[0]}]$ is fully orthogonal ($\boldsymbol{U}'\boldsymbol{U} = \boldsymbol{U}\boldsymbol{U}' = \boldsymbol{I}_n$). Similarly, we can add an m by $m-r$ columnwise orthogonal matrix $\boldsymbol{V}_{[0]} = [\boldsymbol{v}_{r+1}, \cdots, \boldsymbol{v}_m]$ to $\boldsymbol{V}_{[r]}$ to form a fully orthogonal matrix $\boldsymbol{V} = [\boldsymbol{V}_{[r]}, \boldsymbol{V}_{[0]}]$. A complete form of singular value decomposition (SVD) may thus be expressed as

$$\boldsymbol{A} = \boldsymbol{U}\Delta\boldsymbol{V}', \tag{5.24}$$

where

$$\boldsymbol{U}'\boldsymbol{U} = \boldsymbol{U}\boldsymbol{U}' = \boldsymbol{I}_n \text{ and } \boldsymbol{V}'\boldsymbol{V} = \boldsymbol{V}\boldsymbol{V}' = \boldsymbol{I}_m, \tag{5.25}$$

and

$$\boldsymbol{\Delta} = \begin{bmatrix} \boldsymbol{\Delta}_r & \boldsymbol{O} \\ \boldsymbol{O} & \boldsymbol{O} \end{bmatrix}, \tag{5.26}$$

where $\boldsymbol{\Delta}_r$ is as given in (5.17). (In contrast, (5.19) is called the compact (or incomplete) form of SVD.) Premultiplying (5.24) by $\boldsymbol{U}'$, we obtain

$$\boldsymbol{U}'\boldsymbol{A} = \boldsymbol{\Delta}\boldsymbol{V}' \text{ or } \boldsymbol{A}'\boldsymbol{U} = \boldsymbol{V}\boldsymbol{\Delta},$$

and by postmultiplying (5.24) by $\boldsymbol{V}$, we obtain

$$\boldsymbol{A}\boldsymbol{V} = \boldsymbol{U}\boldsymbol{\Delta}.$$

Pre- and postmultiplying (5.24) by $\boldsymbol{U}'$ and $\boldsymbol{V}$, respectively, we obtain

$$\boldsymbol{U}'\boldsymbol{A}\boldsymbol{V} = \boldsymbol{\Delta}. \tag{5.27}$$

When all nonzero (positive) singular values of $\boldsymbol{A}$ (or nonzero eigenvalues of $\boldsymbol{A}'\boldsymbol{A}$) are distinct, $\boldsymbol{U}_{[r]}$ and $\boldsymbol{V}_{[r]}$ are determined uniquely. However, $\boldsymbol{V}_{[0]}$ and $\boldsymbol{U}_{[0]}$ consist of orthonormal basis vectors in $\text{Ker}(\boldsymbol{A})$ and $\text{Sp}(\boldsymbol{A})^{\perp} = \text{Ker}(\boldsymbol{A}')$, respectively, and consequently they are not uniquely determined.

Let us now consider the linear transformation $\boldsymbol{y} = \boldsymbol{A}\boldsymbol{x}$. From (5.24) and (5.25), we have

$$\boldsymbol{y} = \boldsymbol{U}\boldsymbol{\Delta}\boldsymbol{V}'\boldsymbol{x} \text{ or } \boldsymbol{U}'\boldsymbol{y} = \boldsymbol{\Delta}\boldsymbol{V}'\boldsymbol{x}.$$

Let $\tilde{\boldsymbol{y}} = \boldsymbol{U}'\boldsymbol{y}$ and $\tilde{\boldsymbol{x}} = \boldsymbol{V}'\boldsymbol{x}$. Then,

$$\tilde{\boldsymbol{y}} = \boldsymbol{\Delta}\tilde{\boldsymbol{x}}. \tag{5.28}$$

This indicates that the linear transformation $\boldsymbol{y} = \boldsymbol{A}\boldsymbol{x}$ can be viewed, from the perspective of singular value decomposition, as three successive linear transformations,

$$\boldsymbol{x} \xrightarrow{V'} \tilde{\boldsymbol{x}} \xrightarrow{\Delta} \tilde{y} \xrightarrow{U} \boldsymbol{y},$$

an orthogonal transformation ($\boldsymbol{V}'$) from $\boldsymbol{x}$ to $\tilde{\boldsymbol{x}}$, followed by a diagonal transformation (Δ) that only multiplies the elements of $\tilde{\boldsymbol{x}}$ by some constants to obtain $\tilde{\boldsymbol{y}}$, which is further orthogonally transformed (by $\boldsymbol{U}$) to obtain $\boldsymbol{y}$. Note that (5.28) indicates that the transformation matrix corresponding to $\boldsymbol{A}$ is given by Δ when the basis vectors spanning E^n and E^m are chosen to be $\boldsymbol{U}$ and $\boldsymbol{V}$, respectively.

Example 5.1 Find the singular value decomposition of

$$\boldsymbol{A} = \begin{bmatrix} -2 & 1 & 1 \\ 1 & -2 & 1 \\ 1 & 1 & -2 \\ -2 & 1 & 1 \end{bmatrix}.$$

Solution. From $\boldsymbol{A}'\boldsymbol{A} = \begin{bmatrix} 10 & -5 & -5 \\ -5 & 7 & -2 \\ -5 & -2 & 7 \end{bmatrix}$, we obtain

$$\phi(\lambda) = |\lambda \boldsymbol{I}_3 - \boldsymbol{A}'\boldsymbol{A}| = (\lambda - 15)(\lambda - 9)\lambda = 0.$$

Hence, the eigenvalues of $\boldsymbol{A}'\boldsymbol{A}$ are given by $\lambda_1 = 15$, $\lambda_2 = 9$, and $\lambda_3 = 0$, and so the singular values of the matrix $\boldsymbol{A}$ are given by $\mu_1 = \sqrt{15}$, $\mu_2 = 3$, and $\mu_3 = 0$. We thus obtain

$$\boldsymbol{\Delta}_2 = \begin{bmatrix} \sqrt{15} & 0 \\ 0 & 3 \end{bmatrix}.$$

Furthermore, from $\boldsymbol{A}'\boldsymbol{A}\boldsymbol{V}_{[2]} = \boldsymbol{V}_{[2]}\boldsymbol{\Delta}_2^2$ and $\boldsymbol{U}_{[2]} = \boldsymbol{A}\boldsymbol{V}_{[2]}\boldsymbol{\Delta}_2^{-1}$, we obtain

$$\boldsymbol{U}_{[2]} = \begin{bmatrix} \sqrt{\frac{2}{5}} & 0 \\ -\sqrt{\frac{1}{10}} & \frac{\sqrt{2}}{2} \\ -\sqrt{\frac{1}{10}} & -\frac{\sqrt{2}}{2} \\ \sqrt{\frac{2}{5}} & 0 \end{bmatrix} \quad \text{and} \quad \boldsymbol{V}_{[2]} = \begin{bmatrix} -\frac{2}{\sqrt{6}} & 0 \\ \frac{1}{\sqrt{6}} & -\frac{1}{\sqrt{2}} \\ \frac{1}{\sqrt{6}} & \frac{1}{\sqrt{2}} \end{bmatrix}.$$

Thus the SVD of $\boldsymbol{A}$ is given by

$$\begin{aligned} \boldsymbol{A} &= \sqrt{15}\begin{pmatrix} \sqrt{\frac{2}{5}} \\ -\frac{1}{\sqrt{10}} \\ -\frac{1}{\sqrt{10}} \\ \sqrt{\frac{2}{5}} \end{pmatrix}\left(-\frac{2}{\sqrt{6}}, \frac{1}{\sqrt{6}}, \frac{1}{\sqrt{6}}\right) + 3\begin{pmatrix} 0 \\ \frac{\sqrt{2}}{2} \\ -\frac{\sqrt{2}}{2} \\ 0 \end{pmatrix}\left(0, -\frac{1}{\sqrt{2}}, \frac{1}{\sqrt{2}}\right) \\ &= \sqrt{15}\begin{bmatrix} -\frac{2}{\sqrt{15}} & \frac{1}{\sqrt{15}} & \frac{1}{\sqrt{15}} \\ \frac{1}{\sqrt{15}} & -\frac{1}{2\sqrt{15}} & -\frac{1}{2\sqrt{15}} \\ \frac{1}{\sqrt{15}} & -\frac{1}{2\sqrt{15}} & -\frac{1}{2\sqrt{15}} \\ -\frac{2}{\sqrt{15}} & \frac{1}{\sqrt{15}} & \frac{1}{\sqrt{15}} \end{bmatrix} + 3\begin{bmatrix} 0 & 0 & 0 \\ 0 & -\frac{1}{2} & \frac{1}{2} \\ 0 & \frac{1}{2} & -\frac{1}{2} \\ 0 & 0 & 0 \end{bmatrix}. \end{aligned}$$

Example 5.2 We apply the SVD to 10 by 10 data matrices below (the two matrices together show the Chinese characters for "matrix").

Data matrix $\boldsymbol{A}$

0	0	0	1	0	1	1	1	1	1
0	0	1	0	0	0	0	0	0	0
0	1	0	1	0	0	0	0	0	0
1	0	1	0	0	1	1	1	1	1
0	1	1	0	0	0	0	1	0	0,
1	0	1	0	0	0	0	1	0	0
0	0	1	0	0	0	0	1	0	0
0	0	1	0	0	0	0	1	0	0
0	0	1	0	0	0	0	1	0	0
0	0	1	0	0	0	0	1	0	0

Data matrix $\boldsymbol{B}$

1	1	1	1	1	0	1	0	0	1
0	1	0	0	0	0	1	0	0	1
0	1	1	1	1	0	1	0	0	1
0	1	0	0	1	0	1	0	0	1
0	1	0	0	1	0	1	0	0	1.
0	1	1	1	1	0	1	0	0	1
0	1	0	0	1	0	0	0	0	1
0	0	0	0	1	0	0	0	0	1
0	0	0	0	1	0	1	0	0	1
0	1	1	1	1	0	1	1	1	1

We display

$$\boldsymbol{A}_j(\text{and } \boldsymbol{B}_j) = \mu_1 \boldsymbol{u}_1 \boldsymbol{v}_1' + \mu_2 \boldsymbol{u}_2 \boldsymbol{v}_2' + \cdots + \mu_j \boldsymbol{u}_j \boldsymbol{v}_j'$$

in Figure 5.1. (Elements of $\boldsymbol{A}_j$ larger than .8 are indicated by "*", those between .6 and .8 are indicated by "+", and those below .6 are left blank.) In the figure, μ_j is the jth largest singular value and S_j indicates the cumulative contribution up to the jth term defined by

$$S_j = (\lambda_1 + \lambda_2 + \cdots + \lambda_j)/(\lambda_1 + \lambda_2 + \cdots + \lambda_{10}) \times 100(\%).$$

With the coding scheme above, $\boldsymbol{A}$ can be "perfectly" recovered by the first five terms, while $\boldsymbol{B}$ is "almost perfectly" recovered except that in four places "*" is replaced by "+". This result indicates that by analyzing the pattern of data using SVD, a more economical transmission of information is possible than with the original data.

(1) $\boldsymbol{A}_1$ (2) $\boldsymbol{A}_2$ (3) $\boldsymbol{A}_3$ (4) $\boldsymbol{A}_4$ (5) $\boldsymbol{A}_5$

$\mu_1 = 4.24$, $S_1 = 60.06$; $\mu_2 = 2.62$, $S_2 = 82.96$; $\mu_3 = 1.69$, $S_3 = 92.47$; $\mu_4 = 1.11$, $S_4 = 96.59$; $\mu_5 = 0.77$, $S_5 = 98.57$

Figure 5.1: Data matrices $\boldsymbol{A}$ and $\boldsymbol{B}$ and their SVDs. (The μ_j is the singular value and S_j is the cumulative percentage of contribution.)

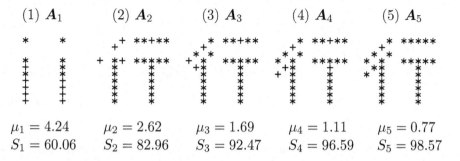

(6) $\boldsymbol{B}_1$ (7) $\boldsymbol{B}_2$ (8) $\boldsymbol{B}_3$ (9) $\boldsymbol{A}_4$ (10) $\boldsymbol{A}_5$

$\mu_1 = 6.07$	$\mu_2 = 2.06$	$\mu_3 = 1.30$	$\mu_4 = 1.25$	$\mu_5 = 1.00$
$S_1 = 80.13$	$S_2 = 88.97$	$S_3 = 92.66$	$S_4 = 96.05$	$S_5 = 98.23$

Figure 5.1: (Continued.)

5.2 SVD and Projectors

In this section, we discuss principles underlying the SVD in more detail.

Lemma 5.2 *Let*

$$\boldsymbol{P}_i = \boldsymbol{u}_i\boldsymbol{u}_i', \ \tilde{\boldsymbol{P}}_i = \boldsymbol{v}_i\boldsymbol{v}_i', \ \textit{and}\ \boldsymbol{Q}_i = \boldsymbol{u}_i\boldsymbol{v}_i'. \tag{5.29}$$

Then the following relations hold:

$$\boldsymbol{P}_i^2 = \boldsymbol{P}_i, \ \ \boldsymbol{P}_i\boldsymbol{P}_j = \boldsymbol{O}\ (i \neq j), \tag{5.30}$$

$$\tilde{\boldsymbol{P}}_i^2 = \tilde{\boldsymbol{P}}_i, \ \ \tilde{\boldsymbol{P}}_i\tilde{\boldsymbol{P}}_j = \boldsymbol{O}\ \ (i \neq j), \tag{5.31}$$

$$\boldsymbol{Q}_i\boldsymbol{Q}_i' = \boldsymbol{P}_i, \ \ \boldsymbol{Q}_i'\boldsymbol{Q}_i = \tilde{\boldsymbol{P}}_i, \tag{5.32}$$

$$\boldsymbol{Q}_i'\boldsymbol{Q}_j = \boldsymbol{O}\ (i \neq j), \ \boldsymbol{Q}_i\boldsymbol{Q}_j' = \boldsymbol{O}\ (i \neq j), \tag{5.33}$$

and

$$\boldsymbol{P}_i'\boldsymbol{Q}_i = \boldsymbol{Q}_i, \ \tilde{\boldsymbol{P}}_i\boldsymbol{Q}_i' = \boldsymbol{Q}_i'. \tag{5.34}$$

(Proof omitted.)

As is clear from the results above, $\boldsymbol{P}_j$ and $\tilde{\boldsymbol{P}}_j$ are both orthogonal projectors of rank 1. When $r < \min(n, m)$, neither $\boldsymbol{P}_1 + \boldsymbol{P}_2 + \cdots + \boldsymbol{P}_r = \boldsymbol{I}_n$ nor $\tilde{\boldsymbol{P}}_1 + \tilde{\boldsymbol{P}}_2 + \cdots + \tilde{\boldsymbol{P}}_r = \boldsymbol{I}_m$ holds. Instead, the following lemma holds.

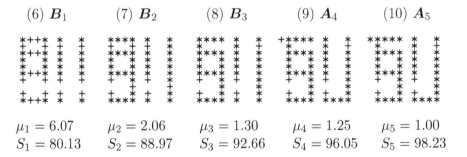

Lemma 5.3 *Let* $V_1 = \mathrm{Sp}(\boldsymbol{A})$, $V_2 = \mathrm{Sp}(\boldsymbol{A}')$, $V_{1j} = \mathrm{Sp}(\boldsymbol{u}_j)$, *and* $V_{2j} = \mathrm{Sp}(\boldsymbol{v}_j)$, *and let* $\boldsymbol{P}_{1j}$ *and* $\boldsymbol{P}_{2j}$ *be the orthogonal projectors onto* V_{1j} *and* V_{2j}, *respectively. Then the following relations hold:*

$$\begin{aligned} V_1 &= V_{11} \dot{\oplus} V_{12} \dot{\oplus} \cdots \dot{\oplus} V_{1r}, \\ V_2 &= V_{21} \dot{\oplus} V_{22} \dot{\oplus} \cdots \dot{\oplus} V_{2r}, \end{aligned} \tag{5.35}$$

and

$$\begin{aligned} \boldsymbol{P}_A &= \boldsymbol{P}_{11} + \boldsymbol{P}_{12} + \cdots + \boldsymbol{P}_{1r}, \\ \boldsymbol{P}_{A'} &= \boldsymbol{P}_{21} + \boldsymbol{P}_{22} + \cdots + \boldsymbol{P}_{2r}. \end{aligned} \tag{5.36}$$

(Proof omitted.)

Theorem 5.3 *Matrix* $\boldsymbol{A}$ *can be decomposed as follows using* $\boldsymbol{P}_j$, $\tilde{\boldsymbol{P}}_j$, *and* $\boldsymbol{Q}_j$ *that satisfy (5.30) through (5.34):*

$$\boldsymbol{A} = (\boldsymbol{P}_1 + \boldsymbol{P}_2 + \cdots + \boldsymbol{P}_r)\boldsymbol{A}, \tag{5.37}$$

$$\boldsymbol{A}' = (\tilde{\boldsymbol{P}}_1 + \tilde{\boldsymbol{P}}_2 + \cdots + \tilde{\boldsymbol{P}}_r)\boldsymbol{A}', \tag{5.38}$$

$$\boldsymbol{A} = \mu_1 \boldsymbol{Q}_1 + \mu_2 \boldsymbol{Q}_2 + \cdots + \mu_r \boldsymbol{Q}_r. \tag{5.39}$$

Proof. (5.37) and (5.38): Clear from Lemma 5.3 and the fact that $\boldsymbol{A} = \boldsymbol{P}_A \boldsymbol{A}$ and $\boldsymbol{A}' = \boldsymbol{P}_{A'}\boldsymbol{A}'$.

(5.39): Note that $\boldsymbol{A} = (\boldsymbol{P}_1 + \boldsymbol{P}_2 + \cdots + \boldsymbol{P}_r)\boldsymbol{A}(\tilde{\boldsymbol{P}}_1 + \tilde{\boldsymbol{P}}_2 + \cdots + \tilde{\boldsymbol{P}}_r)$ and that $\boldsymbol{P}_j \boldsymbol{A} \tilde{\boldsymbol{P}}_i = \boldsymbol{u}_j(\boldsymbol{u}_j'\boldsymbol{A}\boldsymbol{v}_i)\boldsymbol{v}_i' = \mu_i \boldsymbol{u}_j(\boldsymbol{u}_j'\boldsymbol{v}_i)\boldsymbol{v}_i' = \delta_{ij}\mu_i$ (where δ_{ij} is the Kronecker delta that takes the value of unity when $i = j$ and zero otherwise). Hence, we have

$$\begin{aligned} \boldsymbol{A} &= \boldsymbol{P}_1 \boldsymbol{A} \tilde{\boldsymbol{P}}_1 + \boldsymbol{P}_2 \boldsymbol{A} \tilde{\boldsymbol{P}}_2 + \cdots + \boldsymbol{P}_r \boldsymbol{A} \tilde{\boldsymbol{P}}_r \\ &= \boldsymbol{u}_1(\boldsymbol{u}_1'\boldsymbol{A}\boldsymbol{v}_1)\boldsymbol{v}_1' + \boldsymbol{u}_2(\boldsymbol{u}_2'\boldsymbol{A}\boldsymbol{v}_2)\boldsymbol{v}_2' + \cdots + \boldsymbol{u}_r(\boldsymbol{u}_r'\boldsymbol{A}\boldsymbol{v}_r)\boldsymbol{v}_r' \\ &= \mu_1 \boldsymbol{u}_1 \boldsymbol{v}_1' + \mu_2 \boldsymbol{u}_2 \boldsymbol{v}_2' + \cdots + \mu_r \boldsymbol{u}_r \boldsymbol{v}_r' \\ &= \mu_1 \boldsymbol{Q}_1 + \mu_2 \boldsymbol{Q}_2 + \cdots + \mu_r \boldsymbol{Q}_r. \end{aligned}$$

Q.E.D.

Let $\boldsymbol{F}$ and $\boldsymbol{G}$ be matrices of orthonormal basis vectors for $V_1 = \text{Sp}(\boldsymbol{A})$ and $V_2 = \text{Sp}(\boldsymbol{A}')$, respectively. Since $\boldsymbol{F}'\boldsymbol{F} = \boldsymbol{I}_r$ and $\boldsymbol{G}'\boldsymbol{G} = \boldsymbol{I}_r$,

$$\boldsymbol{P}_A = \boldsymbol{P}_F = \boldsymbol{F}(\boldsymbol{F}'\boldsymbol{F})^{-1}\boldsymbol{F}' = \boldsymbol{F}\boldsymbol{F}' \text{ and } \boldsymbol{P}_{A'} = \boldsymbol{P}_G = \boldsymbol{G}(\boldsymbol{G}'\boldsymbol{G})^{-1}\boldsymbol{G}' = \boldsymbol{G}\boldsymbol{G}'.$$

Hence,

$$\boldsymbol{A} = \boldsymbol{P}_F\boldsymbol{A}\boldsymbol{P}_G = \boldsymbol{F}(\boldsymbol{F}'\boldsymbol{A}\boldsymbol{G})\boldsymbol{G}'. \tag{5.40}$$

If we choose $\boldsymbol{F}$ and $\boldsymbol{G}$ in such a way that $\boldsymbol{F}'\boldsymbol{A}\boldsymbol{G}$ is diagonal, we obtain the SVD of $\boldsymbol{A}$.

Corollary (i) *When* $\boldsymbol{x} \in \text{Sp}(\boldsymbol{A})$,

$$\boldsymbol{x} = (\boldsymbol{u}_1, \boldsymbol{x})\boldsymbol{u}_1 + (\boldsymbol{u}_2, \boldsymbol{x})\boldsymbol{u}_2 + \cdots + (\boldsymbol{u}_r, \boldsymbol{x})\boldsymbol{u}_r$$

and

$$||\boldsymbol{x}||^2 = (\boldsymbol{u}_1, \boldsymbol{x})^2 + (\boldsymbol{u}_2, \boldsymbol{x})^2 + \cdots + (\boldsymbol{u}_r, \boldsymbol{x})^2. \tag{5.41}$$

(ii) *When* $\boldsymbol{y} \in \text{Sp}(\boldsymbol{A}')$,

$$\boldsymbol{y} = (\boldsymbol{v}_1, \boldsymbol{y})\boldsymbol{v}_1 + (\boldsymbol{v}_2, \boldsymbol{y})\boldsymbol{v}_2 + \cdots + (\boldsymbol{v}_r, \boldsymbol{y})\boldsymbol{v}_r$$

and

$$||\boldsymbol{y}||^2 = (\boldsymbol{v}_1, \boldsymbol{y})^2 + (\boldsymbol{v}_2, \boldsymbol{y})^2 + \cdots + (\boldsymbol{v}_r, \boldsymbol{y})^2. \tag{5.42}$$

(A proof is omitted.)

Equations (5.41) and (5.42) correspond with Parseval's equality.

We now present a theorem concerning decompositions of symmetric matrices $\boldsymbol{A}'\boldsymbol{A}$ and $\boldsymbol{A}\boldsymbol{A}'$.

Theorem 5.4 *Using the decompositions given in (5.30) through (5.34),* $\boldsymbol{A}\boldsymbol{A}'$ *and* $\boldsymbol{A}'\boldsymbol{A}$ *can be decomposed as*

$$\boldsymbol{A}\boldsymbol{A}' = \lambda_1\boldsymbol{P}_1 + \lambda_2\boldsymbol{P}_2 + \cdots + \lambda_r\boldsymbol{P}_r \tag{5.43}$$

and

$$\boldsymbol{A}'\boldsymbol{A} = \lambda_1\tilde{\boldsymbol{P}}_1 + \lambda_2\tilde{\boldsymbol{P}}_2 + \cdots + \lambda_r\tilde{\boldsymbol{P}}_r, \tag{5.44}$$

where $\lambda_j = \mu_j^2$ *is the* j*th largest eigenvalue of* $\boldsymbol{A}'\boldsymbol{A}$ *(or* $\boldsymbol{A}\boldsymbol{A}'$*).*

Proof. Use (5.37) and (5.38), and the fact that $\boldsymbol{Q}_i\boldsymbol{Q}_i' = \boldsymbol{P}_i$, $\boldsymbol{G}_i'\boldsymbol{G}_i = \tilde{\boldsymbol{P}}_i$, $\boldsymbol{Q}_i'\boldsymbol{Q}_j = \boldsymbol{O}$ $(i \neq j)$, and $\boldsymbol{G}_i\boldsymbol{G}_j' = \boldsymbol{O}$ $(i \neq j)$. Q.E.D.

Decompositions (5.43) and (5.44) above are called the spectral decompositions of $\boldsymbol{A}'\boldsymbol{A}$ and $\boldsymbol{A}\boldsymbol{A}'$, respectively. Theorem 5.4 can further be generalized as follows.

Theorem 5.5 *Let f denote an arbitrary polynomial function of the matrix $\boldsymbol{B} = \boldsymbol{A}'\boldsymbol{A}$, and let $\lambda_1, \lambda_2, \cdots, \lambda_r$ denote nonzero (positive) eigenvalues of $\boldsymbol{B}$. Then,*

$$f(\boldsymbol{B}) = f(\lambda_1)\tilde{\boldsymbol{P}}_1 + f(\lambda_2)\tilde{\boldsymbol{P}}_2 + \cdots + f(\lambda_r)\tilde{\boldsymbol{P}}_r. \tag{5.45}$$

Proof. Let s be an arbitrary natural number. From Lemma 5.2 and the fact that $\tilde{\boldsymbol{P}}_i^2 = \tilde{\boldsymbol{P}}_i$ and $\tilde{\boldsymbol{P}}_i\tilde{\boldsymbol{P}}_j = \boldsymbol{O}$ $(i \neq j)$, it follows that

$$\begin{aligned} \boldsymbol{B}^s &= (\lambda_1\tilde{\boldsymbol{P}}_1 + \lambda_2\tilde{\boldsymbol{P}}_2 + \cdots + \lambda_r\tilde{\boldsymbol{P}}_r)^s \\ &= \lambda_1^s\tilde{\boldsymbol{P}}_1 + \lambda_2^s\tilde{\boldsymbol{P}}_2 + \cdots + \lambda_r^s\tilde{\boldsymbol{P}}_r. \end{aligned}$$

Let s_1 and s_2 be two distinct natural numbers. Then,

$$v\boldsymbol{B}^{s_1} + w\boldsymbol{B}^{s_2} = \sum_{j=1}^{r}(v\lambda_j^{s_1} + w\lambda_j^{s_2})\tilde{\boldsymbol{P}}_j,$$

establishing (5.45). Q.E.D.

Corollary *Let $\boldsymbol{A}$ be an n by m matrix $(n \geq m)$. If $f(\boldsymbol{B}) = f(\boldsymbol{A}'\boldsymbol{A})$ is nonsingular,*

$$(f(\boldsymbol{B}))^{-1} = f(\lambda_1)^{-1}\tilde{\boldsymbol{P}}_1 + f(\lambda_2)^{-1}\tilde{\boldsymbol{P}}_2 + \cdots + f(\lambda_r)^{-1}\tilde{\boldsymbol{P}}_r. \tag{5.46}$$

Proof. Since $\boldsymbol{A}'\boldsymbol{A}$ is nonsingular,

$$\tilde{\boldsymbol{P}}_1 + \tilde{\boldsymbol{P}}_2 + \cdots + \tilde{\boldsymbol{P}}_r = \boldsymbol{I}_m,$$

assuming that the m eigenvalues $\lambda_1, \lambda_2, \cdots, \lambda_m$ are all distinct. Then,

$$\begin{aligned} &(f(\lambda_1)\tilde{\boldsymbol{P}}_1 + f(\lambda_2)\tilde{\boldsymbol{P}}_2 + \cdots + f(\lambda_r)\tilde{\boldsymbol{P}}_r) \\ &\qquad (f(\lambda_1)^{-1}\tilde{\boldsymbol{P}}_1 + f(\lambda_2)^{-1}\tilde{\boldsymbol{P}}_2 + \cdots + f(\lambda_r)^{-1}\tilde{\boldsymbol{P}}_r) = \boldsymbol{I}_m, \end{aligned}$$

leading to (5.46). Q.E.D.

Note If the matrix $\boldsymbol{A}'\boldsymbol{A}$ has identical roots, let $\lambda_1, \lambda_2, \cdots, \lambda_s$ $(s < r)$ denote distinct eigenvalues with their multiplicities indicated by $n_1, n_2, \cdots, n_s$ $(n_1+n_2+\cdots+n_s = r)$. Let $\boldsymbol{U}_i$ denote the matrix of n_i eigenvectors corresponding to λ_i. (The $\mathrm{Sp}(\boldsymbol{U}_i)$ constitutes the eigenspace corresponding to λ_i.) Furthermore, let

$$\boldsymbol{P}_i = \boldsymbol{U}_i\boldsymbol{U}_i', \quad \tilde{\boldsymbol{P}}_i = \boldsymbol{V}_i\boldsymbol{V}_i', \text{ and } \boldsymbol{Q}_i = \boldsymbol{U}_i\boldsymbol{V}_i',$$

analogous to (5.29). Then Lemma 5.3 and Theorems 5.3, 5.4, and 5.5 hold as stated. Note that $\boldsymbol{P}_i$ and $\tilde{\boldsymbol{P}}_i$ are orthogonal projectors of rank n_i, however.

5.3 SVD and Generalized Inverse Matrices

We consider how generalized inverses of the matrix $\boldsymbol{A}$ can be expressed in terms of its SVD given in (5.25).

Lemma 5.4 *Let the SVD of an n by m matrix $\boldsymbol{A}$ be given by (5.25), and let $\boldsymbol{S}_1$, $\boldsymbol{S}_2$, and $\boldsymbol{S}_3$ be arbitrary r by $n-r$, $m-r$ by r, and $m-r$ by $n-r$ matrices, respectively. Then a generalized inverse of $\boldsymbol{A}$ is given by*

$$\boldsymbol{A}^- = \boldsymbol{V}\begin{bmatrix} \boldsymbol{\Delta}_r & \boldsymbol{S}_1 \\ \boldsymbol{S}_2 & \boldsymbol{S}_3 \end{bmatrix}\boldsymbol{U}'. \tag{5.47}$$

Proof. Substituting $\boldsymbol{A} = \boldsymbol{U\Delta V}'$ into $\boldsymbol{AA}^-\boldsymbol{A} = \boldsymbol{A}$, we obtain $\boldsymbol{U\Delta V}'\boldsymbol{A}^-\boldsymbol{U}$ $\boldsymbol{\Delta V}' = \boldsymbol{U\Delta V}'$. Let $\boldsymbol{V}'\boldsymbol{A}^-\boldsymbol{U} = \boldsymbol{A}^*$. Then, $\boldsymbol{\Delta A}^*\boldsymbol{\Delta} = \boldsymbol{\Delta}$, namely $\boldsymbol{A}^* = \boldsymbol{\Delta}^-$, and so $\boldsymbol{A}^- = \boldsymbol{V\Delta}^-\boldsymbol{U}'$. Let

$$\boldsymbol{\Delta}^- = \begin{bmatrix} \boldsymbol{\Delta}_{11} & \boldsymbol{\Delta}_{12} \\ \boldsymbol{\Delta}_{21} & \boldsymbol{\Delta}_{22} \end{bmatrix},$$

where $\boldsymbol{\Delta}_{11}$ is r by r, $\boldsymbol{\Delta}_{12}$ is r by $n-r$, $\boldsymbol{\Delta}_{21}$ is $m-r$ by r, and $\boldsymbol{\Delta}_{22}$ is $m-r$ by $n-r$. Then, since $\boldsymbol{\Delta}$ is as given in (5.26), we have

$$\boldsymbol{\Delta\Delta}^-\boldsymbol{\Delta} = \begin{bmatrix} \boldsymbol{\Delta}_r & \boldsymbol{O} \\ \boldsymbol{O} & \boldsymbol{O} \end{bmatrix} = \boldsymbol{\Delta}.$$

Hence, we have $\boldsymbol{\Delta}_r\boldsymbol{\Delta}_{11}\boldsymbol{\Delta}_r = \boldsymbol{\Delta}_r$. Since $\boldsymbol{\Delta}_r$ is a nonsingular matrix of order r, $\boldsymbol{\Delta}_{11} = \boldsymbol{\Delta}_r^{-1}$, and the remaining submatrices can be arbitrary. Q.E.D.

The following theorem is readily derived from Lemma 5.4.

Theorem 5.6 *We have*

$$\boldsymbol{A}_r^- = \boldsymbol{V}\begin{bmatrix} \boldsymbol{\Delta}_r^{-1} & \boldsymbol{S}_1 \\ \boldsymbol{S}_2 & \boldsymbol{S}_3 \end{bmatrix}\boldsymbol{U}', \tag{5.48}$$

where $\boldsymbol{S}_3 = \boldsymbol{S}_2\boldsymbol{\Delta}_r\boldsymbol{S}_1$ and $\boldsymbol{S}_1$ and $\boldsymbol{S}_2$ are arbitrary r by $n-r$ and $m-r$ by r matrices, respectively;

$$\boldsymbol{A}_m^- = \boldsymbol{V}\begin{bmatrix} \boldsymbol{\Delta}_r^{-1} & \boldsymbol{T}_1 \\ \boldsymbol{O} & \boldsymbol{T}_2 \end{bmatrix}\boldsymbol{U}', \tag{5.49}$$

where $\boldsymbol{T}_1$ and $\boldsymbol{T}_2$ are arbitrary r by $n-r$ and $m-r$ by $n-r$ matrices, respectively;

$$\boldsymbol{A}_\ell^- = \boldsymbol{V}\begin{bmatrix} \boldsymbol{\Delta}_r^{-1} & \boldsymbol{O} \\ \boldsymbol{W}_1 & \boldsymbol{W}_2 \end{bmatrix}\boldsymbol{U}', \tag{5.50}$$

where $\boldsymbol{W}_1$ and $\boldsymbol{W}_2$ are arbitrary $m-r$ by r and $m-r$ by $n-r$ matrices, respectively, and

$$\boldsymbol{A}^+ = \boldsymbol{V}\begin{bmatrix} \boldsymbol{\Delta}_r^{-1} & \boldsymbol{O} \\ \boldsymbol{O} & \boldsymbol{O} \end{bmatrix}\boldsymbol{U}' \tag{5.51}$$

or

$$\boldsymbol{A}^+ = \frac{1}{\mu_1}\boldsymbol{v}_1\boldsymbol{u}_1' + \frac{1}{\mu_2}\boldsymbol{v}_2\boldsymbol{u}_2' + \cdots + \frac{1}{\mu_r}\boldsymbol{v}_r\boldsymbol{u}_r'. \tag{5.52}$$

Proof. (5.48): $\text{rank}(\boldsymbol{A}_r^-) = \text{rank}(\boldsymbol{A})$. Since $\boldsymbol{U}$ and $\boldsymbol{V}$ are nonsingular,

$$\text{rank}(\boldsymbol{A}_r^-) = \text{rank}\begin{bmatrix} \boldsymbol{\Delta}_r^{-1} & \boldsymbol{S}_1 \\ \boldsymbol{S}_2 & \boldsymbol{S}_3 \end{bmatrix} = \text{rank}\begin{bmatrix} \boldsymbol{\Delta}_r^{-1} \\ \boldsymbol{S}_2 \end{bmatrix} = \text{rank}(\boldsymbol{\Delta}_r^-).$$

By Example 3.3, we must have $\boldsymbol{S}_3 = \boldsymbol{S}_2\boldsymbol{\Delta}_r\boldsymbol{S}_1$.

(5.49): Since $\boldsymbol{A}_m^-\boldsymbol{A}$ is symmetric, we have

$$\begin{aligned} \boldsymbol{V}\begin{bmatrix} \boldsymbol{\Delta}_r^{-1} & \boldsymbol{S}_1 \\ \boldsymbol{S}_2 & \boldsymbol{S}_3 \end{bmatrix}\boldsymbol{U}'\boldsymbol{U}\boldsymbol{\Delta}\boldsymbol{V}' &= \begin{bmatrix} \boldsymbol{\Delta}_r^{-1} & \boldsymbol{S}_1 \\ \boldsymbol{S}_2 & \boldsymbol{S}_3 \end{bmatrix}\begin{bmatrix} \boldsymbol{\Delta}_r & \boldsymbol{O} \\ \boldsymbol{O} & \boldsymbol{O} \end{bmatrix}\boldsymbol{V}' \\ &= \boldsymbol{V}\begin{bmatrix} \boldsymbol{I}_r & \boldsymbol{O} \\ \boldsymbol{S}_2\boldsymbol{\Delta}_r & \boldsymbol{O} \end{bmatrix}\boldsymbol{V}'. \end{aligned}$$

To make the matrix above symmetric, it must be that $\boldsymbol{S}_2 = \boldsymbol{O}$.

(5.50): Since $\boldsymbol{A}\boldsymbol{A}_\ell^-$ is symmetric,

$$\boldsymbol{A}\boldsymbol{A}_\ell^- = \boldsymbol{U}\begin{bmatrix} \boldsymbol{\Delta}_r^{-1} & \boldsymbol{S}_1\boldsymbol{\Delta}_r \\ \boldsymbol{O} & \boldsymbol{O} \end{bmatrix}\boldsymbol{U}',$$

and so it must be that $\boldsymbol{S}_1 = \boldsymbol{O}$.

(5.51): Since $\boldsymbol{A}^+$ should satisfy (5.48), (5.49), and (5.50), it holds that $\boldsymbol{S}_3 = \boldsymbol{O}$. Q.E.D.

5.4 Some Properties of Singular Values

As is clear from the argument given in Section 5.1, the following two lemmas hold concerning the singular value $\mu_j(\boldsymbol{A})$ of an n by m matrix $\boldsymbol{A}$ and the eigenvalue $\lambda_j(\boldsymbol{A}'\boldsymbol{A})$ of $\boldsymbol{A}'\boldsymbol{A}$ (or $\boldsymbol{A}\boldsymbol{A}'$).

Lemma 5.5

$$\max_x \frac{||\boldsymbol{A}\boldsymbol{x}||}{||\boldsymbol{x}||} = \mu_1(\boldsymbol{A}). \tag{5.53}$$

Proof. Clear from Lemma 5.1. Q.E.D.

Lemma 5.6 *Let* $\boldsymbol{V}_1 = [\boldsymbol{v}_1, \boldsymbol{v}_2, \cdots, \boldsymbol{v}_s]$ $(s < r)$ *represent the matrix of eigenvectors of* $\boldsymbol{A}'\boldsymbol{A}$ *corresponding to the* s *largest eigenvalues. Then,*

$$\max_{V_1'x=0} \frac{\boldsymbol{x}'\boldsymbol{A}'\boldsymbol{A}\boldsymbol{x}}{\boldsymbol{x}'\boldsymbol{x}} = \lambda_{s+1}(\boldsymbol{A}'\boldsymbol{A}) \tag{5.54}$$

and

$$\max_{V_1'x=0} \frac{||\boldsymbol{A}\boldsymbol{x}||}{||\boldsymbol{x}||} = \mu_{s+1}(\boldsymbol{A}). \tag{5.55}$$

Proof. (5.54): From $\boldsymbol{V}_1'\boldsymbol{x} = \boldsymbol{0}$, we can express $\boldsymbol{x}$ as $\boldsymbol{x} = (\boldsymbol{I}_m - (\boldsymbol{V}_1')^-\boldsymbol{V}_1')\boldsymbol{z}$, where $\boldsymbol{z}$ is an arbitrary m-component vector. On the other hand, $\boldsymbol{V}_1'\boldsymbol{V}_1 = \boldsymbol{I}_s$, which implies $\boldsymbol{V}_1'\boldsymbol{V}_1\boldsymbol{V}_1' = \boldsymbol{V}_1'$, which in turn implies $\boldsymbol{V}_1 \in \{(\boldsymbol{V}_1')^-\}$. That is, $\boldsymbol{x} = (\boldsymbol{I}_m - \boldsymbol{V}_1\boldsymbol{V}_1')\boldsymbol{z}$. Let $\boldsymbol{V}_2 = [\boldsymbol{v}_{s+1}, \cdots, \boldsymbol{v}_r]$,

$$\boldsymbol{\Delta}_1^2 = \begin{bmatrix} \lambda_1 & 0 & \cdots & 0 \\ 0 & \lambda_2 & \cdots & 0 \\ \vdots & \vdots & \ddots & \vdots \\ 0 & 0 & \cdots & \lambda_s \end{bmatrix}, \text{ and } \boldsymbol{\Delta}_2^2 = \begin{bmatrix} \lambda_{s+1} & 0 & \cdots & 0 \\ 0 & \lambda_{s+2} & \cdots & 0 \\ \vdots & \vdots & \ddots & \vdots \\ 0 & 0 & \cdots & \lambda_r \end{bmatrix}.$$

From $\boldsymbol{A}'\boldsymbol{A} = \boldsymbol{V}_1\boldsymbol{\Delta}_1^2\boldsymbol{V}_1' + \boldsymbol{V}_2\boldsymbol{\Delta}_2^2\boldsymbol{V}_2'$, we obtain

$$\boldsymbol{x}'\boldsymbol{A}'\boldsymbol{A}\boldsymbol{x} = \boldsymbol{z}'\boldsymbol{V}_2\boldsymbol{\Delta}_2^2\boldsymbol{V}_2'\boldsymbol{z} = \lambda_{s+1}a_{s+1}^2 + \cdots + \lambda_r a_r^2$$

and

$$\boldsymbol{x}'\boldsymbol{x} = \boldsymbol{z}'\boldsymbol{V}_2\boldsymbol{V}_2'\boldsymbol{z} = a_{s+1}^2 + \cdots + a_r^2,$$

where $\boldsymbol{z}'\boldsymbol{V}_2 = (a_{s+1}, \cdots, a_r)$.

When $a_1, a_2, \cdots, a_r$ are all positive and $b_1 \geq b_2 \geq \cdots \geq b_r > 0$, it holds that

$$b_1 \geq \frac{a_1 b_1 + a_2 b_2 + \cdots + a_r b_r}{a_1 + a_2 + \cdots + a_r} \geq b_r, \tag{5.56}$$

which implies

$$\lambda_r \geq \frac{\boldsymbol{x}'\boldsymbol{A}'\boldsymbol{A}\boldsymbol{x}}{\boldsymbol{x}'\boldsymbol{x}} = \frac{\sum_{j=s+1}^{r} \lambda_j ||a_j||^2}{\sum_{j=s+1}^{r} ||a_j||^2} \geq \lambda_{s+1}.$$

(5.55): This is clear from the proof above by noting that $\mu_j^2 = \lambda_j$ and $\mu_j > 0$. Q.E.D.

An alternative proof. Using the SVD of the matrix $\boldsymbol{A}$, we can give a more direct proof. Since $\boldsymbol{x} \in \text{Sp}(\boldsymbol{V}_2)$, it can be expressed as

$$\boldsymbol{x} = \alpha_{s+1}\boldsymbol{v}_{s+1} + \cdots + \alpha_r \boldsymbol{v}_r = \boldsymbol{V}_2 \boldsymbol{\alpha}_s,$$

where $\alpha_{s+1}, \cdots, \alpha_r$ are appropriate weights. Using the SVD of $\boldsymbol{A}$ in (5.18), we obtain

$$\boldsymbol{A}\boldsymbol{x} = \alpha_{s+1}\mu_{s+1}\boldsymbol{u}_{s+1} + \cdots + \alpha_r \mu_r \boldsymbol{u}_r.$$

On the other hand, since $(\boldsymbol{u}_i, \boldsymbol{u}_j) = 0$ and $(\boldsymbol{v}_i, \boldsymbol{v}_j) = 0$ $(i \neq j)$, we have

$$\frac{||\boldsymbol{A}\boldsymbol{x}||^2}{||\boldsymbol{x}||^2} = \frac{\alpha_{s+1}^2\mu_{s+1}^2 + \cdots + \alpha_r^2\mu_r^2}{\alpha_{s+1}^2 + \cdots + \alpha_r^2},$$

and so

$$\mu_r^2 \leq \frac{||\boldsymbol{A}\boldsymbol{x}||^2}{||\boldsymbol{x}||^2} \leq \mu_{s+1}^2 \Rightarrow \mu_r \leq \frac{||\boldsymbol{A}\boldsymbol{x}||}{||\boldsymbol{x}||} \leq \mu_{s+1}$$

by noting $\mu_{s+1} \geq \mu_{s+2} \geq \cdots \geq \mu_r$ and using (5.56). Q.E.D.

Corollary *If we replace* $\boldsymbol{V}_1$ *by an arbitrary* n *by* s *matrix* $\boldsymbol{B}$ *in (5.55),*

$$\mu_{s+1}(\boldsymbol{A}) \leq \max_{B'x=0} \frac{||\boldsymbol{Ax}||}{||\boldsymbol{x}||} \leq \mu_1(\boldsymbol{A}). \tag{5.57}$$

Proof. The second inequality is obvious. The first inequality can be shown as follows. Since $\boldsymbol{B}'\boldsymbol{x} = \boldsymbol{0}$, $\boldsymbol{x}$ can be expressed as $\boldsymbol{x} = (\boldsymbol{I}_m - (\boldsymbol{B}')^-\boldsymbol{B}')\boldsymbol{z} = (\boldsymbol{I}_m - \boldsymbol{P}_{B'})\boldsymbol{z}$ for an arbitrary m-component vector $\boldsymbol{z}$. Let $\boldsymbol{B}' = [\boldsymbol{v}_1, \cdots, \boldsymbol{v}_s]$. Use

$$\begin{aligned} \boldsymbol{x}'\boldsymbol{A}'\boldsymbol{A}\boldsymbol{x} &= \boldsymbol{z}'(\boldsymbol{I} - \boldsymbol{P}_{B'})\boldsymbol{A}'\boldsymbol{A}(\boldsymbol{I} - \boldsymbol{P}_{B'})\boldsymbol{z} \\ &= \boldsymbol{z}'\Big(\sum_{j=s+1}^{r} \lambda_j \boldsymbol{v}_j \boldsymbol{v}_j'\Big)\boldsymbol{z}. \end{aligned}$$

Q.E.D.

The following theorem can be derived from the lemma and the corollary above.

Theorem 5.7 *Let*

$$\boldsymbol{C} = \begin{bmatrix} \boldsymbol{C}_{11} & \boldsymbol{C}_{12} \\ \boldsymbol{C}_{21} & \boldsymbol{C}_{22} \end{bmatrix},$$

where $\boldsymbol{C}_{11}$ *and* $\boldsymbol{C}_{22}$ *are square matrices of orders* k *and* $m-k$*, respectively, and* $\boldsymbol{C}_{12}$ *and* $\boldsymbol{C}_{21}$ *are* k *by* $m-k$ *and* $m-k$ *by* k *matrices, respectively. Then,*

$$\lambda_j(\boldsymbol{C}) \geq \lambda_j(\boldsymbol{C}_{11}), \;\; j = 1, \cdots, k. \tag{5.58}$$

Proof. Let $\boldsymbol{e}_j$ denote an m-component vector with the jth element being unity and all other elements being zero, and let $\boldsymbol{B} = [\boldsymbol{e}_{k+1}, \cdots, \boldsymbol{e}_m]$. Then $\boldsymbol{B}'\boldsymbol{x} = \boldsymbol{0}$ implies $\boldsymbol{x} = \boldsymbol{0}$ $(k+1 \leq j \leq m)$. Let $\boldsymbol{0}$ denote the $m-k$-component zero vector, and let $\boldsymbol{y} = (\boldsymbol{z}', \boldsymbol{0}')'$. Then,

$$\max_{B'x=0} \frac{\boldsymbol{x}'\boldsymbol{C}\boldsymbol{x}}{\boldsymbol{x}'\boldsymbol{x}} = \max_{y} \frac{\boldsymbol{y}'\boldsymbol{C}\boldsymbol{y}}{\boldsymbol{y}'\boldsymbol{y}} = \max_{z} \frac{\boldsymbol{z}'\boldsymbol{C}_{11}\boldsymbol{z}}{\boldsymbol{z}'\boldsymbol{z}}.$$

Let $\boldsymbol{V}_j$ denote the matrix of eigenvectors corresponding to the j largest eigenvalues of $\boldsymbol{C}$, and let $\boldsymbol{V}_k$ $(k < j)$ denote the matrix of eigenvectors of $\boldsymbol{C}$ corresponding to the k largest eigenvalues. Then,

$$\lambda_{j+1}(\boldsymbol{C}) = \max_{V_j'x=0} \frac{\boldsymbol{x}'\boldsymbol{C}\boldsymbol{x}}{\boldsymbol{x}'\boldsymbol{x}} \geq \max_{V_j'x=0, B'x=0} \frac{\boldsymbol{x}'\boldsymbol{C}\boldsymbol{x}}{\boldsymbol{x}'\boldsymbol{x}} = \max_{V_k'x=0} \frac{\boldsymbol{z}'\boldsymbol{C}_{11}\boldsymbol{z}}{\boldsymbol{z}'\boldsymbol{z}} \geq \lambda_{j+1}(\boldsymbol{C}_{11}).$$

Q.E.D.

Corollary *Let*

$$C = \begin{bmatrix} C_{11} & C_{12} \\ C_{21} & C_{22} \end{bmatrix} = \begin{bmatrix} A_1'A_1 & A_1'A_2 \\ A_2'A_1 & A_2'A_2 \end{bmatrix}.$$

Then,

$$\mu_j(C) \geq \mu_j(A_1) \text{ and } \mu_j(C) \geq \mu_j(A_2)$$

for $j = 1, \cdots, k$.

Proof. Use the fact that $\lambda_j(C) \geq \lambda_j(C_{11}) = \lambda_j(A_1'A_1)$ and that $\lambda_j(C) \geq \lambda_j(C_{22}) = \lambda_j(A_2'A_2)$. Q.E.D.

Lemma 5.7 *Let* A *be an* n *by* m *matrix, and let* B *be an* m *by* n *matrix. Then the following relation holds for nonzero eigenvalues of* AB *and* BA*:*

$$\lambda_j(AB) = \lambda_j(BA). \tag{5.59}$$

(Proof omitted.)

The following corollary is derived from Lemma 5.7.

Corollary *Let* T *denote an orthogonal matrix of order* m *(i.e.,* $T'T = TT' = I_m$*). Then,*

$$\lambda_j(T'A'AT) = \lambda_j(A'A) \ (j = 1, \cdots, m). \tag{5.60}$$

Proof. $\lambda_j(T'A'AT) = \lambda_j(A'ATT') = \lambda_j(A'A)$. Q.E.D.

Let T_r be a columnwise orthogonal matrix (i.e., $T_r'T_r = I_r$). The following inequality holds.

Lemma 5.8 $\lambda_j(\boldsymbol{T}_r'\boldsymbol{A}'\boldsymbol{A}\boldsymbol{T}_r) \le \lambda_j(\boldsymbol{A}'\boldsymbol{A})$ *for* $j = 1, \cdots, r$.

Proof. Let $\boldsymbol{T}_o$ be such that $\boldsymbol{T} = [\boldsymbol{T}_r, \boldsymbol{T}_o]$ is fully orthogonal (i.e., $\boldsymbol{T}'\boldsymbol{T} = \boldsymbol{T}\boldsymbol{T}' = \boldsymbol{I}_n$). Then,

$$\boldsymbol{T}'\boldsymbol{A}'\boldsymbol{A}\boldsymbol{T} = \begin{bmatrix} \boldsymbol{T}_r'\boldsymbol{A}'\boldsymbol{A}\boldsymbol{T}_r & \boldsymbol{T}_r\boldsymbol{A}'\boldsymbol{A}\boldsymbol{T}_o \\ \boldsymbol{T}_o'\boldsymbol{A}'\boldsymbol{A}\boldsymbol{T}_r & \boldsymbol{T}_o'\boldsymbol{A}'\boldsymbol{A}\boldsymbol{T}_o \end{bmatrix}.$$

Hence, from Theorem 5.7 and Lemma 5.6, we obtain

$$\lambda_j(\boldsymbol{A}'\boldsymbol{A}) = \lambda_j(\boldsymbol{T}'\boldsymbol{A}'\boldsymbol{A}\boldsymbol{T}) \ge \lambda_j(\boldsymbol{T}_r'\boldsymbol{A}'\boldsymbol{A}\boldsymbol{T}_r).$$

Q.E.D.

Let $\boldsymbol{V}_{[r]}$ denote the matrix of eigenvectors of $\boldsymbol{A}'\boldsymbol{A}$ corresponding to the r largest eigenvalues, and let $\boldsymbol{T}_r = \boldsymbol{V}_{[r]}$ in the lemma above. Then,

$$\boldsymbol{V}_{[r]}'\boldsymbol{V}\boldsymbol{\Delta}_r^2\boldsymbol{V}'\boldsymbol{V}_{[r]} = \boldsymbol{\Delta}_r^2 = \begin{bmatrix} \lambda_1 & 0 & \cdots & 0 \\ 0 & \lambda_2 & \cdots & 0 \\ \vdots & \vdots & \ddots & \vdots \\ 0 & 0 & \cdots & \lambda_r \end{bmatrix}.$$

That is, the equality holds in the lemma above when $\lambda_j(\boldsymbol{\Delta}_{[r]}^2) = \lambda_j(\boldsymbol{A}'\boldsymbol{A})$ for $j = 1, \cdots, r$.

Let $\boldsymbol{V}_{(r)}$ denote the matrix of eigenvectors of $\boldsymbol{A}'\boldsymbol{A}$ corresponding to the r smallest eigenvalues. We have

$$\boldsymbol{V}_{(r)}'\boldsymbol{V}\boldsymbol{\Delta}_r^2\boldsymbol{V}'\boldsymbol{V}_{(r)} = \boldsymbol{\Delta}_{(r)}^2 = \begin{bmatrix} \lambda_{m-r+1} & 0 & \cdots & 0 \\ 0 & \lambda_{m-r+2} & \cdots & 0 \\ \vdots & \vdots & \ddots & \vdots \\ 0 & 0 & \cdots & \lambda_m \end{bmatrix}.$$

Hence, $\lambda_j(\boldsymbol{\Delta}_{(r)}^2) = \lambda_{m-r+j}(\boldsymbol{A}'\boldsymbol{A})$, and the following theorem holds.

Theorem 5.8 *Let* $\boldsymbol{A}$ *be an* n *by* m *matrix, and let* $\boldsymbol{T}_r$ *be an* m *by* r *columnwise orthogonal matrix. Then,*

$$\lambda_{m-r+j}(\boldsymbol{A}'\boldsymbol{A}) \le \lambda_j(\boldsymbol{T}_r'\boldsymbol{A}'\boldsymbol{A}\boldsymbol{T}_r) \le \lambda_j(\boldsymbol{A}'\boldsymbol{A}). \tag{5.61}$$

(Proof omitted.)

The inequalities above hold even if we replace $\boldsymbol{A}'\boldsymbol{A}$ by any symmetric matrix, as is clear from the proof above. (Theorem 5.8 is called the Poincaré Separation Theorem.)

The following result can be derived from the theorem above (Rao, 1979).

Corollary *Let* $\boldsymbol{A}$ *be an* n *by* m *matrix, and let* $\boldsymbol{B}$ *and* $\boldsymbol{C}$ *denote* n *by* r *and* m *by* k *matrices, respectively, such that* $\boldsymbol{B}'\boldsymbol{B} = \boldsymbol{I}_r$ *and* $\boldsymbol{C}'\boldsymbol{C} = \boldsymbol{I}_k$. *Furthermore, let* $\mu_j(\boldsymbol{A})$ *represent the* j*th largest singular value of* $\boldsymbol{A}$. *Then,*

$$\mu_{j+t}(\boldsymbol{A}) \le \mu_j(\boldsymbol{B}'\boldsymbol{A}\boldsymbol{C}) \le \mu_j(\boldsymbol{A}) \text{ for } j = 1, \cdots, \min(r, k), \tag{5.62}$$

where $t = m + n - r - k$.

Proof. The second inequality holds because $\mu_j^2(\boldsymbol{B}'\boldsymbol{A}\boldsymbol{C}) = \lambda_j(\boldsymbol{B}'\boldsymbol{A}\boldsymbol{C}\boldsymbol{C}'\boldsymbol{A}'\boldsymbol{B}) \le \lambda_j(\boldsymbol{A}\boldsymbol{C}\boldsymbol{C}'\boldsymbol{A}') = \lambda_j(\boldsymbol{C}'\boldsymbol{A}'\boldsymbol{A}\boldsymbol{C}) \le \lambda_j(\boldsymbol{A}'\boldsymbol{A}) = \mu_j^2(\boldsymbol{A})$. The first inequality holds because $\mu_j^2(\boldsymbol{B}'\boldsymbol{A}\boldsymbol{C}) = \lambda_j(\boldsymbol{B}'\boldsymbol{A}\boldsymbol{C}\boldsymbol{C}'\boldsymbol{A}'\boldsymbol{B}) \ge \lambda_{j+m-r}(\boldsymbol{A}\boldsymbol{C}\boldsymbol{C}'\boldsymbol{A}') = \lambda_{j+m-r}(\boldsymbol{C}'\boldsymbol{A}'\boldsymbol{A}\boldsymbol{C}) \ge \lambda_{t+j}(\boldsymbol{A}'\boldsymbol{A}) = \mu_{j+t}^2(\boldsymbol{A})$. Q.E.D.

The following theorem is derived from the result above.

Theorem 5.9 (i) *Let* $\boldsymbol{P}$ *denote an orthogonal projector of order* m *and rank* k. *Then,*

$$\lambda_{m-k+j}(\boldsymbol{A}'\boldsymbol{A}) \le \lambda_j(\boldsymbol{A}'\boldsymbol{P}\boldsymbol{A}) \le \lambda_j(\boldsymbol{A}'\boldsymbol{A}), \quad j = 1, \cdots, k. \tag{5.63}$$

(ii) *Let* $\boldsymbol{P}_1$ *denote an orthogonal projector of order* n *and rank* r, *and let* $\boldsymbol{P}_2$ *denote an orthogonal projector of order* m *and rank* k. *Then,*

$$\mu_{j+t}(\boldsymbol{A}) \le \mu_j(\boldsymbol{P}_1\boldsymbol{A}\boldsymbol{P}_2) \le \mu_j(\boldsymbol{A}), \quad j = 1, \cdots, \min(k, r), \tag{5.64}$$

where $t = m - r + n - k$.

Proof. (i): Decompose $\boldsymbol{P}$ as $\boldsymbol{P} = \boldsymbol{T}_k\boldsymbol{T}_k'$, where $\boldsymbol{T}_k'\boldsymbol{T}_k = \boldsymbol{I}_k$. Since $\boldsymbol{P}^2 = \boldsymbol{P}$, we obtain $\lambda_j(\boldsymbol{A}'\boldsymbol{P}\boldsymbol{A}) = \lambda_j(\boldsymbol{P}\boldsymbol{A}\boldsymbol{A}'\boldsymbol{P}) = \lambda_j(\boldsymbol{T}_k\boldsymbol{T}_k'\boldsymbol{A}\boldsymbol{A}'\boldsymbol{T}_k\boldsymbol{T}_k') = \lambda_j(\boldsymbol{T}_k'\boldsymbol{A}\boldsymbol{A}'\boldsymbol{T}_k\boldsymbol{T}_k'\boldsymbol{T}_k) = \lambda_j(\boldsymbol{T}_k'\boldsymbol{A}\boldsymbol{A}'\boldsymbol{T}_k) \le \lambda_j(\boldsymbol{A}\boldsymbol{A}') = \lambda(\boldsymbol{A}'\boldsymbol{A})$.

(ii): Let $\boldsymbol{P}_1 = \boldsymbol{T}_r\boldsymbol{T}_r'$, where $\boldsymbol{T}_r'\boldsymbol{T}_r = \boldsymbol{I}_r$, and let $\boldsymbol{P}_2 = \boldsymbol{T}_k\boldsymbol{T}_k'$, where $\boldsymbol{T}_k'\boldsymbol{T}_k = \boldsymbol{I}_k$. The rest is similar to (i). Q.E.D.

The following result is derived from the theorem above (Rao, 1980).

Corollary *If* $\boldsymbol{A}'\boldsymbol{A} - \boldsymbol{B}'\boldsymbol{B} \geq \boldsymbol{O}$,

$$\mu_j(\boldsymbol{A}) \geq \mu_j(\boldsymbol{B}) \text{ for } j = 1, \cdots, r;\ r = \min(\text{rank}(\boldsymbol{A}), \text{rank}(\boldsymbol{B})).$$

Proof. Let $\boldsymbol{A}'\boldsymbol{A} - \boldsymbol{B}'\boldsymbol{B} = \boldsymbol{C}'\boldsymbol{C}$. Then,

$$\begin{aligned}\boldsymbol{A}'\boldsymbol{A} = \boldsymbol{B}'\boldsymbol{B} + \boldsymbol{C}'\boldsymbol{C} &= [\boldsymbol{B}', \boldsymbol{C}'] \begin{bmatrix} \boldsymbol{B} \\ \boldsymbol{C} \end{bmatrix} \\ &\geq [\boldsymbol{B}', \boldsymbol{C}'] \begin{bmatrix} \boldsymbol{I} & \boldsymbol{O} \\ \boldsymbol{O} & \boldsymbol{O} \end{bmatrix} \begin{bmatrix} \boldsymbol{B} \\ \boldsymbol{C} \end{bmatrix} = \boldsymbol{B}'\boldsymbol{B}.\end{aligned}$$

Since $\begin{bmatrix} \boldsymbol{I} & \boldsymbol{O} \\ \boldsymbol{O} & \boldsymbol{O} \end{bmatrix}$ is an orthogonal projection matrix, the theorem above applies and $\mu_j(\boldsymbol{A}) \geq \mu_j(\boldsymbol{B})$ follows. Q.E.D.

Example 5.3 Let $\boldsymbol{X}_R$ denote a data matrix of raw scores, and let $\boldsymbol{X}$ denote a matrix of mean deviation scores. From (2.18), we have $\boldsymbol{X} = \boldsymbol{Q}_M\boldsymbol{X}_R$, and

$$\boldsymbol{X}_R = \boldsymbol{P}_M\boldsymbol{X}_R + \boldsymbol{Q}_M\boldsymbol{X}_R = \boldsymbol{P}_M\boldsymbol{X}_R + \boldsymbol{X}.$$

Since $\boldsymbol{X}_R'\boldsymbol{X}_R = \boldsymbol{X}_R'\boldsymbol{P}_M\boldsymbol{X}_R + \boldsymbol{X}'\boldsymbol{X}$, we obtain $\lambda_j(\boldsymbol{X}_R'\boldsymbol{X}_R) \geq \lambda_j(\boldsymbol{X}'\boldsymbol{X})$ (or $\mu_j(\boldsymbol{X}_R) \geq \mu_j(\boldsymbol{X})$). Let

$$\boldsymbol{X}_R = \begin{bmatrix} 0 & 1 & 2 & 3 & 4 \\ 2 & 1 & 1 & 2 & 0 \\ 0 & 2 & 1 & 0 & 2 \\ 0 & 1 & 2 & 2 & 1 \\ 3 & 1 & 2 & 0 & 3 \\ 4 & 3 & 3 & 2 & 7 \end{bmatrix}.$$

Then,

$$\boldsymbol{X} = \begin{bmatrix} -1.5 & -0.5 & 1/6 & 1.5 & 7/6 \\ 0.5 & -0.5 & -5/6 & 0.5 & -17/6 \\ -1.5 & 0.5 & -5/6 & -1.5 & -5/6 \\ -1.5 & -0.5 & 1/6 & 0.5 & -11/6 \\ 1.5 & -0.5 & 1/6 & -1.5 & 1/6 \\ 2.5 & 1.5 & 7/6 & 0.5 & 25/6 \end{bmatrix}$$

and

$$\begin{aligned} \mu_1(\boldsymbol{X}_R) &= 4.813, & \mu_1(\boldsymbol{X}) &= 3.936, \\ \mu_2(\boldsymbol{X}_R) &= 3.953, & \mu_2(\boldsymbol{X}) &= 3.309, \\ \mu_3(\boldsymbol{X}_R) &= 3.724, & \mu_3(\boldsymbol{X}) &= 2.671, \\ \mu_4(\boldsymbol{X}_R) &= 1.645, & \mu_4(\boldsymbol{X}) &= 1.171, \\ \mu_5(\boldsymbol{X}_R) &= 1.066, & \mu_5(\boldsymbol{X}) &= 0.471. \end{aligned}$$

Clearly, $\mu_j(\boldsymbol{X}_R) \geq \mu_j(\boldsymbol{X})$ holds.

The following theorem is derived from Theorem 5.9 and its corollary.

Theorem 5.10 *Let $\boldsymbol{A}$ denote an n by m matrix of rank r, and let $\boldsymbol{B}$ denote a matrix of the same size but of rank k ($k < r$). Furthermore, let $\boldsymbol{A} = \boldsymbol{U}\boldsymbol{\Delta}_r\boldsymbol{V}'$ denote the SVD of $\boldsymbol{A}$, where $\boldsymbol{U} = [\boldsymbol{u}_1, \boldsymbol{u}_2, \cdots, \boldsymbol{u}_r]$, $\boldsymbol{V} = [\boldsymbol{v}_1, \boldsymbol{v}_2, \cdots, \boldsymbol{v}_r]$, and $\boldsymbol{\Delta}_r = \mathrm{diag}(\mu_1, \mu_2, \cdots, \mu_r)$. Then,*

$$\begin{aligned} \mu_j(\boldsymbol{A}-\boldsymbol{B}) &\geq \mu_{j+k}(\boldsymbol{A}), \quad \text{if } j+k \leq r, \\ &\geq 0, \qquad\qquad\quad \text{if } j+k > r, \end{aligned} \tag{5.65}$$

where the equality in (5.65) holds when

$$\boldsymbol{B} = \mu_1\boldsymbol{u}_1\boldsymbol{v}_1' + \mu_2\boldsymbol{u}_2\boldsymbol{v}_2' + \cdots, \mu_k\boldsymbol{u}_k\boldsymbol{v}_k'. \tag{5.66}$$

Proof. (5.65): Let $\boldsymbol{P}_B$ denote the orthogonal projector onto $\mathrm{Sp}(\boldsymbol{B})$. Then, $(\boldsymbol{A}-\boldsymbol{B})'(\boldsymbol{I}_n-\boldsymbol{P}_B)(\boldsymbol{A}-\boldsymbol{B}) = \boldsymbol{A}'(\boldsymbol{I}_n-\boldsymbol{P}_B)\boldsymbol{A}$, and we obtain, using Theorem 5.9,

$$\begin{aligned} \mu_j^2(\boldsymbol{A}-\boldsymbol{B}) &= \lambda_j[(\boldsymbol{A}-\boldsymbol{B})'(\boldsymbol{A}-\boldsymbol{B})] \geq \lambda_j[\boldsymbol{A}'(\boldsymbol{I}_n-\boldsymbol{P}_B)\boldsymbol{A}] \\ &\geq \lambda_{j+k}(\boldsymbol{A}'\boldsymbol{A}) = \mu_{j+k}^2(\boldsymbol{A}), \end{aligned} \tag{5.67}$$

when $k + j \leq r$.

(5.65): The first inequality in (5.67) can be replaced by an equality when $\boldsymbol{A}-\boldsymbol{B} = (\boldsymbol{I}_n-\boldsymbol{P}_B)\boldsymbol{A}$, which implies $\boldsymbol{B} = \boldsymbol{P}_B\boldsymbol{A}$. Let $\boldsymbol{I}_n - \boldsymbol{P}_B = \boldsymbol{T}\boldsymbol{T}'$, where $\boldsymbol{T}$ is an n by $r-k$ matrix such that $\boldsymbol{T}'\boldsymbol{T} = \boldsymbol{I}_{r-k}$. Using the fact that $\boldsymbol{T} = [\boldsymbol{u}_{k+1}, \cdots, \boldsymbol{u}_r] = \boldsymbol{U}_{r-k}$ holds when the second equality in (5.67) holds, we obtain

$$\begin{aligned} \boldsymbol{B} &= \boldsymbol{P}_B\boldsymbol{A} = (\boldsymbol{I}_n - \boldsymbol{U}_{r-k}\boldsymbol{U}_{r-k}')\boldsymbol{A} \\ &= \boldsymbol{U}_{[k]}\boldsymbol{U}_{[k]}'\boldsymbol{U}\boldsymbol{\Delta}_r\boldsymbol{V}' \\ &= \boldsymbol{U}_{[k]}\begin{bmatrix} \boldsymbol{I}_k & \boldsymbol{O} \\ \boldsymbol{O} & \boldsymbol{O} \end{bmatrix}\begin{bmatrix} \boldsymbol{\Delta}_{[k]} & \boldsymbol{O} \\ \boldsymbol{O} & \boldsymbol{\Delta}_{(r-k)} \end{bmatrix}\boldsymbol{V}' \\ &= \boldsymbol{U}_{[k]}\boldsymbol{\Delta}_{[k]}\boldsymbol{V}_{[k]}'. \end{aligned} \tag{5.68}$$

Q.E.D.

Theorem 5.10 implies

$$\lambda_j[(\boldsymbol{A}-\boldsymbol{B})'(\boldsymbol{A}-\boldsymbol{B})] \geq \lambda_{j+k}(\boldsymbol{A}'\boldsymbol{A}) \ \textit{for} \ j+k \geq r. \tag{5.69}$$

Let $\boldsymbol{A}$ and $\boldsymbol{B}$ be n by m matrices of ranks r and k $(< r)$, respectively. Then,

$$\text{tr}(\boldsymbol{A}-\boldsymbol{B})'(\boldsymbol{A}-\boldsymbol{B}) \geq \lambda_{k+1}(\boldsymbol{A}'\boldsymbol{A}) + \cdots + \lambda_r(\boldsymbol{A}'\boldsymbol{A}) \tag{5.70}$$

holds. The equality holds in the inequality above when $\boldsymbol{B}$ is given by (5.68).

5.5 Exercises for Chapter 5

1. Apply the SVD to $\boldsymbol{A} = \begin{bmatrix} 1 & -2 \\ -2 & 1 \\ 1 & 1 \end{bmatrix}$, and obtain $\boldsymbol{A}^+$.

2. Show that the maximum value of $(\boldsymbol{x}'\boldsymbol{A}\boldsymbol{y})^2$ under the condition $||\boldsymbol{x}|| = ||\boldsymbol{y}|| = 1$ is equal to the square of the largest singular value of $\boldsymbol{A}$.

3. Show that $\lambda_j(\boldsymbol{A}+\boldsymbol{A}') \leq 2\mu_j(\boldsymbol{A})$ for an arbitrary square matrix $\boldsymbol{A}$, where $\lambda_j(\boldsymbol{A})$ and $\mu_j(\boldsymbol{A})$ are the jth largest eigenvalue and singular value of $\boldsymbol{A}$, respectively.

4. Let $\boldsymbol{A} = \boldsymbol{U}\boldsymbol{\Delta}\boldsymbol{V}'$ denote the SVD of an arbitrary n by m matrix $\boldsymbol{A}$, and let $\boldsymbol{S}$ and $\boldsymbol{T}$ be orthogonal matrices of orders n and m, respectively. Show that the SVD of $\tilde{\boldsymbol{A}} = \boldsymbol{S}\boldsymbol{A}\boldsymbol{T}$ is given by $\tilde{\boldsymbol{A}} = \tilde{\boldsymbol{U}}\boldsymbol{\Delta}\tilde{\boldsymbol{V}}'$, where $\tilde{\boldsymbol{U}} = \boldsymbol{S}\boldsymbol{U}$ and $\tilde{\boldsymbol{V}} = \boldsymbol{T}\boldsymbol{V}$.

5. Let

$$\boldsymbol{A} = \lambda_1\boldsymbol{P}_1 + \lambda_2\boldsymbol{P}_2 + \cdots + \lambda_n\boldsymbol{P}_n$$

denote the spectral decomposition of $\boldsymbol{A}$, where $\boldsymbol{P}_i^2 = \boldsymbol{P}_i$ and $\boldsymbol{P}_i\boldsymbol{P}_j = \boldsymbol{O}$ $(i \neq j)$. Define

$$e^A = \boldsymbol{I} + \boldsymbol{A} + \frac{1}{2}\boldsymbol{A}^2 + \frac{1}{3!}\boldsymbol{A}^3 + \cdots.$$

Show that

$$e^A = e^{\lambda_1}\boldsymbol{P}_1 + e^{\lambda_2}\boldsymbol{P}_2 + \cdots, + e^{\lambda_n}\boldsymbol{P}_n.$$

6. Show that the necessary and sufficient condition for all the singular values of $\boldsymbol{A}$ to be unity is $\boldsymbol{A}' \in \{\boldsymbol{A}^-\}$.

7. Let $\boldsymbol{A}$, $\boldsymbol{B}$, $\boldsymbol{C}$, $\boldsymbol{X}$, and $\boldsymbol{Y}$ be as defined in Theorem 2.25. Show the following:
(i) $\mu_j(\boldsymbol{A}-\boldsymbol{B}\boldsymbol{X}) \geq \mu_j((\boldsymbol{I}_n - \boldsymbol{P}_B)\boldsymbol{A})$.
(ii) $\mu_j(\boldsymbol{A}-\boldsymbol{Y}\boldsymbol{C}) \geq \mu_j(\boldsymbol{A}(\boldsymbol{I}_n - \boldsymbol{P}_{C'}))$.
(iii) $\mu_j(\boldsymbol{A}-\boldsymbol{B}\boldsymbol{X}-\boldsymbol{Y}\boldsymbol{C}) \geq \mu_j[(\boldsymbol{I}_n - \boldsymbol{P}_B)\boldsymbol{A}(\boldsymbol{I}_n - \boldsymbol{P}_{C'})]$.

8. Let $\boldsymbol{B}$ denote an orthogonal projector of rank r. Show that

$$\sum_{i=1}^{r} \lambda_{n-i+1} \leq \operatorname{tr}(\boldsymbol{AB}) \leq \sum_{i=1}^{r} \lambda_i,$$

where $\boldsymbol{A}$ is a symmetric matrix of order n having eigenvalues $\lambda_1 \geq \lambda_2 \geq \cdots \geq \lambda_n$.

9. Using the SVD of $\boldsymbol{A}$, show that, among the $\boldsymbol{x}$'s that minimize $||\boldsymbol{y} - \boldsymbol{Ax}||^2$, the $\boldsymbol{x}$ that minimizes $||\boldsymbol{x}||^2$ is given by $\boldsymbol{x} = \boldsymbol{A}'\boldsymbol{y}$.

10. Let $\boldsymbol{A}$ be a given n by p matrix whose SVD is given by $\boldsymbol{A} = \boldsymbol{U\Delta V}'$, and let $\phi(\boldsymbol{B}) = ||\boldsymbol{A} - \boldsymbol{B}||^2$. Show that $\boldsymbol{B}$ that minimizes $\phi(\boldsymbol{B})$ subject to $\operatorname{rank}(\boldsymbol{B}) = k$ $(< p)$ is obtained by

$$\boldsymbol{B} = \boldsymbol{U}_k\boldsymbol{\Delta}_k\boldsymbol{V}_k',$$

where $\boldsymbol{U}_k$, $\boldsymbol{\Delta}_k$, and $\boldsymbol{V}_k$ are portions of $\boldsymbol{U}$, $\boldsymbol{\Delta}$, and $\boldsymbol{V}$ pertaining to the k largest singular values of $\boldsymbol{A}$.

11. Let $\boldsymbol{A}$ and $\boldsymbol{B}$ be two matrices of the same size. Show that the orthogonal matrix $\boldsymbol{T}$ of order p that minimizes $\phi(\boldsymbol{T}) = ||\boldsymbol{B} - \boldsymbol{AT}||^2$ is obtained by

$$\boldsymbol{T} = \boldsymbol{UV}',$$

where $\boldsymbol{A}'\boldsymbol{B} = \boldsymbol{U\Delta V}'$ is the SVD of $\boldsymbol{A}'\boldsymbol{B}$. (This problem is called the orthogonal Procrustes rotation problem (Schönemann, 1966). The matrix $\boldsymbol{B}$ is called a target matrix, and $\boldsymbol{A}$ is the matrix to be rotated into a best match with $\boldsymbol{B}$.)

Chapter 6

Various Applications

6.1 Linear Regression Analysis

6.1.1 The method of least squares and multiple regression analysis

Linear regression analysis represents the criterion variable y by the sum of a linear combination of p predictor variables $x_1, x_2, \cdots, x_p$ and an error term ϵ,

$$y_j = \alpha + \beta_1 x_{1j} + \cdots + \beta_p x_{pj} + \epsilon_j \quad (j = 1, \cdots, n), \tag{6.1}$$

where j indexes cases (observation units, subjects, etc.) and n indicates the total number of cases, and where α and β_i $(i = 1, \cdots, p)$ are regression coefficients (parameters) to be estimated. Assume first that the error terms $\epsilon_1, \epsilon_2, \cdots, \epsilon_n$ are mutually independent with an equal variance σ^2. We may obtain the estimates $a, b_1, \cdots, b_p$ of the regression coefficients using the method of least squares (LS) that minimizes

$$\sum_{j=1}^{n} (y_j - a_1 - b_1 x_{1j} - \cdots - b_p x_{pj})^2. \tag{6.2}$$

Differentiating (6.2) with respect to a and setting the results to zero, we obtain

$$a = \bar{y} - b_1 \bar{x}_1 - \cdots - b_p \bar{x}_p. \tag{6.3}$$

Substituting this into (6.2), we may rewrite (6.2) as

$$||\boldsymbol{y} - b_1 \boldsymbol{x}_x - b_2 \boldsymbol{x}_2 - \cdots - b_p \boldsymbol{x}_p||^2 = ||\boldsymbol{y} - \boldsymbol{X}\boldsymbol{b}||^2, \tag{6.4}$$

where $\boldsymbol{X} = [\boldsymbol{x}_1, \boldsymbol{x}_2, \cdots, \boldsymbol{x}_p]$ and $\boldsymbol{x}_i$ is the vector of mean deviation scores. The $\boldsymbol{b} = (b_1, b_2, \cdots, b_p)'$ that minimizes the criterion above is obtained by solving

$$\boldsymbol{P}_X \boldsymbol{y} = \boldsymbol{X}\boldsymbol{b}, \tag{6.5}$$

where $\boldsymbol{P}_X$ is the orthogonal projector onto $\mathrm{Sp}(\boldsymbol{X})$ and

$$\boldsymbol{b} = \boldsymbol{X}_\ell^- \boldsymbol{y} + (\boldsymbol{I}_p - \boldsymbol{X}_\ell^- \boldsymbol{X})\boldsymbol{z},$$

where $\boldsymbol{z}$ is an arbitrary p-component vector. Assume that $\boldsymbol{x}_1, \boldsymbol{x}_2, \cdots, \boldsymbol{x}_p$ are linearly independent. From (4.30), we get

$$\boldsymbol{P}_X = \boldsymbol{P}_{1\cdot(1)} + \boldsymbol{P}_{2\cdot(2)} + \cdots + \boldsymbol{P}_{p\cdot(p)},$$

where $\boldsymbol{P}_{j\cdot(j)}$ is the projector onto $\mathrm{Sp}(\boldsymbol{x}_j)$ along $\mathrm{Sp}(\boldsymbol{X}_{(j)}) \dot{\oplus} \mathrm{Sp}(\boldsymbol{X})^\perp$, where $\mathrm{Sp}(\boldsymbol{X}_{(j)}) = \mathrm{Sp}([\boldsymbol{x}_1, \cdots, \boldsymbol{x}_{j-1}, \boldsymbol{x}_{j+1}, \cdots, \boldsymbol{x}_p])$. From (4.27), we obtain

$$\boldsymbol{b}_j \boldsymbol{x}_j = \boldsymbol{P}_{j\cdot(j)} \boldsymbol{y} = \boldsymbol{x}_j (\boldsymbol{x}_j' \boldsymbol{Q}_{(j)} \boldsymbol{x}_j)^{-1} \boldsymbol{x}_j' \boldsymbol{Q}_{(j)} \boldsymbol{y}, \tag{6.6}$$

where $\boldsymbol{Q}_{(j)}$ is the orthogonal projector onto $\mathrm{Sp}(\boldsymbol{X}_{(j)})^\perp$ and the estimate b_j of the parameter β_j is given by

$$b_j = (\boldsymbol{x}_j' \boldsymbol{Q}_{(j)} \boldsymbol{x}_j)^{-1} \boldsymbol{x}_j' \boldsymbol{Q}_{(j)} \boldsymbol{y} = (\boldsymbol{x}_j)^-_{\ell(X_{(j)})} \boldsymbol{y}, \tag{6.7}$$

where $(\boldsymbol{x}_j)^-_{\ell(X_{(j)})}$ is a $\boldsymbol{X}_{(j)}$-constrained (least squares) g-inverse of $\boldsymbol{x}_j$. Let $\tilde{\boldsymbol{x}}_j = \boldsymbol{Q}_{(j)} \boldsymbol{x}_j$. The formula above can be rewritten as

$$b_j = (\tilde{\boldsymbol{x}}_j, \boldsymbol{y}) / ||\tilde{\boldsymbol{x}}_j||^2. \tag{6.8}$$

This indicates that b_j represents the regression coefficient when the effects of $\boldsymbol{X}_{(j)}$ are eliminated from $\boldsymbol{x}_j$; that is, it can be considered as the regression coefficient for $\tilde{\boldsymbol{x}}_j$ as the explanatory variable. In this sense, it is called the partial regression coefficient. It is interesting to note that b_j is obtained by minimizing

$$||\boldsymbol{y} - b_j \boldsymbol{x}_j||^2_{Q_{(j)}} = (\boldsymbol{y} - b_j \boldsymbol{x}_j)' \boldsymbol{Q}_{(j)} (\boldsymbol{y} - b_j \boldsymbol{x}_j). \tag{6.9}$$

(See Figure 6.1.)

When the vectors in $\boldsymbol{X} = [\boldsymbol{x}_1, \boldsymbol{x}_2, \cdots, \boldsymbol{x}_p]$ are not linearly independent, we may choose $\boldsymbol{X}_1, \boldsymbol{X}_2, \cdots, \boldsymbol{X}_m$ in such a way that $\mathrm{Sp}(\boldsymbol{X})$ is a direct-sum of the m subspaces $\mathrm{Sp}(\boldsymbol{X}_j)$. That is,

$$\mathrm{Sp}(\boldsymbol{X}) = \mathrm{Sp}(\boldsymbol{X}_1) \oplus \mathrm{Sp}(\boldsymbol{X}_2) \oplus \cdots \oplus \mathrm{Sp}(\boldsymbol{X}_m) \quad (m < p). \tag{6.10}$$

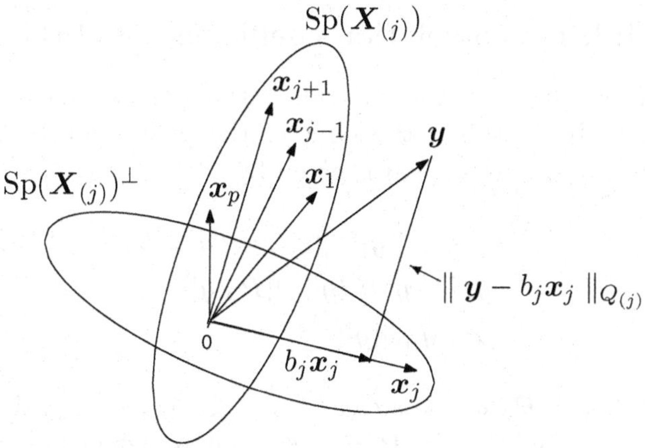

Figure 6.1: Geometric representation of a partial correlation coefficient.

Let $\boldsymbol{b}_j$ denote the vector of partial regression coefficients corresponding to $\boldsymbol{X}_j$. Then, $\boldsymbol{X}_j\boldsymbol{b}_j = \boldsymbol{P}_{X_j \cdot X_{(j)}}$; that is,

$$\boldsymbol{X}_j\boldsymbol{b}_j = \boldsymbol{X}_j(\boldsymbol{X}_j'\boldsymbol{Q}_{(j)}\boldsymbol{X}_j)^-\boldsymbol{X}_j'\boldsymbol{Q}_{(j)}\boldsymbol{y}, \tag{6.11}$$

where $\boldsymbol{Q}_{(j)}$ is the orthogonal projector onto $\text{Sp}(\boldsymbol{X}_1) \oplus \cdots \oplus \text{Sp}(\boldsymbol{X}_{j-1}) \oplus \text{Sp}(\boldsymbol{X}_{j+1}) \oplus \cdots \oplus \text{Sp}(\boldsymbol{X}_m)$.

If $\boldsymbol{X}_j'\boldsymbol{X}_j$ is nonsingular,

$$\boldsymbol{b}_j = (\boldsymbol{X}_j'\boldsymbol{Q}_{(j)}\boldsymbol{X}_j)^{-1}\boldsymbol{X}_j'\boldsymbol{Q}_{(j)}\boldsymbol{y} = (\boldsymbol{X}_j)^{-1}_{\ell(X_{(j)})}\boldsymbol{y}, \tag{6.12}$$

where $(\boldsymbol{X}_j)^{-1}_{\ell(X_{(j)})}$ is the $\boldsymbol{X}_{(j)}$-constrained least squares g-inverse of $\boldsymbol{X}_j$. If, on the other hand, $\boldsymbol{X}_j'\boldsymbol{X}_j$ is singular, $\boldsymbol{b}_j$ is not uniquely determined. In this case, $\boldsymbol{b}_j$ may be constrained to satisfy

$$\boldsymbol{C}_j\boldsymbol{b}_j = \boldsymbol{0} \Leftrightarrow \boldsymbol{b}_j = \boldsymbol{Q}_{C_j}\boldsymbol{z}, \tag{6.13}$$

where $\boldsymbol{z}$ is arbitrary and $\boldsymbol{C}_j$ is such that $E^{k_j} = \text{Sp}(\boldsymbol{X}_j') \oplus \text{Sp}(\boldsymbol{C}_j')$ and $k_j = \text{rank}(\boldsymbol{X}_j) + \text{rank}(\boldsymbol{C}_j)$. From (4.97), we obtain

$$\boldsymbol{X}_j\boldsymbol{b}_j = \boldsymbol{P}_{X_j \cdot X_{(j)}}\boldsymbol{y} = \boldsymbol{X}_j(\boldsymbol{X}_j)^+_{X_{(j)} \cdot C_j}\boldsymbol{y}. \tag{6.14}$$

Premultiplying the equation above by $(\boldsymbol{X}_j)^+_{X_{(j)} \cdot C_j}$, we obtain

$$\begin{aligned} \boldsymbol{b}_j &= (\boldsymbol{X}_j)^+_{X_{(j)} \cdot C_j}\boldsymbol{y} \\ &= (\boldsymbol{X}_j'\boldsymbol{X}_j + \boldsymbol{C}_j'\boldsymbol{C}_j)^{-1}\boldsymbol{X}_j'\boldsymbol{X}_j\boldsymbol{X}_j'(\boldsymbol{X}_j\boldsymbol{X}_j' + \boldsymbol{X}_{(j)}\boldsymbol{X}_{(j)}')^{-1}\boldsymbol{y}. \end{aligned} \tag{6.15}$$

6.1.2 Multiple correlation coefficients and their partitions

The correlation between the criterion variable y and its estimate $\hat{y}$ obtained as described above (this is the same as the correlation between y_R and $\hat{y}_R$, where $_R$ indicates raw scores) is given by

$$\begin{aligned} r_{y\hat{y}} &= (\boldsymbol{y}, \hat{\boldsymbol{y}})/(||\boldsymbol{y}|| \cdot ||\hat{\boldsymbol{y}}||) = (\boldsymbol{y}, \boldsymbol{X}\boldsymbol{b})/(||\boldsymbol{y}|| \cdot ||\boldsymbol{X}\boldsymbol{b}||) \\ &= (\boldsymbol{y}, \boldsymbol{P}_X\boldsymbol{y})/(||\boldsymbol{y}|| \cdot ||\boldsymbol{P}_X\boldsymbol{y}||) \\ &= ||\boldsymbol{P}_X\boldsymbol{y}||/||\boldsymbol{y}|| \end{aligned} \tag{6.16}$$

since $\hat{\boldsymbol{y}} = \boldsymbol{X}\boldsymbol{b} = \boldsymbol{P}_X\boldsymbol{y}$. It is clear from (2.56) that $r_{y\hat{y}}$ does not exceed 1. It is equal to 1 only when $\boldsymbol{P}_x\boldsymbol{y} = \boldsymbol{y}$, that is, when $\boldsymbol{y} \in \text{Sp}(\boldsymbol{X})$. The $r_{y\hat{y}}$ is often denoted as $R_{X \cdot y}$, which is called the multiple correlation coefficient in predicting the criterion variable $\boldsymbol{y}$ from the set of predictor variables $\boldsymbol{X} = [\boldsymbol{x}_1, \boldsymbol{x}_2, \cdots, \boldsymbol{x}_p]$. Its square, $R^2_{X \cdot y}$, is often called the coefficient of determination, and can be expanded as

$$\begin{aligned} R^2_{X \cdot y} &= \boldsymbol{y}'\boldsymbol{X}(\boldsymbol{X}'\boldsymbol{X})^-\boldsymbol{X}'\boldsymbol{y}/\boldsymbol{y}'\boldsymbol{y} \\ &= \boldsymbol{c}'_{Xy}\boldsymbol{C}^-_{XX}\boldsymbol{c}_{Xy}/s^2_y \\ &= \boldsymbol{r}'_{Xy}\boldsymbol{R}^-_{XX}\boldsymbol{r}_{Xy}, \end{aligned}$$

where $\boldsymbol{c}_{Xy}$ and $\boldsymbol{r}_{Xy}$ are the covariance and the correlation vectors between $\boldsymbol{X}$ and $\boldsymbol{y}$, respectively, $\boldsymbol{C}_{XX}$ and $\boldsymbol{R}_{XX}$ are covariance and correlation matrices of $\boldsymbol{X}$, respectively, and s^2_y is the variance of $\boldsymbol{y}$. When $p = 2$, $R^2_{X \cdot y}$ is expressed as

$$R^2_{X \cdot y} = (r_{yx_1}, r_{yx_2}) \begin{bmatrix} 1 & r_{x_1x_2} \\ r_{x_2x_1} & 1 \end{bmatrix}^- \begin{pmatrix} r_{yx_1} \\ r_{yx_2} \end{pmatrix}.$$

If $r_{x_1x_2} \neq 1$, $R^2_{X \cdot y}$ can further be expressed as

$$R^2_{X \cdot y} = \frac{r^2_{yx_1} + r^2_{yx_2} - 2r_{x_1x_2}r_{yx_1}r_{yx_2}}{1 - r^2_{x_1x_2}}.$$

The multiple regression coefficient $R_{X \cdot y}$ satisfies the following relation.

Theorem 6.1 *If* $\text{Sp}(\boldsymbol{X}) \supset \text{Sp}(\boldsymbol{X}_1)$,

$$R_{X \cdot y} \geq R_{X_1 \cdot y}. \tag{6.17}$$

Proof. Use (6.16) and (2.63). Q.E.D.

Theorem 6.2 *Let* $\boldsymbol{X} = [\boldsymbol{X}_1, \boldsymbol{X}_2]$, *that is,* $\text{Sp}(\boldsymbol{X}) = \text{Sp}(\boldsymbol{X}_1) + \text{Sp}(\boldsymbol{X}_2)$. *Then,*

$$R^2_{X\cdot y} = R^2_{X_1\cdot y} + R^2_{X_2[X_1]\cdot y}, \tag{6.18}$$

where $R^2_{X_2[X_1]\cdot y}$ *indicates the coefficient of determination (or the square of the multiple correlation coefficient) in predicting the criterion variable* $\boldsymbol{y}$ *from the predictor variables* $\boldsymbol{Q}_{X_1}\boldsymbol{X}_2$, *where* $\boldsymbol{Q}_{X_1} = \boldsymbol{I}_n - \boldsymbol{P}_{X_1}$.

Proof. Use the decomposition given in (4.37); that is, $\boldsymbol{P}_X = \boldsymbol{P}_{X_1\cup X_2} = \boldsymbol{P}_{X_1} + \boldsymbol{P}_{X_2[X_1]}$. Q.E.D.

Let us expand $R^2_{X_2[X_1]\cdot y}$. Let $\boldsymbol{Q}_{X_1}$ denote the orthogonal projector onto $\text{Sp}(\boldsymbol{X}_1)^\perp$, and $\boldsymbol{P}_{Q_{X_1}X_2}$ the orthogonal projector onto $\text{Sp}(\boldsymbol{Q}_{X_1}\boldsymbol{X}_2)$. Then,

$$\begin{aligned} R^2_{X_2[X_1]\cdot y} &= \boldsymbol{y}'\boldsymbol{P}_{Q_{X_1}X_2}\boldsymbol{y}/\boldsymbol{y}'\boldsymbol{y} \\ &= \boldsymbol{y}'\boldsymbol{Q}_{X_1}\boldsymbol{X}_2(\boldsymbol{X}_2'\boldsymbol{Q}_{X_1}\boldsymbol{X}_2)^-\boldsymbol{X}_2'\boldsymbol{Q}_{X_1}\boldsymbol{y}/\boldsymbol{y}'\boldsymbol{y} \\ &= (\boldsymbol{c}_{02} - \boldsymbol{c}_{01}\boldsymbol{C}_{11}^-\boldsymbol{c}_{12})(\boldsymbol{C}_{22} - \boldsymbol{C}_{21}\boldsymbol{C}_{11}^-\boldsymbol{C}_{12})^- \\ &\qquad \times(\boldsymbol{c}_{20} - \boldsymbol{C}_{21}\boldsymbol{C}_{11}^-\boldsymbol{c}_{10})/s_y^2, \end{aligned} \tag{6.19}$$

where $\boldsymbol{c}_{i0}$ ($\boldsymbol{c}_{i0} = \boldsymbol{c}_{0i}'$) is the vector of covariances between $\boldsymbol{X}_i$ and $\boldsymbol{y}$, and $\boldsymbol{C}_{ij}$ is the matrix of covariances between $\boldsymbol{X}_i$ and $\boldsymbol{X}_j$. The formula above can also be stated in terms of correlation vectors and matrices:

$$R^2_{X_2[X_1]\cdot y} = (\boldsymbol{r}_{02} - \boldsymbol{r}_{01}\boldsymbol{R}_{11}^-\boldsymbol{r}_{12})(\boldsymbol{R}_{22} - \boldsymbol{R}_{21}\boldsymbol{R}_{11}^-\boldsymbol{R}_{12})^-(\boldsymbol{r}_{20} - \boldsymbol{R}_{21}\boldsymbol{R}_{11}^-\boldsymbol{r}_{10}).$$

The $R^2_{X_2[X_1]\cdot y}$ is sometimes called a partial coefficient of determination.

When $R^2_{X_2[X_1]\cdot y} = 0$, $\boldsymbol{y}'\boldsymbol{P}_{X_2[X_1]}\boldsymbol{y} = 0 \Leftrightarrow \boldsymbol{P}_{X_2[X_1]}\boldsymbol{y} = \boldsymbol{0} \Leftrightarrow \boldsymbol{X}_2'\boldsymbol{Q}_{X_1}\boldsymbol{y} = \boldsymbol{0} \Leftrightarrow \boldsymbol{c}_{20} = \boldsymbol{C}_{21}\boldsymbol{C}_{11}^-\boldsymbol{c}_{10} \Leftrightarrow \boldsymbol{r}_{20} = \boldsymbol{R}_{21}\boldsymbol{R}_{11}^-\boldsymbol{r}_{10}$. This means that the partial correlation coefficients between $\boldsymbol{y}$ and $\boldsymbol{X}_2$ eliminating the effects of $\boldsymbol{X}_1$ are zero.

Let $\boldsymbol{X} = [\boldsymbol{x}_1, \boldsymbol{x}_2]$ and $\boldsymbol{Y} = \boldsymbol{y}$. If $r^2_{x_1x_2} \neq 1$,

$$\begin{aligned} R^2_{x_1x_2\cdot y} &= \frac{r^2_{yx_1} + r^2_{yx_2} - 2r_{x_1x_2}r_{yx_1}r_{yx_2}}{1 - r^2_{x_1x_2}} \\ &= r^2_{yx_1} + \frac{(r_{yx_2} - r_{yx_1}r_{x_1x_2})^2}{1 - r^2_{x_1x_2}}. \end{aligned}$$

Hence, $R^2_{x_1x_2\cdot y} = r^2_{yx_1}$ when $r_{yx_2} = r_{yx_1}r_{x_1x_2}$; that is, when the partial correlation between y and x_2 eliminating the effect of x_1 is zero.

Let $\boldsymbol{X}$ be partitioned into m subsets, namely $\mathrm{Sp}(\boldsymbol{X}) = \mathrm{Sp}(\boldsymbol{X}_1) + \cdots + \mathrm{Sp}(\boldsymbol{X}_m)$. Then the following decomposition holds:

$$R^2_{X\cdot y} = R^2_{X_1\cdot y} + R^2_{X_2[X_1]\cdot y} + R^2_{X_3[X_1X_2]\cdot y} + \cdots + R^2_{X_m[X_1X_2\cdots X_{m-1}]\cdot y}. \tag{6.20}$$

The decomposition of the form above exists in $m!$ different ways depending on how the m subsets of variables are ordered. The forward inclusion method for variable selection in multiple regression analysis selects the variable sets $\boldsymbol{X}_{j1}$, $\boldsymbol{X}_{j2}$, and $\boldsymbol{X}_{j3}$ in such a way that $R^2_{X_{j1}\cdot y}$, $R_{X_{j2}[X_{j1}]\cdot y}$, and $R^2_{X_{j3}[X_{j1}X_{j2}]\cdot y}$ are successively maximized.

Note When $X_j = \boldsymbol{x}_j$ in (6.20), $R_{x_j[x_1x_2\cdots x_{j-1}]\cdot y}$ is the correlation between $\boldsymbol{x}_j$ and $\boldsymbol{y}$ eliminating the effects of $\boldsymbol{X}_{[j-1]} = [\boldsymbol{x}_1, \boldsymbol{x}_2, \cdots, \boldsymbol{x}_{j-1}]$ from the former. This is called the part correlation, and is different from the partial correlation between $\boldsymbol{x}_j$ and $\boldsymbol{y}$ eliminating the effects of $\boldsymbol{X}_{[j-1]}$ from both, which is equal to the correlation between $\boldsymbol{Q}_{X_{[j-1]}}\boldsymbol{x}_j$ and $\boldsymbol{Q}_{X_{[j-1]}}\boldsymbol{y}$.

6.1.3 The Gauss-Markov model

In the previous subsection, we described the method of estimating parameters in linear regression analysis from a geometric point of view, while in this subsection we treat n variables y_i $(i = 1, \cdots, n)$ as random variables from a certain population. In this context, it is not necessary to relate explanatory variables $x_1, \cdots, x_p$ to the matrix $\boldsymbol{R}_{XX}$ of correlation coefficients or regard $\boldsymbol{x}_1, \cdots, \boldsymbol{x}_p$ as vectors having zero means. We may consequently deal with

$$\boldsymbol{y} = \beta_1\boldsymbol{x}_1 + \cdots + \beta_p\boldsymbol{x}_p + \boldsymbol{\epsilon} = \boldsymbol{X\beta} + \boldsymbol{\epsilon}, \tag{6.21}$$

derived from (6.1) by setting $\alpha = 0$. We assume that the error term ϵ_j $(j = 1, \cdots, n)$ in the regression equation has zero expectation, namely

$$\mathrm{E}(\boldsymbol{\epsilon}) = \boldsymbol{0}, \tag{6.22}$$

and the covariance matrix $\mathrm{Cov}(\epsilon_i, \epsilon_j) = \sigma^2 g_{ij}$. Let $\boldsymbol{G} = [g_{ij}]$. Then,

$$\mathrm{V}(\boldsymbol{\epsilon}) = \mathrm{E}(\boldsymbol{\epsilon\epsilon}') = \sigma^2\boldsymbol{G}, \tag{6.23}$$

where $\boldsymbol{G}$ is a *pd* matrix of order n. It follows that

$$\mathrm{E}(\boldsymbol{y}) = \boldsymbol{X\beta} \tag{6.24}$$

and

$$\mathrm{V}(\boldsymbol{y}) = \mathrm{E}(\boldsymbol{y} - \boldsymbol{X\beta})(\boldsymbol{y} - \boldsymbol{X\beta})' = \sigma^2 \boldsymbol{G}. \tag{6.25}$$

The random vector $\boldsymbol{y}$ that satisfies the conditions above is generally said to follow the Gauss-Markov model $(\boldsymbol{y}, \boldsymbol{X\beta}, \sigma^2\boldsymbol{G})$.

Assume that $\mathrm{rank}(\boldsymbol{X}) = p$ and that $\boldsymbol{G}$ is nonsingular. Then there exists a nonsingular matrix $\boldsymbol{T}$ of order n such that $\boldsymbol{G} = \boldsymbol{TT}'$. Let $\tilde{\boldsymbol{y}} = \boldsymbol{T}^{-1}\boldsymbol{y}$, $\tilde{\boldsymbol{X}} = \boldsymbol{T}^{-1}\boldsymbol{X}$, and $\tilde{\boldsymbol{\epsilon}} = \boldsymbol{T}^{-1}\boldsymbol{\epsilon}$. Then, (6.21) can be rewritten as

$$\tilde{\boldsymbol{y}} = \tilde{\boldsymbol{X}}\boldsymbol{\beta} + \tilde{\boldsymbol{\epsilon}} \tag{6.26}$$

and

$$\mathrm{V}(\tilde{\boldsymbol{\epsilon}}) = \mathrm{V}(\boldsymbol{T}^{-1}\boldsymbol{\epsilon}) = \boldsymbol{T}^{-1}\mathrm{V}(\boldsymbol{\epsilon})(\boldsymbol{T}^{-1})' = \sigma^2\boldsymbol{I}_n.$$

Hence, the least squares estimate of $\boldsymbol{\beta}$ is given by

$$\hat{\boldsymbol{\beta}} = (\tilde{\boldsymbol{X}}'\tilde{\boldsymbol{X}})^{-1}\tilde{\boldsymbol{X}}'\tilde{\boldsymbol{y}} = (\boldsymbol{X}'\boldsymbol{G}^{-1}\boldsymbol{X})^{-1}\boldsymbol{X}'\boldsymbol{G}\boldsymbol{y}. \tag{6.27}$$

(See the previous section for the least squares method.) The estimate of $\boldsymbol{\beta}$ can also be obtained more directly by minimizing

$$||\boldsymbol{y} - \boldsymbol{X\beta})||^2_{G^{-1}} = (\boldsymbol{y} - \boldsymbol{X\beta})'\boldsymbol{G}^{-1}(\boldsymbol{y} - \boldsymbol{X\beta}). \tag{6.28}$$

The $\hat{\boldsymbol{\beta}}$ obtained by minimizing (6.28) (identical to the one given in (6.27)) is called the generalized least squares estimate of $\boldsymbol{\beta}$. We obtain as the prediction vector

$$\boldsymbol{X}\hat{\boldsymbol{\beta}} = \boldsymbol{X}(\boldsymbol{X}'\boldsymbol{G}^{-1}\boldsymbol{X})^{-1}\boldsymbol{X}'\boldsymbol{G}^{-1}\boldsymbol{y} = \boldsymbol{P}_{X/G^{-1}}\boldsymbol{y}. \tag{6.29}$$

Lemma 6.1 *For $\hat{\boldsymbol{\beta}}$ given in (6.27), it holds that*

$$\mathrm{E}(\hat{\boldsymbol{\beta}}) = \boldsymbol{\beta} \tag{6.30}$$

and

$$\mathrm{V}(\hat{\boldsymbol{\beta}}) = \sigma^2(\boldsymbol{X}'\boldsymbol{G}^{-1}\boldsymbol{X})^{-1}. \tag{6.31}$$

Proof. (6.30): Since $\hat{\boldsymbol{\beta}} = (\boldsymbol{X}'\boldsymbol{G}^{-1}\boldsymbol{X})^{-1}\boldsymbol{X}'\boldsymbol{G}^{-1}\boldsymbol{y} = (\boldsymbol{X}'\boldsymbol{G}^{-1}\boldsymbol{X})^{-1}\boldsymbol{X}'\boldsymbol{G}^{-1} \times (\boldsymbol{X\beta} + \boldsymbol{\epsilon}) = \boldsymbol{\beta} + (\boldsymbol{X}'\boldsymbol{G}^{-1}\boldsymbol{X})^{-1}\boldsymbol{X}'\boldsymbol{G}^{-1}\boldsymbol{\epsilon}$, and $\mathrm{E}(\boldsymbol{\epsilon}) = \boldsymbol{0}$, we get $\mathrm{E}(\hat{\boldsymbol{\beta}}) = \boldsymbol{\beta}$.

(6.31): From $\hat{\boldsymbol{\beta}} - \boldsymbol{\beta} = (\boldsymbol{X}'\boldsymbol{G}^{-1}\boldsymbol{X})^{-1}\boldsymbol{X}'\boldsymbol{G}^{-1}\boldsymbol{\epsilon}$, we have $\mathrm{V}(\hat{\boldsymbol{\beta}}) = \mathrm{E}(\hat{\boldsymbol{\beta}} - \boldsymbol{\beta})(\hat{\boldsymbol{\beta}} - \boldsymbol{\beta})' = (\boldsymbol{X}'\boldsymbol{G}^{-1}\boldsymbol{X})^{-1}\boldsymbol{X}'\boldsymbol{G}^{-1}\mathrm{E}(\boldsymbol{\epsilon\epsilon}')\boldsymbol{G}^{-1}\boldsymbol{X}(\boldsymbol{X}'\boldsymbol{G}^{-1}\boldsymbol{X})^{-1} = \sigma^2(\boldsymbol{X}'\boldsymbol{G}^{-1}\boldsymbol{X})^{-1}\boldsymbol{X}'\boldsymbol{G}^{-1}\boldsymbol{G}\boldsymbol{G}^{-1}\boldsymbol{X}(\boldsymbol{X}'\boldsymbol{G}^{-1}\boldsymbol{X})^{-1} = \sigma^2(\boldsymbol{X}'\boldsymbol{G}^{-1}\boldsymbol{X})^{-1}$. Q.E.D.

Theorem 6.3 *Let $\hat{\boldsymbol{\beta}}^*$ denote an arbitrary linear unbiased estimator of $\boldsymbol{\beta}$. Then $V(\hat{\boldsymbol{\beta}}^*) - V(\hat{\boldsymbol{\beta}})$ is an nnd matrix.*

Proof. Let $\boldsymbol{S}$ be a p by n matrix such that $\hat{\boldsymbol{\beta}}^* = \boldsymbol{S}\boldsymbol{y}$. Then, $\boldsymbol{\beta} = \mathrm{E}(\hat{\boldsymbol{\beta}}^*) = \boldsymbol{S}\mathrm{E}(\boldsymbol{y}) = \boldsymbol{S}\boldsymbol{X}\boldsymbol{\beta} \Rightarrow \boldsymbol{S}\boldsymbol{X} = \boldsymbol{I}_p$. Let $\boldsymbol{P}_{X/G^{-1}} = \boldsymbol{X}(\boldsymbol{X}'\boldsymbol{G}^{-1}\boldsymbol{X})^{-1}\boldsymbol{X}'\boldsymbol{G}^{-1}$ and $\boldsymbol{Q}_{X/G^{-1}} = \boldsymbol{I}_n - \boldsymbol{P}_{X/G^{-1}}$. From

$$\mathrm{E}(\boldsymbol{P}_{X/G^{-1}}(\boldsymbol{y} - \boldsymbol{X}\boldsymbol{\beta})(\boldsymbol{y} - \boldsymbol{X}\boldsymbol{\beta})'\boldsymbol{Q}'_{X/G^{-1}}) = \boldsymbol{P}_{X/G^{-1}}\mathrm{V}(\boldsymbol{y})\boldsymbol{Q}'_{X/G^{-1}}$$
$$= \sigma^2\boldsymbol{X}(\boldsymbol{X}'\boldsymbol{G}^{-1}\boldsymbol{X})^{-1}\boldsymbol{X}'\boldsymbol{G}^{-1}\boldsymbol{G}(\boldsymbol{I}_n - \boldsymbol{G}^{-1}\boldsymbol{X}(\boldsymbol{X}'\boldsymbol{G}^{-1}\boldsymbol{X})^{-1}\boldsymbol{X}') = \boldsymbol{O},$$

we obtain

$$\begin{aligned}\mathrm{V}(\hat{\boldsymbol{\beta}}^*) &= \mathrm{V}(\boldsymbol{S}\boldsymbol{y}) = \boldsymbol{S}\mathrm{V}(\boldsymbol{y})\boldsymbol{S}' = \boldsymbol{S}\mathrm{V}(\boldsymbol{P}_{X/G^{-1}}\boldsymbol{y} + \boldsymbol{Q}_{X/G^{-1}}\boldsymbol{y})\boldsymbol{S}' \\ &= \boldsymbol{S}\mathrm{V}(\boldsymbol{P}_{X/G^{-1}}\boldsymbol{y})\boldsymbol{S}' + \boldsymbol{S}\mathrm{V}(\boldsymbol{Q}_{X/G^{-1}}\boldsymbol{y})\boldsymbol{S}'.\end{aligned}$$

Since the first term in the equation above is equal to

$$\boldsymbol{S}\mathrm{V}(\boldsymbol{P}_{X/G^{-1}}\boldsymbol{y})\boldsymbol{S}'$$
$$= (\boldsymbol{S}\boldsymbol{X}(\boldsymbol{X}'\boldsymbol{G}^{-1}\boldsymbol{X})^{-1}\boldsymbol{X}'\boldsymbol{G}^{-1}\boldsymbol{G}\boldsymbol{G}^{-1}\boldsymbol{X}'(\boldsymbol{X}'\boldsymbol{G}^{-1}\boldsymbol{X})^{-1}\boldsymbol{X}'\boldsymbol{S}')\sigma^2$$
$$= \sigma^2(\boldsymbol{X}'\boldsymbol{G}^{-1}\boldsymbol{X})^{-1} = \mathrm{V}(\hat{\boldsymbol{\beta}}),$$

and since the second term is *nnd*, $\mathrm{V}(\hat{\boldsymbol{\beta}}^*) - \mathrm{V}(\hat{\boldsymbol{\beta}})$ is also *nnd*. Q.E.D.

This indicates that the generalized least squares estimator $\hat{\boldsymbol{\beta}}$ given in (6.27) is unbiased and has a minimum variance. Among linear unbiased estimators, the one having the minimum variance is called the best linear unbiased estimator (BLUE), and Theorem 6.3 is called the Gauss-Markov Theorem.

Lemma 6.2 *Let*

$$\boldsymbol{d}'\boldsymbol{y} = d_1y_1 + d_2y_2 + \cdots + d_ny_n$$

represent a linear combination of n random variables in $\boldsymbol{y} = (y_1, y_2, \cdots, y_n)'$. Then the following four conditions are equivalent:

$$\boldsymbol{d}'\boldsymbol{y} \text{ is an unbiased estimator of } \boldsymbol{c}'\boldsymbol{\beta}, \tag{6.32}$$

$$\boldsymbol{c} \in \mathrm{Sp}(\boldsymbol{X}'), \tag{6.33}$$

$$\boldsymbol{c}'\boldsymbol{X}^-\boldsymbol{X} = \boldsymbol{c}', \tag{6.34}$$

$$\boldsymbol{c}'(\boldsymbol{X}'\boldsymbol{X})^-\boldsymbol{X}'\boldsymbol{X} = \boldsymbol{c}'. \tag{6.35}$$

Proof. (6.32) → (6.33): Since $\mathrm{E}(\boldsymbol{d}'\boldsymbol{y}) = \boldsymbol{d}'\mathrm{E}(\boldsymbol{y}) = \boldsymbol{d}'\boldsymbol{X\beta} = \boldsymbol{c}'\boldsymbol{\beta}$ has to hold for any $\boldsymbol{\beta}$, it must hold that $\boldsymbol{d}'\boldsymbol{X} = \boldsymbol{c}' \Rightarrow \boldsymbol{c} = \boldsymbol{X}'\boldsymbol{d} \Rightarrow \boldsymbol{c} \in \mathrm{Sp}(\boldsymbol{X}')$.

(6.33) → (6.34): Since $\boldsymbol{c} \in \mathrm{Sp}(\boldsymbol{X}')$, and an arbitrary projector onto $\mathrm{Sp}(\boldsymbol{X}')$ can be expressed as $\boldsymbol{X}'(\boldsymbol{X}')^-$, we have $\boldsymbol{X}'(\boldsymbol{X}')^-\boldsymbol{c} = \boldsymbol{c}$. Note that $(\boldsymbol{X}^-)' \in \{(\boldsymbol{X}')^-\}$ since $\boldsymbol{XX}^-\boldsymbol{X} = \boldsymbol{X} \Rightarrow \boldsymbol{X}'(\boldsymbol{X}^-)'\boldsymbol{X}' = \boldsymbol{X}'$, from which it follows that $\boldsymbol{X}'(\boldsymbol{X}')^-\boldsymbol{c} = \boldsymbol{c} \Rightarrow \boldsymbol{X}'(\boldsymbol{X}^-)'\boldsymbol{c} = \boldsymbol{c} \Rightarrow \boldsymbol{c}' = \boldsymbol{c}'\boldsymbol{X}^-\boldsymbol{X}$.

(6.34) → (6.35): Use the fact that $(\boldsymbol{X}'\boldsymbol{X})^-\boldsymbol{X}' \in \{\boldsymbol{X}^-\}$ since $\boldsymbol{X}(\boldsymbol{X}'\boldsymbol{X})^-\boldsymbol{X}'\boldsymbol{X} = \boldsymbol{X}$ by (3.13).

(6.35) → (6.33): This is trivial. (Transpose both sides.)

(6.33) → (6.32): Set $\boldsymbol{c} = \boldsymbol{X}'\boldsymbol{d}$. Q.E.D.

When any one of the four conditions in Lemma 6.2 is satisfied, a linear combination $\boldsymbol{c}'\boldsymbol{\beta}$ of $\boldsymbol{\beta}$ is said to be unbiased-estimable or simply estimable. Clearly, $\boldsymbol{X\beta}$ is estimable, and so if $\hat{\boldsymbol{\beta}}$ is the BLUE of $\boldsymbol{\beta}$, $\boldsymbol{X}\hat{\boldsymbol{\beta}}$ is the BLUE of $\boldsymbol{X\beta}$.

Let us now derive the BLUE $\boldsymbol{X}\hat{\boldsymbol{\beta}}$ of $\boldsymbol{X\beta}$ when the covariance matrix $\boldsymbol{G}$ of the error terms $\boldsymbol{\epsilon} = (\epsilon_1, \epsilon_2, \cdots, \epsilon_n)'$ is not necessarily nonsingular.

Theorem 6.4 *When $\boldsymbol{G}$ in the Gauss-Markov model is not necessarily nonsingular, the BLUE of $\boldsymbol{X\beta}$ can be expressed as*

$$\boldsymbol{X}\hat{\boldsymbol{\beta}} = \boldsymbol{Py}, \tag{6.36}$$

where $\boldsymbol{P}$ is a square matrix that satisfies

$$\boldsymbol{PX} = \boldsymbol{X} \tag{6.37}$$

and

$$\boldsymbol{PGZ} = \boldsymbol{O}, \tag{6.38}$$

where $\boldsymbol{Z}$ is such that $\mathrm{Sp}(\boldsymbol{Z}) = \mathrm{Sp}(\boldsymbol{X})^\perp$.

Proof. First, let $\boldsymbol{Py}$ denote an unbiased estimator of $\boldsymbol{X\beta}$. Then, $\mathrm{E}(\boldsymbol{Py}) = \boldsymbol{P}\mathrm{E}(\boldsymbol{y}) = \boldsymbol{PX\beta} = \boldsymbol{X\beta} \Rightarrow \boldsymbol{PX} = \boldsymbol{X}$. On the other hand, since

$$\begin{aligned} \mathrm{V}(\boldsymbol{Py}) &= \mathrm{E}(\boldsymbol{Py} - \boldsymbol{X\beta})(\boldsymbol{Py} - \boldsymbol{X\beta})' = \mathrm{E}(\boldsymbol{P\epsilon\epsilon}'\boldsymbol{P}') \\ &= \boldsymbol{P}\mathrm{V}(\boldsymbol{\epsilon})\boldsymbol{P}' = \sigma^2\boldsymbol{PGP}', \end{aligned}$$

the sum of the variances of the elements of $\boldsymbol{Py}$ is equal to $\sigma^2\mathrm{tr}(\boldsymbol{PGP}')$. To minimize $\mathrm{tr}(\boldsymbol{PGP}')$ subject to $\boldsymbol{PX} = \boldsymbol{X}$, we define

$$f(\boldsymbol{P}, \boldsymbol{L}) = \frac{1}{2}\mathrm{tr}(\boldsymbol{PGP}') - \mathrm{tr}((\boldsymbol{PX} - \boldsymbol{X})\boldsymbol{L}),$$

where $\boldsymbol{L}$ is a matrix of Lagrangean multipliers. We differentiate f with respect to $\boldsymbol{P}$ and set the results equal to zero,

$$\boldsymbol{G}\boldsymbol{P}' = \boldsymbol{X}\boldsymbol{L} \Rightarrow \boldsymbol{Z}'\boldsymbol{G}\boldsymbol{P}' = \boldsymbol{Z}'\boldsymbol{X}\boldsymbol{L} = \boldsymbol{O} \Rightarrow \boldsymbol{P}\boldsymbol{G}\boldsymbol{Z} = \boldsymbol{O},$$

showing that the BLUE of $\boldsymbol{X}\boldsymbol{\beta}$ can be expressed as $\boldsymbol{P}\boldsymbol{y}$ using $\boldsymbol{P}$ satisfying (6.37) and (6.38). Q.E.D.

Lemma 6.3 *The following relations hold:*

$$\text{Sp}([\boldsymbol{X}, \boldsymbol{G}]) = \text{Sp}(\boldsymbol{X}) \oplus \text{Sp}(\boldsymbol{G}\boldsymbol{Z}), \tag{6.39}$$

where $\boldsymbol{Z}$ *is such that* $\text{Sp}(\boldsymbol{Z}) = \text{Sp}(\boldsymbol{X})^{\perp}$, *and*

$$\boldsymbol{y} \in \text{Sp}([\boldsymbol{X}, \boldsymbol{G}]) \text{ with probability 1.} \tag{6.40}$$

Proof. (6.39): $\boldsymbol{X}\boldsymbol{a} + \boldsymbol{G}\boldsymbol{Z}\boldsymbol{b} = \boldsymbol{0} \Rightarrow \boldsymbol{Z}'\boldsymbol{X}\boldsymbol{a} + \boldsymbol{Z}'\boldsymbol{G}\boldsymbol{Z}\boldsymbol{b} = \boldsymbol{Z}'\boldsymbol{G}\boldsymbol{Z}\boldsymbol{b} = \boldsymbol{0} \Rightarrow \boldsymbol{G}\boldsymbol{Z}\boldsymbol{b} = \boldsymbol{0}$, and, by Theorem 1.4, $\text{Sp}(\boldsymbol{X})$ and $\text{Sp}(\boldsymbol{G}\boldsymbol{Z})$ are disjoint.

(6.40): There exists a vector $\boldsymbol{w}$ that satisfies $\boldsymbol{w}'\boldsymbol{G} = \boldsymbol{0}'$ and $\boldsymbol{w}'\boldsymbol{X} = \boldsymbol{0}'$. Let $\boldsymbol{w} \in \text{Sp}([\boldsymbol{X}, \boldsymbol{G}])$. Then, $\text{E}(\boldsymbol{w}'\boldsymbol{y}) = 0$ and $\text{V}(\boldsymbol{w}'\boldsymbol{y}) = \sigma^2\boldsymbol{w}'\boldsymbol{G}\boldsymbol{w} = 0$, implying that $\boldsymbol{w}'\boldsymbol{y} = 0$ with probability 1. Q.E.D.

The lemma above indicates that $\text{Sp}(\boldsymbol{X})$ and $\text{Sp}(\boldsymbol{G}\boldsymbol{Z})$ are disjoint. Let $\boldsymbol{P}_{X \cdot GZ}$ denote the projector onto $\text{Sp}(\boldsymbol{X})$ along $\text{Sp}(\boldsymbol{G}\boldsymbol{Z})$ when $\text{Sp}(\boldsymbol{X}) \oplus \text{Sp}(\boldsymbol{G}\boldsymbol{Z}) = E^n$. Then,

$$\boldsymbol{P}_{X \cdot GZ} = \boldsymbol{X}(\boldsymbol{X}'(\boldsymbol{I}_n - \boldsymbol{P}_{GZ})\boldsymbol{X})^{-}\boldsymbol{X}'(\boldsymbol{I}_n - \boldsymbol{P}_{GZ}). \tag{6.41}$$

On the other hand, let $\boldsymbol{Z} = \boldsymbol{I}_n - \boldsymbol{P}_X$. We have

$$\begin{aligned} \boldsymbol{P}_{GZ \cdot X} &= \boldsymbol{G}\boldsymbol{Z}(\boldsymbol{Z}\boldsymbol{G}(\boldsymbol{I}_n - \boldsymbol{P}_X)\boldsymbol{G}\boldsymbol{Z})^{-}\boldsymbol{Z}\boldsymbol{G}(\boldsymbol{I}_n - \boldsymbol{P}_X) \\ &= \boldsymbol{G}\boldsymbol{Z}(\boldsymbol{Z}\boldsymbol{G}\boldsymbol{Z}\boldsymbol{G}\boldsymbol{Z})^{-}\boldsymbol{Z}\boldsymbol{G}\boldsymbol{Z}. \end{aligned}$$

Since $\text{Sp}(\boldsymbol{X}) \oplus \text{Sp}(\boldsymbol{G}\boldsymbol{Z}) = E^n$, it holds that $\dim(\text{Sp}(\boldsymbol{G}\boldsymbol{Z})) = \dim(\text{Sp}(\boldsymbol{Z})) \Rightarrow \text{rank}(\boldsymbol{G}\boldsymbol{Z}) = \text{rank}(\boldsymbol{Z})$, and so $\boldsymbol{Z}(\boldsymbol{Z}\boldsymbol{G}\boldsymbol{Z})^{-}\boldsymbol{Z}\boldsymbol{G}\boldsymbol{Z} = \boldsymbol{Z}$. This indicates that $(\boldsymbol{Z}\boldsymbol{G}\boldsymbol{Z})^{-}\boldsymbol{Z}(\boldsymbol{Z}\boldsymbol{G}\boldsymbol{Z})^{-}$ is a g-inverse of the symmetric matrix $\boldsymbol{Z}\boldsymbol{G}\boldsymbol{Z}\boldsymbol{G}\boldsymbol{Z}$, and so we obtain

$$\boldsymbol{P}_{GZ \cdot X} = \boldsymbol{G}\boldsymbol{Z}(\boldsymbol{Z}\boldsymbol{G}\boldsymbol{Z})^{-}\boldsymbol{Z}. \tag{6.42}$$

Let $\boldsymbol{T}$ be

$$\boldsymbol{T} = \boldsymbol{X}\boldsymbol{U}\boldsymbol{X}' + \boldsymbol{G}, \tag{6.43}$$

where $\boldsymbol{U}$ is an arbitrary matrix such that rank($\boldsymbol{T}$) = rank($[\boldsymbol{X}, \boldsymbol{G}]$). Then, $\boldsymbol{P}_{X \cdot GZ}\boldsymbol{G}\boldsymbol{Z} = \boldsymbol{O} \Rightarrow \boldsymbol{P}_{X \cdot GZ}(\boldsymbol{G}+\boldsymbol{X}\boldsymbol{U}\boldsymbol{X}')\boldsymbol{Z} = \boldsymbol{P}_{X \cdot GZ}\boldsymbol{T}\boldsymbol{Z} = \boldsymbol{O} \Rightarrow \boldsymbol{P}_{X \cdot GZ}\boldsymbol{T} = \boldsymbol{K}\boldsymbol{X}' \Rightarrow \boldsymbol{P}_{X \cdot GZ} = \boldsymbol{K}\boldsymbol{X}'\boldsymbol{T}^{-1}$. Substituting this into $\boldsymbol{P}_{X \cdot GZ}\boldsymbol{X} = \boldsymbol{X}$, we obtain $\boldsymbol{K}\boldsymbol{X}'\boldsymbol{T}^{-1}\boldsymbol{X} = \boldsymbol{X} \Rightarrow \boldsymbol{K} = \boldsymbol{X}(\boldsymbol{X}'\boldsymbol{T}^{-1}\boldsymbol{X})^{-}$, and so

$$\boldsymbol{P}_{X \cdot GZ} = \boldsymbol{X}(\boldsymbol{X}'\boldsymbol{T}^{-1}\boldsymbol{X})^{-}\boldsymbol{X}'\boldsymbol{T}^{-1}, \tag{6.44}$$

where $\boldsymbol{T}$ is as defined in (6.43). The following theorem can be derived.

Theorem 6.5 *Let* Sp($[\boldsymbol{X}, \boldsymbol{G}]$) $= E^n$, *and let* $\hat{\boldsymbol{\beta}}$ *denote the BLUE of* $\boldsymbol{\beta}$. *Then,* $\tilde{\boldsymbol{y}} = \boldsymbol{X}\hat{\boldsymbol{\beta}}$ *is given by one of the following expressions:*

(i) $\boldsymbol{X}(\boldsymbol{X}'\boldsymbol{Q}_{GZ}\boldsymbol{X})^{-}\boldsymbol{X}'\boldsymbol{Q}_{GZ}\boldsymbol{y}$,

(ii) $(\boldsymbol{I}_n - \boldsymbol{G}\boldsymbol{Z}(\boldsymbol{Z}\boldsymbol{G}\boldsymbol{Z})^{-}\boldsymbol{Z})\boldsymbol{y}$,

(iii) $\boldsymbol{X}(\boldsymbol{X}'\boldsymbol{T}^{-1}\boldsymbol{X})^{-}\boldsymbol{X}'\boldsymbol{T}^{-1}\boldsymbol{y}$.

(Proof omitted.)

Corollary *Let* $\boldsymbol{A}$ *be an arbitrary square matrix of order* n. *When* Sp($\boldsymbol{X}$) $\oplus$ Sp($\boldsymbol{G}$) *does not cover the entire space of* E^n, *a generalized projection onto* Sp($\boldsymbol{X}$) *along* Sp($\boldsymbol{G}\boldsymbol{Z}$) *is given by*

(i) $\boldsymbol{I}_n - \boldsymbol{G}\boldsymbol{Z}(\boldsymbol{Z}\boldsymbol{G}\boldsymbol{Z})^{-}\boldsymbol{Z} + \boldsymbol{A}(\boldsymbol{I}_n - \boldsymbol{Z}\boldsymbol{G}\boldsymbol{Z}(\boldsymbol{Z}\boldsymbol{G}\boldsymbol{Z})^{-})\boldsymbol{Z}$,

(ii) $\boldsymbol{X}(\boldsymbol{X}'\boldsymbol{T}^{-}\boldsymbol{X})^{-}\boldsymbol{X}'\boldsymbol{T}^{-} + \boldsymbol{A}(\boldsymbol{I}_n - \boldsymbol{T}\boldsymbol{T}^{-})$.

(Proof omitted.)

6.2 Analysis of Variance

6.2.1 One-way design

In the regression models discussed in the previous section, the criterion variable y and the explanatory variables $x_1, x_2, \cdots, x_m$ both are usually continuous. In this section, we consider the situation in which one of the m predictor variables takes the value of one and the remaining $m - 1$ variables are all zeroes. That is, when the subject (the case) k belongs to group j,

$$x_{kj} = 1 \text{ and } x_{ki} = 0 \quad (i \neq j; i = 1, \cdots, m; k = 1, \cdots, n). \tag{6.45}$$

Such variables are called dummy variables. Let n_j subjects belong to group j (and $\sum_{j=1}^{m} n_j = n$). Define

$$
\boldsymbol{G} = \begin{array}{c} \begin{matrix} x_1 & x_2 & \cdots & x_m \end{matrix} \\ \begin{bmatrix} 1 & 0 & \cdots & 0 \\ \vdots & \vdots & \ddots & \vdots \\ 1 & 0 & \cdots & 0 \\ 0 & 1 & \cdots & 0 \\ \vdots & \vdots & \ddots & \vdots \\ 0 & 1 & \cdots & 0 \\ \vdots & \vdots & \ddots & \vdots \\ 0 & 0 & \cdots & 1 \\ \vdots & \vdots & \ddots & \vdots \\ 0 & 0 & \cdots & 1 \end{bmatrix} \end{array}. \tag{6.46}
$$

(There are ones in the first n_1 rows in the first column, in the next n_2 rows in the second column, and so on, and in the last n_m rows in the last column.) A matrix of the form above is called a matrix of dummy variables.

The $\boldsymbol{G}$ above indicates which one of m groups (corresponding to columns) each of n subjects (corresponding to rows) belongs to. A subject (row) belongs to the group indicated by one in a column. Consequently, the row sums are equal to one, that is,

$$
\boldsymbol{G}\boldsymbol{1}_m = \boldsymbol{1}_n. \tag{6.47}
$$

Let y_{ij} $(i = 1, \cdots, m; j = 1, \cdots, n_j)$ denote an observation in a survey obtained from one of n subjects belonging to one of m groups. In accordance with the assumption made in (6.45), a one-way analysis of variance (ANOVA) model can be written as

$$
y_{ij} = \mu + \alpha_i + \epsilon_{ij}, \tag{6.48}
$$

where μ is the population mean, α_i is the main effect of the ith level (ith group) of the factor, and ϵ_{ij} is the error (disturbance) term. We estimate μ by the sample mean $\bar{x}$, and so if each y_{ij} has been "centered" in such a way that its mean is equal to 0, we may write (6.48) as

$$
y_{ij} = \alpha_i + \epsilon_{ij}. \tag{6.49}
$$

Estimating the parameter vector $\boldsymbol{\alpha} = (\alpha_1, \alpha_2, \cdots, \alpha_m)'$ by the least squares (LS) method, we obtain

$$
\min_{\alpha} ||\boldsymbol{y} - \boldsymbol{G}\boldsymbol{\alpha}||^2 = ||(\boldsymbol{I}_n - \boldsymbol{P}_G)\boldsymbol{y}||^2, \tag{6.50}
$$

where $\boldsymbol{P}_G$ denotes the orthogonal projector onto Sp($\boldsymbol{G}$). Let $\hat{\boldsymbol{\alpha}}$ denote the $\boldsymbol{\alpha}$ that satisfies the equation above. Then,

$$\boldsymbol{P}_G\boldsymbol{y} = \boldsymbol{G}\hat{\boldsymbol{\alpha}}. \tag{6.51}$$

Premultiplying both sides of the equation above by $(\boldsymbol{G}'\boldsymbol{G})^{-1}\boldsymbol{G}'$, we obtain

$$\hat{\boldsymbol{\alpha}} = (\boldsymbol{G}'\boldsymbol{G})^{-1}\boldsymbol{G}'\boldsymbol{y}. \tag{6.52}$$

Noting that

$$(\boldsymbol{G}'\boldsymbol{G})^{-1} = \begin{bmatrix} \frac{1}{n_1} & 0 & \cdots & 0 \\ 0 & \frac{1}{n_2} & \cdots & 0 \\ \vdots & \vdots & \ddots & \vdots \\ 0 & 0 & \cdots & \frac{1}{n_m} \end{bmatrix}, \text{ and } \boldsymbol{G}'\boldsymbol{y} = \begin{pmatrix} \sum_j y_{1j} \\ \sum_j y_{2j} \\ \vdots \\ \sum_j y_{mj} \end{pmatrix},$$

we obtain

$$\hat{\boldsymbol{\alpha}} = \begin{pmatrix} \bar{y}_1 \\ \bar{y}_2 \\ \vdots \\ \bar{y}_m \end{pmatrix}.$$

Let $\boldsymbol{y}_R$ denote the vector of raw observations that may not have zero mean. Then, by $\boldsymbol{y} = \boldsymbol{Q}_M\boldsymbol{y}_R$, where $\boldsymbol{Q}_M = \boldsymbol{I}_n - (1/n)\boldsymbol{1}_n\boldsymbol{1}_n'$, we have

$$\hat{\boldsymbol{\alpha}} = \begin{pmatrix} \bar{y}_1 - \bar{y} \\ \bar{y}_2 - \bar{y} \\ \vdots \\ \bar{y}_m - \bar{y} \end{pmatrix}. \tag{6.53}$$

The vector of observations $\boldsymbol{y}$ is decomposed as

$$\boldsymbol{y} = \boldsymbol{P}_G\boldsymbol{y} + (\boldsymbol{I}_n - \boldsymbol{P}_G)\boldsymbol{y},$$

and because $\boldsymbol{P}_G(\boldsymbol{I}_n - \boldsymbol{P}_G) = \boldsymbol{O}$, the total variation in $\boldsymbol{y}$ is decomposed into the sum of between-group (the first term on the right-hand side of the equation below) and within-group (the second term) variations according to

$$\boldsymbol{y}'\boldsymbol{y} = \boldsymbol{y}'\boldsymbol{P}_G\boldsymbol{y} + \boldsymbol{y}'(\boldsymbol{I}_n - \boldsymbol{P}_G)\boldsymbol{y}. \tag{6.54}$$

6.2.2 Two-way design

Consider the situation in which subjects are classified by two factors such as gender and age group. The model in such cases is called a two-way ANOVA model. Let us assume that there are m_1 and m_2 levels in the two factors, and define matrices of dummy variables $\boldsymbol{G}_1$ and $\boldsymbol{G}_2$ of size n by m_1 and n by m_2, respectively. Clearly, it holds that

$$\boldsymbol{G}_1\boldsymbol{1}_{m_1} = \boldsymbol{G}_2\boldsymbol{1}_{m_2} = \boldsymbol{1}_n. \tag{6.55}$$

Let $V_j = \mathrm{Sp}(\boldsymbol{G}_j)$ $(j = 1, 2)$. Let $\boldsymbol{P}_{1+2}$ denote the orthogonal projector onto $V_1 + V_2$, and let $\boldsymbol{P}_j$ $(j = 1, 2)$ denote the orthogonal projector onto V_j. Then, if $\boldsymbol{P}_1\boldsymbol{P}_2 = \boldsymbol{P}_2\boldsymbol{P}_1$,

$$\boldsymbol{P}_{1+2} = (\boldsymbol{P}_1 - \boldsymbol{P}_1\boldsymbol{P}_2) + (\boldsymbol{P}_2 - \boldsymbol{P}_1\boldsymbol{P}_2) + \boldsymbol{P}_1\boldsymbol{P}_2 \tag{6.56}$$

by Theorem 2.18. Here, $\boldsymbol{P}_1\boldsymbol{P}_2 = \boldsymbol{P}_2\boldsymbol{P}_1$ is the orthogonal projector onto $V_1 \cap V_2 = \mathrm{Sp}(\boldsymbol{G}_1) \cap \mathrm{Sp}(\boldsymbol{G}_2)$ and $\mathrm{Sp}(\boldsymbol{G}_1) \cap \mathrm{Sp}(\boldsymbol{G}_2) = \mathrm{Sp}(\boldsymbol{1}_n)$. Let $\boldsymbol{P}_0 = \boldsymbol{1}_n\boldsymbol{1}_n'/n$ denote the orthogonal projector onto $\mathrm{Sp}(\boldsymbol{1}_n)$. Then,

$$\boldsymbol{P}_1\boldsymbol{P}_2 = \boldsymbol{P}_0 \Leftrightarrow \boldsymbol{G}_1'\boldsymbol{G}_2 = \frac{1}{n}(\boldsymbol{G}_1'\boldsymbol{1}_n\boldsymbol{1}_n'\boldsymbol{G}_2), \tag{6.57}$$

where

$$\boldsymbol{G}_1'\boldsymbol{G}_2 = \begin{bmatrix} n_{11} & n_{12} & \cdots & n_{1m_2} \\ n_{21} & n_{22} & \cdots & n_{2m_2} \\ \vdots & \vdots & \ddots & \vdots \\ n_{m_11} & n_{m_12} & \cdots & n_{m_1m_2} \end{bmatrix},$$

$$\boldsymbol{G}_1'\boldsymbol{1}_n = \begin{pmatrix} n_{1.} \\ n_{2.} \\ \vdots \\ n_{m_1.} \end{pmatrix}, \text{ and } \boldsymbol{G}_2'\boldsymbol{1}_n = \begin{pmatrix} n_{.1} \\ n_{.2} \\ \vdots \\ n_{.m_2} \end{pmatrix}.$$

Here $n_{i.} = \sum_j n_{ij}$, $n_{.j} = \sum_i n_{ij}$, and n_{ij} is the number of subjects in the ith level of factor 1 and in the jth level of factor 2. (In the standard ANOVA terminology, n_{ij} indicates the cell size of the (i, j)th cell.) The (i, j)th element of (6.57) can be written as

$$n_{ij} = \frac{1}{n}n_{i.}n_{.j}, \quad (i = 1, \cdots, m_1; j = 1, \cdots, m_2). \tag{6.58}$$

Let $\boldsymbol{y}$ denote the vector of observations on the criterion variable in mean deviation form, and let $\boldsymbol{y}_R$ denote the vector of raw scores. Then $\boldsymbol{P}_0\boldsymbol{y} = \boldsymbol{P}_0\boldsymbol{Q}_M\boldsymbol{y}_R = \boldsymbol{P}_0(\boldsymbol{I}_n - \boldsymbol{P}_0)\boldsymbol{y}_R = \boldsymbol{0}$, and so

$$\boldsymbol{y} = \boldsymbol{P}_1\boldsymbol{y} + \boldsymbol{P}_2\boldsymbol{y} + (\boldsymbol{I}_n - \boldsymbol{P}_1 - \boldsymbol{P}_2)\boldsymbol{y}.$$

Hence, the total variation can be decomposed into

$$\boldsymbol{y}'\boldsymbol{y} = \boldsymbol{y}'\boldsymbol{P}_1\boldsymbol{y} + \boldsymbol{y}'\boldsymbol{P}_2\boldsymbol{y} + \boldsymbol{y}'(\boldsymbol{I}_n - \boldsymbol{P}_1 - \boldsymbol{P}_2)\boldsymbol{y}. \tag{6.59}$$

When (6.58) does not hold, we have from Theorem 4.5

$$\begin{aligned} \boldsymbol{P}_{1+2} &= \boldsymbol{P}_1 + \boldsymbol{P}_{2[1]} \\ &= \boldsymbol{P}_2 + \boldsymbol{P}_{1[2]}, \end{aligned}$$

where $\boldsymbol{P}_{2[1]} = \boldsymbol{Q}_1\boldsymbol{G}_2(\boldsymbol{G}_2'\boldsymbol{Q}_1\boldsymbol{G}_2)^-\boldsymbol{G}_2'\boldsymbol{Q}_1$, $\boldsymbol{P}_{1[2]} = \boldsymbol{Q}_2\boldsymbol{G}_1(\boldsymbol{G}_1'\boldsymbol{Q}_2\boldsymbol{G}_1)^-\boldsymbol{G}_1'\boldsymbol{Q}_2$, and $\boldsymbol{Q}_j = \boldsymbol{I} - \boldsymbol{P}_j$ $(j = 1, 2)$. In this case, the total variation is decomposed as

$$\boldsymbol{y}'\boldsymbol{y} = \boldsymbol{y}'\boldsymbol{P}_1\boldsymbol{y} + \boldsymbol{y}'\boldsymbol{P}_{2[1]}\boldsymbol{y} + \boldsymbol{y}'(\boldsymbol{I}_n - \boldsymbol{P}_{1+2})\boldsymbol{y} \tag{6.60}$$

or

$$\boldsymbol{y}'\boldsymbol{y} = \boldsymbol{y}'\boldsymbol{P}_2\boldsymbol{y} + \boldsymbol{y}'\boldsymbol{P}_{1[2]}\boldsymbol{y} + \boldsymbol{y}'(\boldsymbol{I}_n - \boldsymbol{P}_{1+2})\boldsymbol{y}. \tag{6.61}$$

The first term in (6.60), $\boldsymbol{y}'\boldsymbol{P}_1\boldsymbol{y}$, represents the main effect of factor 1 under the assumption that there is no main effect of factor 2, and is called the unadjusted sum of squares, while the second term, $\boldsymbol{y}'\boldsymbol{P}_{2[1]}\boldsymbol{y}$, represents the main effect of factor 2 after the main effect of factor 1 is eliminated, and is called the adjusted sum of squares. The third term is the residual sum of squares. From (6.60) and (6.61), it follows that

$$\boldsymbol{y}'\boldsymbol{P}_{2[1]}\boldsymbol{y} = \boldsymbol{y}'\boldsymbol{P}_2\boldsymbol{y} + \boldsymbol{y}'\boldsymbol{P}_{1[2]}\boldsymbol{y} - \boldsymbol{y}'\boldsymbol{P}_1\boldsymbol{y}.$$

Let us now introduce a matrix of dummy variables $\boldsymbol{G}_{12}$ having factorial combinations of all levels of factor 1 and factor 2. There are m_1m_2 levels represented in this matrix, where m_1 and m_2 are the number of levels of the two factors. Let $\boldsymbol{P}_{12}$ denote the orthogonal projector onto $\text{Sp}(\boldsymbol{G}_{12})$. Since $\text{Sp}(\boldsymbol{G}_{12}) \supset \text{Sp}(\boldsymbol{G}_1)$ and $\text{Sp}(\boldsymbol{G}_{12}) \supset \text{Sp}(\boldsymbol{G}_2)$, we have

$$\boldsymbol{P}_{12}\boldsymbol{P}_1 = \boldsymbol{P}_1 \text{ and } \boldsymbol{P}_{12}\boldsymbol{P}_2 = \boldsymbol{P}_2. \tag{6.62}$$

Note Suppose that there are two and three levels in factors 1 and 2, respectively. Assume further that factor 1 represents gender and factor 2 represents level of education. Let m and f stand for male and female, and let e, j, and s stand for elementary, junior high, and senior high schools, respectively. Then $\boldsymbol{G}_1$, $\boldsymbol{G}_2$, and $\boldsymbol{G}_{12}$ might look like

$$
\boldsymbol{G}_1 = \begin{array}{c} \begin{matrix} m & f \end{matrix} \\ \begin{bmatrix} 1 & 0 \\ 1 & 0 \\ 1 & 0 \\ 1 & 0 \\ 1 & 0 \\ 1 & 0 \\ 0 & 1 \\ 0 & 1 \\ 0 & 1 \\ 0 & 1 \\ 0 & 1 \\ 0 & 1 \end{bmatrix} \end{array}, \quad
\boldsymbol{G}_2 = \begin{array}{c} \begin{matrix} e & j & s \end{matrix} \\ \begin{bmatrix} 1 & 0 & 0 \\ 1 & 0 & 0 \\ 0 & 1 & 0 \\ 0 & 1 & 0 \\ 0 & 0 & 1 \\ 0 & 0 & 1 \\ 1 & 0 & 0 \\ 1 & 0 & 0 \\ 0 & 1 & 0 \\ 0 & 1 & 0 \\ 0 & 0 & 1 \\ 0 & 0 & 1 \end{bmatrix} \end{array}, \text{ and }
\boldsymbol{G}_{12} = \begin{array}{c} \begin{matrix} m & m & m & f & f & f \\ e & j & s & e & j & s \end{matrix} \\ \begin{bmatrix} 1 & 0 & 0 & 0 & 0 & 0 \\ 1 & 0 & 0 & 0 & 0 & 0 \\ 0 & 1 & 0 & 0 & 0 & 0 \\ 0 & 1 & 0 & 0 & 0 & 0 \\ 0 & 0 & 1 & 0 & 0 & 0 \\ 0 & 0 & 1 & 0 & 0 & 0 \\ 0 & 0 & 0 & 1 & 0 & 0 \\ 0 & 0 & 0 & 1 & 0 & 0 \\ 0 & 0 & 0 & 0 & 1 & 0 \\ 0 & 0 & 0 & 0 & 1 & 0 \\ 0 & 0 & 0 & 0 & 0 & 1 \\ 0 & 0 & 0 & 0 & 0 & 1 \end{bmatrix} \end{array}.
$$

It is clear that $\text{Sp}(\boldsymbol{G}_{12}) \supset \text{Sp}(\boldsymbol{G}_1)$ and $\text{Sp}(\boldsymbol{G}_{12}) \supset \text{Sp}(\boldsymbol{G}_2)$.

From Theorem 2.18, we have

$$\boldsymbol{P}_{12} = (\boldsymbol{P}_{12} - \boldsymbol{P}_{1+2}) + (\boldsymbol{P}_{1+2} - \boldsymbol{P}_0) + \boldsymbol{P}_0. \tag{6.63}$$

The three terms on the right-hand side of the equation above are mutually orthogonal. Let

$$\boldsymbol{P}_{1\otimes 2} = \boldsymbol{P}_{12} - \boldsymbol{P}_{1+2} \tag{6.64}$$

and

$$\boldsymbol{P}_{1\oplus 2} = \boldsymbol{P}_{1+2} - \boldsymbol{P}_0 \tag{6.65}$$

denote the first two terms in (6.63). Then (6.64) represents interaction effects between factors 1 and 2 and (6.65) the main effects of the two factors.

6.2.3 Three-way design

Let us now consider the three-way ANOVA model in which there is a third factor with m_3 levels in addition to factors 1 and 2 with m_1 and m_2 levels. Let $\boldsymbol{G}_3$ denote the matrix of dummy variables corresponding to the third factor. Let $\boldsymbol{P}_3$ denote the orthogonal projector onto $V_3 = \text{Sp}(\boldsymbol{G}_3)$, and let $\boldsymbol{P}_{1+2+3}$ denote the orthogonal projector onto $V_1 + V_2 + V_3$. Then, under the condition that

$$\boldsymbol{P}_1\boldsymbol{P}_2 = \boldsymbol{P}_2\boldsymbol{P}_1, \;\; \boldsymbol{P}_1\boldsymbol{P}_3 = \boldsymbol{P}_3\boldsymbol{P}_1, \text{ and } \boldsymbol{P}_2\boldsymbol{P}_3 = \boldsymbol{P}_3\boldsymbol{P}_2,$$

the decomposition in (2.43) holds. Let

$$\text{Sp}(\boldsymbol{G}_1) \cap \text{Sp}(\boldsymbol{G}_2) = \text{Sp}(\boldsymbol{G}_1) \cap \text{Sp}(\boldsymbol{G}_3) = \text{Sp}(\boldsymbol{G}_2) \cap \text{Sp}(\boldsymbol{G}_3) = \text{Sp}(\boldsymbol{1}_n).$$

Then,

$$\boldsymbol{P}_1\boldsymbol{P}_2 = \boldsymbol{P}_2\boldsymbol{P}_3 = \boldsymbol{P}_1\boldsymbol{P}_3 = \boldsymbol{P}_0, \tag{6.66}$$

where $\boldsymbol{P}_0 = \frac{1}{n}\mathbf{1}_n\mathbf{1}_n'$. Hence, (2.43) reduces to

$$\boldsymbol{P}_{1+2+3} = (\boldsymbol{P}_1 - \boldsymbol{P}_0) + (\boldsymbol{P}_2 - \boldsymbol{P}_0) + (\boldsymbol{P}_3 - \boldsymbol{P}_0) + \boldsymbol{P}_0. \tag{6.67}$$

Thus, the total variation in $\boldsymbol{y}$ is decomposed as

$$\boldsymbol{y}'\boldsymbol{y} = \boldsymbol{y}'\boldsymbol{P}_1\boldsymbol{y} + \boldsymbol{y}'\boldsymbol{P}_2\boldsymbol{y} + \boldsymbol{y}'\boldsymbol{P}_3\boldsymbol{y} + \boldsymbol{y}'(\boldsymbol{I}_n - \boldsymbol{P}_1 - \boldsymbol{P}_2 - \boldsymbol{P}_3)\boldsymbol{y}. \tag{6.68}$$

Equation (6.66) means

$$n_{ij.} = \frac{1}{n} n_{i..}n_{.j.} \quad (i = 1, \cdots, m_1; j = 1, \cdots, m_2), \tag{6.69}$$

$$n_{i.k} = \frac{1}{n} n_{i..}n_{..k}, \quad (i = 1, \cdots, m_1; k = 1, \cdots, m_3), \tag{6.70}$$

$$n_{.jk} = \frac{1}{n} n_{.j.}n_{..k}, \quad (j = 1, \cdots, m_2; k = 1, \cdots, m_3), \tag{6.71}$$

where n_{ijk} is the number of replicated observations in the (i, j, k)th cell, $n_{ij.} = \sum_k n_{ijk}$, $n_{i.k} = \sum_j n_{ijk}$, $n_{.jk} = \sum_i n_{ijk}$, $n_{i..} = \sum_{j,k} n_{ijk}$, $n_{.j.} = \sum_{i,k} n_{ijk}$, and $n_{..k} = \sum_{i,j} n_{ijk}$.

When (6.69) through (6.71) do not hold, the decomposition

$$\boldsymbol{y}'\boldsymbol{y} = \boldsymbol{y}'\boldsymbol{P}_i\boldsymbol{y} + \boldsymbol{y}'\boldsymbol{P}_{j[i]}\boldsymbol{y} + \boldsymbol{y}'\boldsymbol{P}_{k[ij]}\boldsymbol{y} + \boldsymbol{y}'(\boldsymbol{I}_n - \boldsymbol{P}_{1+2+3})\boldsymbol{y} \tag{6.72}$$

holds, where i, j, and k can take any one of the values 1, 2, and 3 (so there will be six different decompositions, depending on which indices take which values) and where $\boldsymbol{P}_{j[i]}$ and $\boldsymbol{P}_{k[ij]}$ are orthogonal projectors onto $\text{Sp}(\boldsymbol{Q}_i\boldsymbol{G}_j)$ and $\text{Sp}(\boldsymbol{Q}_{i+j}\boldsymbol{G}_k)$.

Following the note just before (6.63), construct matrices of dummy variables, $\boldsymbol{G}_{12}$, $\boldsymbol{G}_{13}$, and $\boldsymbol{G}_{23}$, and their respective orthogonal projectors, $\boldsymbol{P}_{12}$, $\boldsymbol{P}_{13}$, and $\boldsymbol{P}_{23}$. Assume further that

$$\text{Sp}(\boldsymbol{G}_{12}) \cap \text{Sp}(\boldsymbol{G}_{23}) = \text{Sp}(\boldsymbol{G}_2), \quad \text{Sp}(\boldsymbol{G}_{13}) \cap \text{Sp}(\boldsymbol{G}_{23}) = \text{Sp}(\boldsymbol{G}_3),$$

and

$$\text{Sp}(\boldsymbol{G}_{12}) \cap \text{Sp}(\boldsymbol{G}_{13}) = \text{Sp}(\boldsymbol{G}_1).$$

Then,

$$\boldsymbol{P}_{12}\boldsymbol{P}_{13} = \boldsymbol{P}_1, \;\; \boldsymbol{P}_{12}\boldsymbol{P}_{23} = \boldsymbol{P}_2, \text{ and } \boldsymbol{P}_{13}\boldsymbol{P}_{23} = \boldsymbol{P}_3. \tag{6.73}$$

Let $\boldsymbol{P}_{[3]} = \boldsymbol{P}_{12+13+23}$ denote the orthogonal projector onto $\text{Sp}(\boldsymbol{G}_{12}) + \text{Sp}(\boldsymbol{G}_{13}) + \text{Sp}(\boldsymbol{G}_{23})$. By Theorem 2.20 and (2.43), it holds under (6.73) that

$$\boldsymbol{P}_{[3]} = \boldsymbol{P}_{1\otimes 2} + \boldsymbol{P}_{2\otimes 3} + \boldsymbol{P}_{1\otimes 3} + \boldsymbol{P}_{\tilde{1}} + \boldsymbol{P}_{\tilde{2}} + \boldsymbol{P}_{\tilde{3}} + \boldsymbol{P}_{0}, \tag{6.74}$$

where $\boldsymbol{P}_{i\otimes j} = \boldsymbol{P}_{ij} - \boldsymbol{P}_i - \boldsymbol{P}_j + \boldsymbol{P}_0$ and $\boldsymbol{P}_{\tilde{i}} = \boldsymbol{P}_i - \boldsymbol{P}_0$. Hence, the total variation in $\boldsymbol{y}$ is decomposed as

$$\begin{aligned}\boldsymbol{y}'\boldsymbol{y} &= \boldsymbol{y}'\boldsymbol{P}_{1\otimes 2}\boldsymbol{y} + \boldsymbol{y}'\boldsymbol{P}_{2\otimes 3}\boldsymbol{y} \\ &\quad + \boldsymbol{y}'\boldsymbol{P}_{1\otimes 3}\boldsymbol{y} + \boldsymbol{y}'\boldsymbol{P}_{\tilde{1}}\boldsymbol{y} + \boldsymbol{y}'\boldsymbol{P}_{\tilde{2}}\boldsymbol{y} + \boldsymbol{y}'\boldsymbol{P}_{\tilde{3}}\boldsymbol{y} + \boldsymbol{y}'(\boldsymbol{I}_n - \boldsymbol{P}_{[3]})\boldsymbol{y}.\end{aligned}$$

Equation (6.73) corresponds with

$$n_{ijk} = \frac{1}{n_{i..}} n_{ij.} n_{i.k} = \frac{1}{n_{.j.}} n_{ij.} n_{.jk} = \frac{1}{n_{..k}} n_{i.k} n_{.jk}, \tag{6.75}$$

but since

$$n_{ijk} = \frac{1}{n^2} n_{i..} n_{.j.} n_{..k} \tag{6.76}$$

follows from (6.69) through (6.71), the necessary and sufficient condition for the decomposition in (6.74) to hold is that (6.69) through (6.71) and (6.76) hold simultaneously.

6.2.4 Cochran's theorem

Let us assume that each element of an n-component random vector of criterion variables $\boldsymbol{y} = (y_1, y_2, \cdots, y_n)'$ has zero mean and unit variance, and is distributed independently of the others; that is, $\boldsymbol{y}$ follows the multivariate normal distribution $\mathcal{N}(\boldsymbol{0}, \boldsymbol{I}_n)$ with $\text{E}(\boldsymbol{y}) = \boldsymbol{0}$ and $\text{V}(\boldsymbol{y}) = \boldsymbol{I}_n$. It is well known that

$$||\boldsymbol{y}||^2 = y_1^2 + y_2^2 + \cdots + y_n^2$$

follows the chi-square distribution with n degrees of freedom (df).

Lemma 6.4 *Let $\boldsymbol{y} \sim \mathcal{N}(\boldsymbol{0}, \boldsymbol{I})$ (that is, the n-component vector $\boldsymbol{y} = (y_1, y_2, \cdots, y_n)'$ follows the multivariate normal distribution with mean $\boldsymbol{0}$ and variance $\boldsymbol{I}$), and let $\boldsymbol{A}$ be symmetric (i.e., $\boldsymbol{A}' = \boldsymbol{A}$). Then, the necessary and sufficient condition for*

$$Q = \sum_i \sum_j a_{ij} y_i y_j = \boldsymbol{y}'\boldsymbol{A}\boldsymbol{y}$$

to follow the chi-square distribution with $k = rank(\boldsymbol{A})$ degrees of freedom is

$$\boldsymbol{A}^2 = \boldsymbol{A}. \tag{6.77}$$

Proof. (Necessity) The moment generating function for $\boldsymbol{y}'\boldsymbol{A}\boldsymbol{y}$ is given by

$$\begin{aligned}\phi(t) = \mathrm{E}(e^{tQ}) &= \int \cdots \int \frac{1}{(2\pi)^{n/2}} \exp\left\{(\boldsymbol{y}'\boldsymbol{A}\boldsymbol{y})t - \frac{1}{2}\boldsymbol{y}'\boldsymbol{y}\right\} dy_1 \cdots dy_n \\ &= |\boldsymbol{I}_n - 2t\boldsymbol{A}|^{-1/2} = \prod_{i=1}^{n}(1-2t\lambda_i)^{-1/2},\end{aligned}$$

where λ_i is the ith largest eigenvalue of $\boldsymbol{A}$. From $\boldsymbol{A}^2 = \boldsymbol{A}$ and $\mathrm{rank}(\boldsymbol{A}) = k$, we have $\lambda_1 = \lambda_2 = \cdots = \lambda_k = 1$ and $\lambda_{k+1} = \cdots = \lambda_n = 0$. Hence, $\phi(t) = (1-2t)^{-\frac{1}{2}k}$, which indicates that $\phi(t)$ is the moment generating function of the chi-square distribution with k degrees of freedom.

(Sufficiency) $\phi(t) = (1-2t)^{-k/2} = \prod_{i=1}^{n}(1-2\lambda_i t)^{-1/2} \Rightarrow \lambda_i = 1$ $(i = 1, \cdots, k)$, $\lambda_i = 0$ $(i = k+1, \cdots, n)$, which implies $\boldsymbol{A}^2 = \boldsymbol{A}$. Q.E.D.

Let us now consider the case in which $\boldsymbol{y} \sim \mathcal{N}(\boldsymbol{0}, \sigma^2\boldsymbol{G})$. Let $\mathrm{rank}(\boldsymbol{G}) = r$. Then there exists an n by r matrix $\boldsymbol{T}$ such that $\boldsymbol{G} = \boldsymbol{T}\boldsymbol{T}'$. Define $\boldsymbol{z}$ so that $\boldsymbol{y} = \boldsymbol{T}\boldsymbol{z}$. Then, $\boldsymbol{z} \sim \mathcal{N}(\boldsymbol{0}, \sigma^2\boldsymbol{I}_r)$. Hence, the necessary and sufficient condition for

$$Q = \boldsymbol{y}'\boldsymbol{A}\boldsymbol{y} = \boldsymbol{z}'(\boldsymbol{T}'\boldsymbol{A}\boldsymbol{T})\boldsymbol{z}$$

to follow the chi-square distribution is $(\boldsymbol{T}'\boldsymbol{A}\boldsymbol{T})^2 = \boldsymbol{T}'\boldsymbol{A}\boldsymbol{T}$ from Lemma 6.4. Pre- and postmultiplying both sides of this equation by $\boldsymbol{T}$ and $\boldsymbol{T}'$, respectively, we obtain

$$\boldsymbol{GAGAG} = \boldsymbol{GAG} \Rightarrow (\boldsymbol{GA})^3 = (\boldsymbol{GA})^2.$$

We also have

$$\mathrm{rank}(\boldsymbol{T}'\boldsymbol{A}\boldsymbol{T}) = \mathrm{tr}(\boldsymbol{T}'\boldsymbol{A}\boldsymbol{T}) = \mathrm{tr}(\boldsymbol{A}\boldsymbol{T}\boldsymbol{T}') = \mathrm{tr}(\boldsymbol{AG}),$$

from which the following lemma can be derived.

Lemma 6.5 *Let $\boldsymbol{y} \sim \mathcal{N}(\boldsymbol{0}, \sigma^2\boldsymbol{G})$. The necessary and sufficient condition for $Q = \boldsymbol{y}'\boldsymbol{A}\boldsymbol{y}$ to follow the chi-square distribution with $k = \mathrm{tr}(\boldsymbol{AG})$ degrees of freedom is*

$$\boldsymbol{GAGAG} = \boldsymbol{GAG} \tag{6.78}$$

or

$$(\boldsymbol{GA})^3 = (\boldsymbol{GA})^2. \tag{6.79}$$

(A proof is omitted.)

Lemma 6.6 *Let* $\boldsymbol{A}$ *and* $\boldsymbol{B}$ *be square matrices. The necessary and sufficient condition for* $\boldsymbol{y}'\boldsymbol{A}\boldsymbol{y}$ *and* $\boldsymbol{y}'\boldsymbol{B}\boldsymbol{y}$ *to be mutually independent is*

$$\boldsymbol{AB} = \boldsymbol{O}, \quad \textit{if } \boldsymbol{y} \sim \mathcal{N}(\boldsymbol{0}, \sigma^2 \boldsymbol{I}_n), \tag{6.80}$$

or

$$\boldsymbol{GAGBG} = \boldsymbol{O}, \quad \textit{if } \boldsymbol{y} \sim \mathcal{N}(\boldsymbol{0}, \sigma^2 \boldsymbol{G}). \tag{6.81}$$

Proof. (6.80): Let $Q_1 = \boldsymbol{y}'\boldsymbol{A}\boldsymbol{y}$ and $Q_2 = \boldsymbol{y}'\boldsymbol{B}\boldsymbol{y}$. Their joint moment generating function is given by $\phi(\boldsymbol{A}, \boldsymbol{B}) = |\boldsymbol{I}_n - 2\boldsymbol{A}t_1 - 2\boldsymbol{B}t_2|^{-1/2}$, while their marginal moment functions are given by $\phi(\boldsymbol{A}) = |\boldsymbol{I}_n - 2\boldsymbol{A}t_1|^{-1/2}$ and $\phi(\boldsymbol{B}) = |\boldsymbol{I}_n - 2\boldsymbol{B}t_2|^{-1/2}$, so that $\phi(\boldsymbol{A}, \boldsymbol{B}) = \phi(\boldsymbol{A})\phi(\boldsymbol{B})$, which is equivalent to $\boldsymbol{AB} = \boldsymbol{O}$.

(6.81): Let $\boldsymbol{G} = \boldsymbol{T}\boldsymbol{T}'$, and introduce $\boldsymbol{z}$ such that $\boldsymbol{y} = \boldsymbol{T}\boldsymbol{z}$ and $\boldsymbol{z} \sim \mathcal{N}(\boldsymbol{0}, \sigma^2 \boldsymbol{I}_n)$. The necessary and sufficient condition for $\boldsymbol{y}'\boldsymbol{A}\boldsymbol{y} = \boldsymbol{z}'\boldsymbol{T}'\boldsymbol{A}\boldsymbol{T}\boldsymbol{z}$ and $\boldsymbol{y}'\boldsymbol{B}\boldsymbol{y} = \boldsymbol{z}'\boldsymbol{T}'\boldsymbol{B}\boldsymbol{T}\boldsymbol{z}$ to be independent is given, from (6.80), by

$$\boldsymbol{T}'\boldsymbol{A}\boldsymbol{T}\boldsymbol{T}'\boldsymbol{B}\boldsymbol{T} = \boldsymbol{O} \Leftrightarrow \boldsymbol{GAGBG} = \boldsymbol{O}.$$

Q.E.D.

From these lemmas and Theorem 2.13, the following theorem, called Cochran's Theorem, can be derived.

Theorem 6.7 *Let* $\boldsymbol{y} \sim \mathcal{N}(\boldsymbol{0}, \sigma^2 \boldsymbol{I}_n)$*, and let* $\boldsymbol{P}_j$ $(j = 1, \cdots, k)$ *be a square matrix of order* n *such that*

$$\boldsymbol{P}_1 + \boldsymbol{P}_2 + \cdots + \boldsymbol{P}_k = \boldsymbol{I}_n.$$

The necessary and sufficient condition for the quadratic forms $\boldsymbol{y}'\boldsymbol{P}_1\boldsymbol{y}, \boldsymbol{y}'\boldsymbol{P}_2 \times \boldsymbol{y}, \cdots, \boldsymbol{y}'\boldsymbol{P}_k\boldsymbol{y}$ *to be independently distributed according to the chi-square distribution with degrees of freedom equal to* $n_1 = \mathrm{tr}(\boldsymbol{P}_1), n_2 = \mathrm{tr}(\boldsymbol{P}_2), \cdots, n_k = \mathrm{tr}(\boldsymbol{P}_k)$*, respectively, is that one of the following conditions holds:*

$$\boldsymbol{P}_i\boldsymbol{P}_j = \boldsymbol{O}, \quad (i \neq j), \tag{6.82}$$

$$\boldsymbol{P}_j^2 = \boldsymbol{P}_j, \tag{6.83}$$

$$\text{rank}(\boldsymbol{P}_1) + \text{rank}(\boldsymbol{P}_2) + \cdots + \text{rank}(\boldsymbol{P}_k) = n. \tag{6.84}$$

(Proof omitted.)

Corollary *Let $\boldsymbol{y} \sim \mathcal{N}(\boldsymbol{0}, \sigma^2\boldsymbol{G})$, and let $\boldsymbol{P}_j$ $(j = 1, \cdots, k)$ be such that*

$$\boldsymbol{P}_1 + \boldsymbol{P}_2 + \cdots + \boldsymbol{P}_k = \boldsymbol{I}_n.$$

The necessary and sufficient condition for the quadratic form $\boldsymbol{y}'\boldsymbol{P}_j\boldsymbol{y}$ $(j = 1, \cdots, k)$ to be independently distributed according to the chi-square distribution with $k_j = \text{tr}(\boldsymbol{G}\boldsymbol{P}_j\boldsymbol{G})$ degrees of freedom is that one of the three conditions (6.85) through (6.87) plus the fourth condition (6.88) simultaneously hold:

$$\boldsymbol{G}\boldsymbol{P}_i\boldsymbol{G}\boldsymbol{P}_j\boldsymbol{G} = \boldsymbol{O}, \quad (i \neq j), \tag{6.85}$$

$$(\boldsymbol{G}\boldsymbol{P}_j)^3 = (\boldsymbol{G}\boldsymbol{P}_j)^2, \tag{6.86}$$

$$\text{rank}(\boldsymbol{G}\boldsymbol{P}_1\boldsymbol{G}) + \cdots + \text{rank}(\boldsymbol{G}\boldsymbol{P}_k\boldsymbol{G}) = \text{rank}(\boldsymbol{G}^2), \tag{6.87}$$

$$\boldsymbol{G}^3 = \boldsymbol{G}^2. \tag{6.88}$$

Proof. Transform

$$\boldsymbol{y}'\boldsymbol{y} = \boldsymbol{y}'\boldsymbol{P}_1\boldsymbol{y} + \boldsymbol{y}'\boldsymbol{P}_2\boldsymbol{y} + \cdots + \boldsymbol{y}'\boldsymbol{P}_k\boldsymbol{y}$$

by $\boldsymbol{y} = \boldsymbol{T}\boldsymbol{z}$, where $\boldsymbol{T}$ is such that $\boldsymbol{G} = \boldsymbol{T}\boldsymbol{T}'$ and $\boldsymbol{z} \sim \mathcal{N}(\boldsymbol{0}, \sigma^2\boldsymbol{I}_n)$. Then, use

$$\boldsymbol{z}'\boldsymbol{T}'\boldsymbol{T}\boldsymbol{z} = \boldsymbol{z}'\boldsymbol{T}'\boldsymbol{P}_1\boldsymbol{T}\boldsymbol{z} + \boldsymbol{z}'\boldsymbol{T}'\boldsymbol{P}_2\boldsymbol{T}\boldsymbol{z} + \cdots + \boldsymbol{z}'\boldsymbol{T}'\boldsymbol{P}_k\boldsymbol{T}\boldsymbol{z}.$$

Q.E.D.

Note When the population mean of $\boldsymbol{y}$ is not zero, namely $\boldsymbol{y} \sim \mathcal{N}(\boldsymbol{\mu}, \sigma^2\boldsymbol{I}_n)$, Theorem 6.7 can be modified by replacing the "condition that $\boldsymbol{y}'\boldsymbol{P}_j\boldsymbol{y}$ follows the independent chi-square" with the "condition that $\boldsymbol{y}'\boldsymbol{P}_j\boldsymbol{y}$ follows the independent noncentral chi-square with the noncentrality parameter $\boldsymbol{\mu}'\boldsymbol{P}_j\boldsymbol{\mu}$," and everything else holds the same. A similar modification can be made for $\boldsymbol{y} \sim \mathcal{N}(\boldsymbol{\mu}, \sigma^2\boldsymbol{G})$ in the corollary to Theorem 6.7.

6.3 Multivariate Analysis

Utilizing the notion of projection matrices, relationships among various techniques of multivariate analysis, methods for variable selection, and so on can be systematically investigated.

6.3.1 Canonical correlation analysis

Let $\boldsymbol{X} = [\boldsymbol{x}_1, \boldsymbol{x}_2, \cdots, \boldsymbol{x}_p]$ and $\boldsymbol{Y} = [\boldsymbol{y}_1, \boldsymbol{y}_2, \cdots, \boldsymbol{y}_q]$ denote matrices of observations on two sets of variables. It is not necessarily assumed that vectors in those matrices are linearly independent, although it is assumed that they are columnwise centered. We consider forming two sets of linear composite scores,

$$\boldsymbol{f} = a_1\boldsymbol{x}_1 + a_2\boldsymbol{x}_2 + \cdots + a_p\boldsymbol{x}_p = \boldsymbol{X}\boldsymbol{a}$$

and

$$\boldsymbol{g} = b_1\boldsymbol{y}_1 + b_2\boldsymbol{y}_2 + \cdots + b_q\boldsymbol{y}_q = \boldsymbol{Y}\boldsymbol{b},$$

in such a way that their correlation

$$\begin{aligned} r_{fg} &= (\boldsymbol{f}, \boldsymbol{g})/(||\boldsymbol{f}|| \cdot ||\boldsymbol{g}||) \\ &= (\boldsymbol{X}\boldsymbol{a}, \boldsymbol{Y}\boldsymbol{b})/(||\boldsymbol{X}\boldsymbol{a}|| \cdot ||\boldsymbol{Y}\boldsymbol{b}||) \end{aligned}$$

is maximized. This is equivalent to maximizing $\boldsymbol{a}'\boldsymbol{X}'\boldsymbol{Y}\boldsymbol{b}$ subject to the constraints that

$$\boldsymbol{a}'\boldsymbol{X}'\boldsymbol{X}\boldsymbol{a} = \boldsymbol{b}'\boldsymbol{Y}'\boldsymbol{Y}\boldsymbol{b} = 1. \tag{6.89}$$

We define

$$\begin{aligned} &f(\boldsymbol{a}, \boldsymbol{b}, \lambda_1, \lambda_2) \\ &= \boldsymbol{a}'\boldsymbol{X}'\boldsymbol{Y}\boldsymbol{b} - \frac{\lambda_1}{2}(\boldsymbol{a}'\boldsymbol{X}'\boldsymbol{X}\boldsymbol{a} - 1) - \frac{\lambda_2}{2}(\boldsymbol{b}'\boldsymbol{Y}'\boldsymbol{Y}\boldsymbol{b} - 1), \end{aligned}$$

differentiate it with respect to $\boldsymbol{a}$ and $\boldsymbol{b}$, and set the result equal to zero. Then the following two equations can be derived:

$$\boldsymbol{X}'\boldsymbol{Y}\boldsymbol{b} = \lambda_1\boldsymbol{X}'\boldsymbol{X}\boldsymbol{a} \text{ and } \boldsymbol{Y}'\boldsymbol{X}\boldsymbol{a} = \lambda_2\boldsymbol{Y}'\boldsymbol{Y}\boldsymbol{b}. \tag{6.90}$$

Premultiplying the equations above by $\boldsymbol{a}'$ and $\boldsymbol{b}'$, respectively, we obtain $\lambda_1 = \lambda_2$ by (6.89). We may let $\lambda_1 = \lambda_2 = \sqrt{\lambda}$. Furthermore, by premultiplying (6.90) by $\boldsymbol{X}(\boldsymbol{X}'\boldsymbol{X})^-$ and $\boldsymbol{Y}(\boldsymbol{Y}'\boldsymbol{Y})^-$, respectively, we get

$$\boldsymbol{P}_X\boldsymbol{Y}\boldsymbol{b} = \sqrt{\lambda}\boldsymbol{X}\boldsymbol{a} \text{ and } \boldsymbol{P}_Y\boldsymbol{X}\boldsymbol{a} = \sqrt{\lambda}\boldsymbol{Y}\boldsymbol{b}, \tag{6.91}$$

where $\boldsymbol{P}_X = \boldsymbol{X}(\boldsymbol{X}'\boldsymbol{X})^-\boldsymbol{X}'$ and $\boldsymbol{P}_Y = \boldsymbol{Y}(\boldsymbol{Y}'\boldsymbol{Y})^-\boldsymbol{Y}'$ are the orthogonal projectors onto $\text{Sp}(\boldsymbol{X})$ and $\text{Sp}(\boldsymbol{Y})$, respectively. The linear composites that are to be obtained should satisfy the relationships depicted in Figure 6.2.

Substituting one equation into the other in (6.91), we obtain

$$(\boldsymbol{P}_X\boldsymbol{P}_Y)\boldsymbol{X}\boldsymbol{a} = \lambda\boldsymbol{X}\boldsymbol{a} \tag{6.92}$$

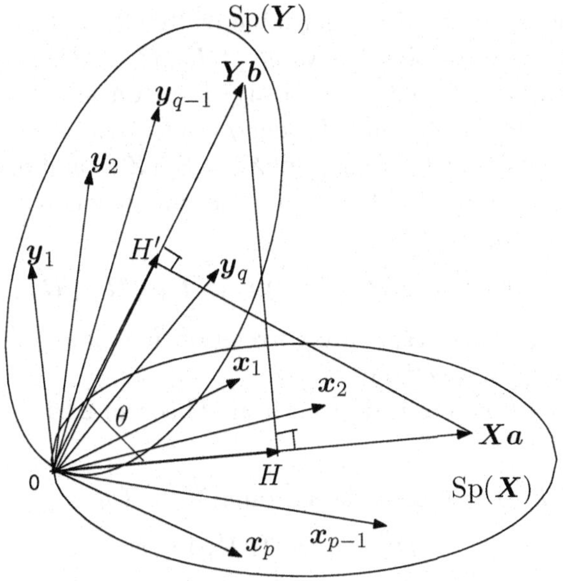

Figure 6.2: Vector representation of canonical correlation analysis. (The vectors $\overrightarrow{0H'}$ and $\overrightarrow{0H}$ are, respectively, $\boldsymbol{P}_Y\boldsymbol{Xa}$ and $\boldsymbol{P}_X\boldsymbol{Yb}$, and the angle between the two vectors is designated as θ.)

or

$$(\boldsymbol{P}_Y\boldsymbol{P}_X)\boldsymbol{Yb} = \lambda\boldsymbol{Yb}. \tag{6.93}$$

Theorem 6.8 *No eigenvalues of $\boldsymbol{P}_X\boldsymbol{P}_Y$ are larger than 1.*

Proof. Since $\boldsymbol{P}_Y$ is an orthogonal projector, its eigenvalues are either 1 or 0. Let $\lambda_j(\boldsymbol{A})$ denote the jth eigenvalue of $\boldsymbol{A}$. From Theorem 5.9, we have

$$1 \geq \lambda_j(\boldsymbol{P}_X) = \lambda_j(\boldsymbol{P}_X\boldsymbol{P}_X) \geq \lambda_j(\boldsymbol{P}_X\boldsymbol{P}_Y\boldsymbol{P}_X) = \lambda_j(\boldsymbol{P}_X\boldsymbol{P}_Y).$$

Q.E.D.

Let $\lambda_1, \lambda_2, \cdots, \lambda_r$ denote all the positive eigenvalues that satisfy (6.93). Then

$$\mathrm{tr}(\boldsymbol{P}_X\boldsymbol{P}_Y) = \mathrm{tr}(\boldsymbol{P}_Y\boldsymbol{P}_X) = \lambda_1 + \lambda_2 + \cdots + \lambda_r \leq r.$$

Furthermore, from $\boldsymbol{a}'\boldsymbol{X}'\boldsymbol{Yb} = \sqrt{\lambda}$, the canonical correlation coefficient defined as the largest correlation between $\boldsymbol{f} = \boldsymbol{Xa}$ and $\boldsymbol{g} = \boldsymbol{Yb}$ is equal to the square root of the largest eigenvalue of (6.92) or (6.93) (that is, $\sqrt{\lambda}$), which is also the largest singular value of $\boldsymbol{P}_X\boldsymbol{P}_Y$. When $\boldsymbol{a}$ and $\boldsymbol{b}$ are the eigenvectors that satisfy (6.92) or (6.93), $\boldsymbol{f} = \boldsymbol{X}\boldsymbol{a}$ and $\boldsymbol{g} = \boldsymbol{Y}\boldsymbol{b}$ are called canonical variates. Let $\boldsymbol{Z}_X$ and $\boldsymbol{Z}_Y$ denote matrices of standardized scores corresponding to $\boldsymbol{X}$ and $\boldsymbol{Y}$. Then, $\text{Sp}(\boldsymbol{X}) = \text{Sp}(\boldsymbol{Z}_X)$ and $\text{Sp}(\boldsymbol{Y}) = \text{Sp}(\boldsymbol{Z}_Y)$, so that $\text{tr}(\boldsymbol{P}_X\boldsymbol{P}_Y) = \text{tr}(\boldsymbol{P}_{Z_X}\boldsymbol{P}_{Z_Y})$, and the sum of squares of canonical correlations is equal to

$$R^2_{X\cdot Y} = \text{tr}(\boldsymbol{P}_X\boldsymbol{P}_Y) = \text{tr}(\boldsymbol{P}_{Z_X}\boldsymbol{P}_{Z_Y}) = \text{tr}(\boldsymbol{R}_{YX}\boldsymbol{R}^-_{XX}\boldsymbol{R}_{XY}\boldsymbol{R}^-_{YY}), \qquad (6.94)$$

where $\boldsymbol{R}_{XX}$, $\boldsymbol{R}_{XY}$, and $\boldsymbol{R}_{YY}$ are correlation matrices for $\boldsymbol{X}$, between $\boldsymbol{X}$ and $\boldsymbol{Y}$, and for $\boldsymbol{Y}$, respectively.

The following theorem is derived from Theorem 2.24.

Theorem 6.9 *Let* $r = \min(\text{rank}(\boldsymbol{X}), \text{rank}(\boldsymbol{Y}))$. *Then,*

$$D^2_{XY} = \text{tr}(\boldsymbol{P}_X\boldsymbol{P}_Y) \leq r, \qquad (6.95)$$

where D^2_{XY} *is called the generalized coefficient of determination and indicates the overall strength of the relationship between* $\boldsymbol{X}$ *and* $\boldsymbol{Y}$.

(Proof omitted.)

When $\boldsymbol{Y}$ consists of a single variable $\boldsymbol{y}$,

$$D^2_{XY} = \text{tr}(\boldsymbol{P}_X\boldsymbol{P}_y) = \boldsymbol{y}'\boldsymbol{P}_X\boldsymbol{y}/\boldsymbol{y}'\boldsymbol{y} = R^2_{X\cdot y}$$

coincides with the coefficient of determination, which is equal to the squared multiple correlation coefficient in multiple regression analysis in which $\boldsymbol{X}$ contains the explanatory variables and $\boldsymbol{y}$ is the criterion variable. When $\boldsymbol{X}$ also consists of a single variable $\boldsymbol{x}$,

$$D^2_{XY} = \text{tr}(\boldsymbol{P}_x\boldsymbol{P}_y) = (\boldsymbol{x}, \boldsymbol{y})^2/(||\boldsymbol{x}||^2||\boldsymbol{y}||^2) = r^2_{xy}; \qquad (6.96)$$

that is, D^2_{XY} is equal to the square of the correlation coefficient between $\boldsymbol{x}$ and $\boldsymbol{y}$.

Note The $\text{tr}(\boldsymbol{P}_x\boldsymbol{P}_y)$ above gives the most general expression of the squared correlation coefficient when both $\boldsymbol{x}$ and $\boldsymbol{y}$ are mean centered. When the variance of either $\boldsymbol{x}$ or $\boldsymbol{y}$ is zero, or both variances are zero, we have $\boldsymbol{x}$ and/or $\boldsymbol{y} = \boldsymbol{0}$, and a g-inverse of zero can be an arbitrary number, so

$$\begin{aligned} r^2_{xy} &= \text{tr}(\boldsymbol{P}_x\boldsymbol{P}_y) = \text{tr}(\boldsymbol{x}(\boldsymbol{x}'\boldsymbol{x})^-\boldsymbol{x}'\boldsymbol{y}(\boldsymbol{y}'\boldsymbol{y})^-\boldsymbol{y}') \\ &= k(\boldsymbol{x}'\boldsymbol{y})^2 = 0, \end{aligned}$$

where k is arbitrary. That is, $r_{xy} = 0$.

Assume that there are r positive eigenvalues that satisfy (6.92), and let

$$\boldsymbol{XA} = [\boldsymbol{X}\boldsymbol{a}_1, \boldsymbol{X}\boldsymbol{a}_2, \cdots, \boldsymbol{X}\boldsymbol{a}_r] \text{ and } \boldsymbol{YB} = [\boldsymbol{Y}\boldsymbol{b}_1, \boldsymbol{Y}\boldsymbol{b}_2, \cdots, \boldsymbol{Y}\boldsymbol{b}_r]$$

denote the corresponding r pairs of canonical variates. Then the following two properties hold (Yanai, 1981).

Theorem 6.10

$$\boldsymbol{P}_{XA} = (\boldsymbol{P}_X\boldsymbol{P}_Y)(\boldsymbol{P}_X\boldsymbol{P}_Y)^-_\ell \tag{6.97}$$

and

$$\boldsymbol{P}_{YB} = (\boldsymbol{P}_Y\boldsymbol{P}_X)(\boldsymbol{P}_Y\boldsymbol{P}_X)^-_\ell. \tag{6.98}$$

Proof. From (6.92), $\text{Sp}(\boldsymbol{XA}) \supset \text{Sp}(\boldsymbol{P}_X\boldsymbol{P}_Y)$. On the other hand, from $\text{rank}(\boldsymbol{P}_X\boldsymbol{P}_Y) = \text{rank}(\boldsymbol{XA}) = r$, we have $\text{Sp}(\boldsymbol{XA}) = \text{Sp}(\boldsymbol{P}_X\boldsymbol{P}_Y)$. By the note given after the corollary to Theorem 2.13, (6.97) holds; (6.98) is similar. Q.E.D.

The theorem above leads to the following.

Theorem 6.11

$$\boldsymbol{P}_{XA}\boldsymbol{P}_Y = \boldsymbol{P}_X\boldsymbol{P}_Y, \tag{6.99}$$

$$\boldsymbol{P}_X\boldsymbol{P}_{YB} = \boldsymbol{P}_X\boldsymbol{P}_Y, \tag{6.100}$$

and

$$\boldsymbol{P}_{XA}\boldsymbol{P}_{YB} = \boldsymbol{P}_X\boldsymbol{P}_Y. \tag{6.101}$$

Proof. (6.99): From $\text{Sp}(\boldsymbol{XA}) \subset \text{Sp}(\boldsymbol{X})$, $\boldsymbol{P}_{XA}\boldsymbol{P}_X = \boldsymbol{P}_{XA}$, from which it follows that $\boldsymbol{P}_{XA}\boldsymbol{P}_Y = \boldsymbol{P}_{XA}\boldsymbol{P}_X\boldsymbol{P}_Y = (\boldsymbol{P}_X\boldsymbol{P}_Y)(\boldsymbol{P}_X\boldsymbol{P}_Y)^-_\ell\boldsymbol{P}_X\boldsymbol{P}_Y = \boldsymbol{P}_X\boldsymbol{P}_Y$.

(6.100): Noting that $\boldsymbol{A}'\boldsymbol{A}\boldsymbol{A}^-_\ell = \boldsymbol{A}'$, we obtain $\boldsymbol{P}_X\boldsymbol{P}_{YB} = \boldsymbol{P}_X\boldsymbol{P}_Y\boldsymbol{P}_{YB}$ $= (\boldsymbol{P}_Y\boldsymbol{P}_X)'(\boldsymbol{P}_Y\boldsymbol{P}_X)(\boldsymbol{P}_Y\boldsymbol{P}_X)^-_\ell = (\boldsymbol{P}_Y\boldsymbol{P}_X)' = \boldsymbol{P}_X\boldsymbol{P}_Y$.

(6.101): $\boldsymbol{P}_{XA}\boldsymbol{P}_{YB} = \boldsymbol{P}_{XA}\boldsymbol{P}_Y\boldsymbol{P}_{YB} = \boldsymbol{P}_X\boldsymbol{P}_Y\boldsymbol{P}_{YB} = \boldsymbol{P}_X\boldsymbol{P}_{YB} = \boldsymbol{P}_X\boldsymbol{P}_Y$. Q.E.D.

Corollary 1

$$(\boldsymbol{P}_X - \boldsymbol{P}_{XA})\boldsymbol{P}_Y = \boldsymbol{O} \text{ and } (\boldsymbol{P}_Y - \boldsymbol{P}_{YB})\boldsymbol{P}_X = \boldsymbol{O},$$

and

$$(\boldsymbol{P}_X - \boldsymbol{P}_{XA})(\boldsymbol{P}_Y - \boldsymbol{P}_{YB}) = \boldsymbol{O}.$$

(Proof omitted.)

The corollary above indicates that $V_{X[XA]}$ and V_Y, V_X and $V_{Y[YB]}$, and $V_{X[XA]}$ and $V_{Y[YB]}$ are mutually orthogonal, where $V_{X[XA]} = \mathrm{Sp}(\boldsymbol{X}) \cap \mathrm{Sp}(\boldsymbol{XA})^{\perp}$ and $V_{Y[YB]} = \mathrm{Sp}(\boldsymbol{Y}) \cap \mathrm{Sp}(\boldsymbol{YB})^{\perp}$. However, $\mathrm{Sp}(\boldsymbol{XA})$ and $\mathrm{Sp}(\boldsymbol{YB})$ are not orthogonal, and their degree of relationship is indicated by the size of the canonical correlation coefficients (ρ_c). (See Figure 6.3(c).)

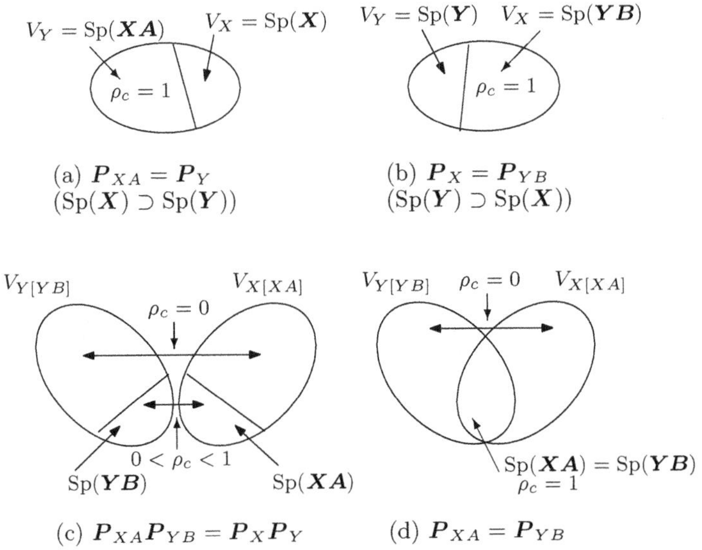

Figure 6.3: Geometric representation of canonical correlation analysis.

Corollary 2

$$\boldsymbol{P}_{XA} = \boldsymbol{P}_{YB} \Leftrightarrow \boldsymbol{P}_X\boldsymbol{P}_Y = \boldsymbol{P}_Y\boldsymbol{P}_X, \tag{6.102}$$

$$\boldsymbol{P}_{XA} = \boldsymbol{P}_Y \Leftrightarrow \boldsymbol{P}_X\boldsymbol{P}_Y = \boldsymbol{P}_Y, \tag{6.103}$$

and

$$\boldsymbol{P}_X = \boldsymbol{P}_{YB} \Leftrightarrow \boldsymbol{P}_X\boldsymbol{P}_Y = \boldsymbol{P}_X. \tag{6.104}$$

Proof. A proof is straightforward using (6.97) and (6.98), and (6.99) through (6.101). (It is left as an exercise.) Q.E.D.

In all of the three cases above, all the canonical correlations (ρ_c) between $\boldsymbol{X}$ and $\boldsymbol{Y}$ are equal to one. In the case of (6.102), however, zero canonical correlations may exist. These should be clear from Figures 6.3(d), (a), and (b), depicting the situations corresponding to (6.102), (6.103), and (6.104), respectively.

We next show a theorem concerning a decomposition of canonical correlation coefficients.

Theorem 6.12 *Let $\boldsymbol{X}$ and $\boldsymbol{Y}$ both be decomposed into two subsets, namely $\boldsymbol{X} = [\boldsymbol{X}_1, \boldsymbol{X}_2]$ and $\boldsymbol{Y} = [\boldsymbol{Y}_3, \boldsymbol{Y}_4]$. Then, the sum of squares of canonical correlations between $\boldsymbol{X}$ and $\boldsymbol{Y}$, namely $R^2_{X \cdot Y} = \mathrm{tr}(\boldsymbol{P}_X \boldsymbol{P}_Y)$, is decomposed as*

$$\mathrm{tr}(\boldsymbol{P}_X \boldsymbol{P}_Y) = R^2_{1\cdot 3} + R^2_{2[1]\cdot 3} + R^2_{1\cdot 4[3]} + R^2_{2[1]\cdot 4[3]}, \tag{6.105}$$

where

$$\begin{aligned}
R^2_{1\cdot 3} &= \mathrm{tr}(\boldsymbol{P}_1 \boldsymbol{P}_3) = \mathrm{tr}(\boldsymbol{R}_{11}^- \boldsymbol{R}_{13} \boldsymbol{R}_{33}^- \boldsymbol{R}_{31}), \\
R^2_{2[1]\cdot 3} &= \mathrm{tr}(\boldsymbol{P}_{2[1]} \boldsymbol{P}_3) \\
&= \mathrm{tr}[(\boldsymbol{R}_{32} - \boldsymbol{R}_{31}\boldsymbol{R}_{11}^-\boldsymbol{R}_{12})(\boldsymbol{R}_{22} - \boldsymbol{R}_{21}\boldsymbol{R}_{11}^-\boldsymbol{R}_{12})^- \\
&\qquad \times (\boldsymbol{R}_{23} - \boldsymbol{R}_{21}\boldsymbol{R}_{11}^-\boldsymbol{R}_{13})\boldsymbol{R}_{33}^-], \\
R^2_{1\cdot 4[3]} &= \mathrm{tr}(\boldsymbol{P}_1 \boldsymbol{P}_{4[3]}) \\
&= \mathrm{tr}[(\boldsymbol{R}_{14} - \boldsymbol{R}_{13}\boldsymbol{R}_{33}^-\boldsymbol{R}_{34})(\boldsymbol{R}_{44} - \boldsymbol{R}_{43}\boldsymbol{R}_{33}^-\boldsymbol{R}_{34})^- \\
&\qquad \times (\boldsymbol{R}_{41} - \boldsymbol{R}_{43}\boldsymbol{R}_{33}^-\boldsymbol{R}_{31})\boldsymbol{R}_{11}^-], \\
R^2_{2[1]\cdot 4[3]} &= \mathrm{tr}(\boldsymbol{P}_{2[1]} \boldsymbol{P}_{4[3]}) \\
&= \mathrm{tr}[(\boldsymbol{R}_{22} - \boldsymbol{R}_{21}\boldsymbol{R}_{11}^-\boldsymbol{R}_{12})^- \boldsymbol{S} (\boldsymbol{R}_{44} - \boldsymbol{R}_{43}\boldsymbol{R}_{33}^-\boldsymbol{R}_{34})^- \boldsymbol{S}'],
\end{aligned}$$

where $\boldsymbol{S} = \boldsymbol{R}_{24} - \boldsymbol{R}_{21}\boldsymbol{R}_{11}^-\boldsymbol{R}_{14} - \boldsymbol{R}_{23}\boldsymbol{R}_{33}^-\boldsymbol{R}_{34} + \boldsymbol{R}_{21}\boldsymbol{R}_{11}^-\boldsymbol{R}_{13}\boldsymbol{R}_{33}^-\boldsymbol{R}_{34}$.

Proof. From (4.33), we have

$$\mathrm{tr}(\boldsymbol{P}_X \boldsymbol{P}_Y) = \mathrm{tr}((\boldsymbol{P}_1 + \boldsymbol{P}_{2[1]})(\boldsymbol{P}_3 + \boldsymbol{P}_{4[3]})),$$

from which Theorem 6.12 follows immediately. To obtain an explicit expression of the right-hand side of (6.105), note that

$$\boldsymbol{P}_{2[1]} = \boldsymbol{Q}_{X_1}\boldsymbol{X}_2(\boldsymbol{X}_2'\boldsymbol{Q}_{X_1}\boldsymbol{X}_2)^-\boldsymbol{X}_2'\boldsymbol{Q}_{X_1}$$

and

$$\boldsymbol{P}_{4[3]} = \boldsymbol{Q}_{Y_3}\boldsymbol{Y}_4(\boldsymbol{Y}_4'\boldsymbol{Q}_{Y_3}\boldsymbol{Y}_4)^-\boldsymbol{Y}_4'\boldsymbol{Q}_{Y_3}.$$

Q.E.D.

Corollary *Let $\boldsymbol{X} = [\boldsymbol{x}_1, \boldsymbol{x}_2]$ and $\boldsymbol{Y} = [\boldsymbol{y}_3, \boldsymbol{y}_4]$. If $r^2_{x_1x_2} \neq 1$ and $r^2_{y_3y_4} \neq 1$, then*

$$\mathrm{tr}(\boldsymbol{P}_X \boldsymbol{P}_Y) = r^2_{1\cdot 3} + r^2_{2[1]\cdot 3} + r^2_{1\cdot 4[3]} + r^2_{2[1]\cdot 4[3]}, \tag{6.106}$$

where

$$r_{2[1]\cdot 3} = \frac{r_{x_2y_3} - r_{x_1x_2}r_{x_1y_3}}{\sqrt{1 - r^2_{x_1x_2}}}, \tag{6.107}$$

$$r_{1\cdot 4[3]} = \frac{r_{x_1y_4} - r_{x_1y_3}r_{y_3y_4}}{\sqrt{1 - r^2_{y_3y_4}}}, \tag{6.108}$$

and

$$r_{2[1]\cdot 4[3]} = \frac{r_{x_2y_4} - r_{x_1x_2}r_{x_1y_4} - r_{x_2y_3}r_{y_3y_4} + r_{x_1x_2}r_{y_3y_4}r_{x_1y_3}}{\sqrt{(1 - r^2_{x_1x_2})(1 - r^2_{y_3y_4})}}. \tag{6.109}$$

(Proof omitted.)

Note Coefficients (6.107) and (6.108) are called part correlation coefficients, and (6.109) is called a bipartial correlation coefficient. Furthermore, $R^2_{2[1]\cdot 3}$ and $R^2_{1\cdot 4[3]}$ in (6.105) correspond with squared part canonical correlations, and $R^2_{2[1]\cdot 4[3]}$ with a bipartial canonical correlation.

To perform the forward variable selection in canonical correlation analysis using (6.105), let $\boldsymbol{R}^2_{[j+1]\cdot[k+1]}$ denote the sum of squared canonical correlation coefficients between $\boldsymbol{X}_{[j+1]} = [\boldsymbol{x}_{j+1}, \boldsymbol{X}_{[j]}]$ and $\boldsymbol{Y}_{[k+1]} = [\boldsymbol{y}_{k+1}, \boldsymbol{Y}_{[k]}]$, where $\boldsymbol{X}_{[j]} = [\boldsymbol{x}_1, \boldsymbol{x}_2, \cdots, \boldsymbol{x}_j]$ and $\boldsymbol{Y}_{[k]} = [\boldsymbol{y}_1, \boldsymbol{y}_2, \cdots, \boldsymbol{y}_k]$. We decompose $\boldsymbol{R}^2_{[j+1]\cdot[k+1]}$ as

$$R^2_{[j+1]\cdot[k+1]} = R^2_{[j]\cdot[k]} + R^2_{j+1[j]\cdot k} + R^2_{j\cdot k+1[k]} + R^2_{j+1[j]\cdot k+1[k]} \tag{6.110}$$

and choose $\boldsymbol{x}_{j+1}$ and $\boldsymbol{y}_{k+1}$ so as to maximize $R^2_{j+1[j]\cdot k}$ and $R^2_{j\cdot k+1[k]}$.

Example 6.1 We have applied canonical correlation analysis to $\boldsymbol{X} = [\boldsymbol{x}_1, \boldsymbol{x}_2, \cdots, \boldsymbol{x}_{10}]$ and $\boldsymbol{Y} = [\boldsymbol{y}_1, \boldsymbol{y}_2, \cdots, \boldsymbol{y}_{10}]$. We present ten canonical correlation coefficients in Table 6.1, the corresponding weight vectors to derive canonical variates in Table 6.2, and the results obtained by the forward selection procedure above in Table 6.3. The A, B, and C in Table 6.3 indicate $R^2_{j+1[j]\cdot k}$, $R^2_{j\cdot k+1[k]}$, and $R^2_{j+1[j]\cdot k+1[k]}$ (Yanai, 1980), respectively.

6.3.2 Canonical discriminant analysis

Let us now replace one of the two sets of variables in canonical correlation analysis, say $\boldsymbol{Y}$, by an n by m matrix of dummy variables defined in (1.54).

Table 6.1: Canonical correlations.

	1	2	3	4	5
Coeff.	0.831	0.671	0.545	0.470	0.249
Cum.	0.831	1.501	2.046	2.516	2.765
	6	7	8	9	10
Coeff.	0.119	0.090	0.052	0.030	0.002
Cum.	2.884	2.974	3.025	3.056	3.058

Define the centering operator $\boldsymbol{Q}_M = \boldsymbol{I}_n - \boldsymbol{P}_M$ (defined earlier in (2.18)), where $\boldsymbol{P}_M = \frac{1}{n}\boldsymbol{1}_n\boldsymbol{1}_n'$ with $\boldsymbol{1}_n$ being the n-component vector of ones. The $\boldsymbol{Q}_M$ is the orthogonal projector onto the null space of $\boldsymbol{1}_n$, and let

$$\tilde{\boldsymbol{G}} = \boldsymbol{Q}_M\boldsymbol{G}. \tag{6.111}$$

Let $\boldsymbol{P}_{\tilde{G}}$ denote the orthogonal projector onto $\text{Sp}(\tilde{\boldsymbol{G}})$. From $\text{Sp}(\boldsymbol{G}) \supset \text{Sp}(\boldsymbol{1}_n)$, we have

$$\boldsymbol{P}_{\tilde{G}} = \boldsymbol{P}_G - \boldsymbol{P}_M$$

by Theorem 2.11. Let $\boldsymbol{X}_R$ denote a data matrix of raw scores (not column-wise centered, and consequently column means are not necessarily zero). From (2.20), we have

$$\boldsymbol{X} = \boldsymbol{Q}_M\boldsymbol{X}_R.$$

Applying canonical correlation analysis to $\boldsymbol{X}$ and $\tilde{\boldsymbol{G}}$, we obtain

$$(\boldsymbol{P}_X\boldsymbol{P}_{\tilde{G}})\boldsymbol{X}\boldsymbol{a} = \lambda\boldsymbol{X}\boldsymbol{a} \tag{6.112}$$

by (6.92). Since $\boldsymbol{P}_G - \boldsymbol{P}_M = \boldsymbol{P}_G - \boldsymbol{P}_G\boldsymbol{P}_M = \boldsymbol{P}_G\boldsymbol{Q}_M$, we have $\boldsymbol{P}_{\tilde{G}}\boldsymbol{X}\boldsymbol{a} = \boldsymbol{P}_G\boldsymbol{Q}_M\boldsymbol{Q}_M\boldsymbol{X}_R\boldsymbol{a} = \boldsymbol{P}_G\boldsymbol{X}\boldsymbol{a}$, so that (6.112) can be rewritten as

$$(\boldsymbol{P}_X\boldsymbol{P}_G)\boldsymbol{X}\boldsymbol{a} = \lambda\boldsymbol{X}\boldsymbol{a}.$$

Premultiplying both sides of the equation above by $\boldsymbol{X}'$, we obtain

$$(\boldsymbol{X}'\boldsymbol{P}_G\boldsymbol{X})\boldsymbol{a} = \lambda\boldsymbol{X}'\boldsymbol{X}\boldsymbol{a}. \tag{6.113}$$

Since $\boldsymbol{X}'\boldsymbol{P}_G\boldsymbol{X} = \boldsymbol{X}_R'\boldsymbol{Q}_M\boldsymbol{P}_G\boldsymbol{Q}_M\boldsymbol{X}_R = \boldsymbol{X}_R'(\boldsymbol{P}_G - \boldsymbol{P}_M)\boldsymbol{X}_R$, $\boldsymbol{C}_A = \boldsymbol{X}'\boldsymbol{P}_G\boldsymbol{X}/n$ represents the between-group covariance matrix. Let $\boldsymbol{C}_{XX} = \boldsymbol{X}'\boldsymbol{X}/n$ denote the total covariance matrix. Then, (6.113) can be further rewritten as

$$\boldsymbol{C}_A\boldsymbol{a} = \lambda\boldsymbol{C}_{XX}\boldsymbol{a}. \tag{6.114}$$

Table 6.2: Weight vectors corresponding to the first eight canonical variates.

	1	2	3	4	5	6	7	8
x_1	−.272	.144	−.068	−.508	−.196	−.243	.036	.218
x_2	.155	.249	−.007	−.020	.702	−.416	.335	.453
x_3	.105	.681	.464	.218	−.390	.097	.258	−.309
x_4	.460	−.353	−.638	.086	−.434	−.048	.652	.021
x_5	.169	−.358	.915	.063	−.091	−.549	.279	.576
x_6	−.139	.385	−.172	−.365	−.499	.351	−.043	.851
x_7	.483	−.074	.500	−.598	.259	.016	.149	−.711
x_8	−.419	−.175	−.356	.282	.526	.872	.362	−.224
x_9	−.368	.225	.259	.138	.280	−.360	−.147	−.571
x_{10}	.254	.102	.006	.353	.498	.146	−.338	.668
y_1	−.071	.174	−.140	.054	.253	.135	−.045	.612
y_2	.348	.262	−.250	.125	.203	−1.225	−.082	−.215
y_3	.177	.364	.231	.201	−.469	−.111	−.607	.668
y_4	−.036	.052	−.111	−.152	−.036	−.057	.186	.228
y_5	.156	.377	−.038	−.428	.073	−.311	.015	−.491
y_6	.024	−.259	.238	.041	−.052	.085	.037	.403
y_7	−.425	−.564	.383	−.121	.047	−.213	−.099	.603
y_8	−.095	−.019	.058	.009	.083	.056	−.022	−.289
y_9	−.358	−.232	.105	.205	−.007	.513	1.426	−.284
y_{10}	.249	.050	.074	−.066	.328	.560	.190	−.426

This is called canonical discriminant analysis. In general, (6.114) has $\text{rank}(\boldsymbol{C}_A) = m - 1$ positive eigenvalues as solutions. The eigenvalue λ in (6.114) is equal to $s^2_{f_A}/s^2_f = ||\boldsymbol{P}_G\boldsymbol{X}\boldsymbol{a}||^2/||\boldsymbol{X}\boldsymbol{a}||^2$, where $s^2_{f_A} = \boldsymbol{a}'\boldsymbol{C}_A\boldsymbol{a}$ is the between-group variance of the composite variable $\boldsymbol{f} = \boldsymbol{X}\boldsymbol{a}$ and $s^2_f = ||\boldsymbol{X}\boldsymbol{a}||^2/n = \boldsymbol{a}'(\boldsymbol{X}'\boldsymbol{X}/n)\boldsymbol{a} = \boldsymbol{a}'\boldsymbol{C}_{XX}\boldsymbol{a}$ is the total variance of $\boldsymbol{f}$. λ is clearly smaller than 1 (see (2.56)).

Let $\boldsymbol{C}_{XX} = \boldsymbol{Q}\boldsymbol{\Delta}^2\boldsymbol{Q}'$ denote the spectral decomposition of $\boldsymbol{C}_{XX}$. Substituting this into (6.114) and premultiplying both sides by $\boldsymbol{\Delta}^{-1}\boldsymbol{Q}'$, and since $\boldsymbol{Q}'\boldsymbol{Q} = \boldsymbol{Q}\boldsymbol{Q}' = \boldsymbol{I}_p$, we obtain

$$(\boldsymbol{\Delta}^{-1}\boldsymbol{Q}'\boldsymbol{C}_A\boldsymbol{Q}\boldsymbol{\Delta}^{-1})\boldsymbol{\Delta}\boldsymbol{Q}'\boldsymbol{a} = \lambda\boldsymbol{\Delta}\boldsymbol{Q}'\boldsymbol{a},$$

from which it can be seen that λ is an eigenvalue of $\boldsymbol{\Delta}^{-1}\boldsymbol{Q}'\boldsymbol{C}_A\boldsymbol{Q}\boldsymbol{\Delta}^{-1}$ and that its square root is a singular value of $\boldsymbol{P}_G\boldsymbol{X}\boldsymbol{Q}\boldsymbol{\Delta}^{-1}$.

Table 6.3: Forward variable selection in canonical correlation analysis.

Step	X	Y	A	B	C	Cum. sum
1	x_5	y_7	–	–	–	0.312
2	x_2	y_6	.190	.059	.220	0.781
3	x_{10}	y_3	.160	.149	.047	1.137
4	x_8	y_9	.126	.162	.029	1.454
5	x_7	y_1	.143	.084	.000	1.681
6	x_4	y_{10}	.139	.153	.038	2.012
7	x_2	y_5	.089	.296	.027	2.423
8	x_1	y_4	.148	.152	.064	2.786
9	x_6	y_8	.134	.038	.000	2.957
10	x_9	y_2	.080	.200	.000	3.057

When the number of groups to be discriminated is 2 in (6.114) (that is, when $m = 2$), $\boldsymbol{C}_A$ becomes a matrix of rank 1, and its nonzero eigenvalue is given by

$$\lambda = \frac{n_1 n_2}{n^2}(\bar{\boldsymbol{x}}_1 - \bar{\boldsymbol{x}}_2)'\boldsymbol{C}_{XX}^{-}(\bar{\boldsymbol{x}}_1 - \bar{\boldsymbol{x}}_2), \tag{6.115}$$

where $\bar{\boldsymbol{x}}_1$ and $\bar{\boldsymbol{x}}_2$ are mean vectors of p variables in groups 1 and 2, respectively. See Takeuchi, Yanai, and Mukherjee (1982, pp. 162–165).

Let both $\boldsymbol{X}$ and $\boldsymbol{Y}$ in canonical correlation analysis be matrices of dummy variables. (Denote them by $\boldsymbol{G}_1$ and $\boldsymbol{G}_2$.) Let

$$\tilde{\boldsymbol{G}}_1 = \boldsymbol{Q}_M \boldsymbol{G}_1 \text{ and } \tilde{\boldsymbol{G}}_2 = \boldsymbol{Q}_M \boldsymbol{G}_2$$

denote the columnwise centered matrices corresponding to $\boldsymbol{G}_1$ and $\boldsymbol{G}_2$. Then, since $\boldsymbol{P}_{\tilde{G}_1} = \boldsymbol{P}_{G_1} - \boldsymbol{P}_M = \boldsymbol{P}_{G_1}\boldsymbol{Q}_M$ and $\boldsymbol{P}_{\tilde{G}_2} = \boldsymbol{P}_{G_2} - \boldsymbol{P}_M = \boldsymbol{P}_{G_2}\boldsymbol{Q}_M$, the sum of squared canonical correlation coefficients is given by

$$s = \operatorname{tr}(\boldsymbol{P}_{\tilde{G}_1}\boldsymbol{P}_{\tilde{G}_2}) = \operatorname{tr}(\boldsymbol{P}_{G_1}\boldsymbol{Q}_M\boldsymbol{P}_{G_2}\boldsymbol{Q}_M) = \operatorname{tr}(\boldsymbol{S}\boldsymbol{S}'), \tag{6.116}$$

where $\boldsymbol{S} = (\boldsymbol{G}_1'\boldsymbol{G}_1)^{-1/2}\boldsymbol{G}_1'\boldsymbol{Q}_M\boldsymbol{G}_2(\boldsymbol{G}_2'\boldsymbol{G}_2)^{-1/2}$.

Let $\boldsymbol{S} = [s_{ij}]$, $\boldsymbol{G}_1'\boldsymbol{G}_2 = [n_{ij}]$, $n_{i.} = \sum_j n_{ij}$, and $n_{.j} = \sum_i n_{ij}$. Since

$$s_{ij} = \frac{n_{ij} - \frac{1}{n}n_{i.}n_{.j}}{\sqrt{n_{i.}}\sqrt{n_{.j}}},$$

we obtain

$$s = \sum_i \sum_j s_{ij}^2 = \frac{1}{n} \left\{ \sum_i \sum_j \frac{\left(n_{ij} - \frac{1}{n} n_{i.} n_{.j}\right)^2}{\frac{1}{n} n_{i.} n_{.j}} \right\} = \frac{1}{n} \chi^2. \tag{6.117}$$

This indicates that (6.116) is equal to $1/n$ times the chi-square statistic often used in tests for contingency tables. Let $\mu_1(\boldsymbol{S}), \mu_2(\boldsymbol{S}), \cdots$ denote the singular values of $\boldsymbol{S}$. From (6.116), we obtain

$$\chi^2 = n \sum_j \mu_j^2(\boldsymbol{S}). \tag{6.118}$$

6.3.3 Principal component analysis

In this subsection, we describe the relationship between principal component analysis (PCA) and singular value decomposition (SVD), and extend the former in several ways using projectors.

Let $\boldsymbol{A} = [\boldsymbol{a}_1, \boldsymbol{a}_2, \cdots, \boldsymbol{a}_p]$, where $\mathrm{Sp}(\boldsymbol{A}) \subset \boldsymbol{E}^n$. Let $\boldsymbol{P}_f$ denote the orthogonal projector onto $\mathrm{Sp}(\boldsymbol{f})$, where $\boldsymbol{f}$ is a linear combination of the columns of $\boldsymbol{A}$,

$$\boldsymbol{f} = w_1 \boldsymbol{a}_1 + w_2 \boldsymbol{a}_2 + \cdots + w_p \boldsymbol{a}_p = \boldsymbol{A}\boldsymbol{w}, \tag{6.119}$$

and let $\boldsymbol{P}_f \boldsymbol{a}_j$ denote the projection of $\boldsymbol{a}_j$ onto $\mathrm{Sp}(\boldsymbol{f})$. The sum of squared norms of the latter is given by

$$\begin{aligned} s &= \sum_{j=1}^p ||\boldsymbol{P}_f \boldsymbol{a}_j||^2 = \sum_{j=1}^p \boldsymbol{a}_j' \boldsymbol{P}_f \boldsymbol{a}_j = \mathrm{tr}(\boldsymbol{A}' \boldsymbol{P}_f \boldsymbol{A}) \\ &= \mathrm{tr}(\boldsymbol{A}'\boldsymbol{f}(\boldsymbol{f}'\boldsymbol{f})^{-1}\boldsymbol{f}'\boldsymbol{A}) = \boldsymbol{f}'\boldsymbol{A}\boldsymbol{A}'\boldsymbol{f}/\boldsymbol{f}'\boldsymbol{f} = ||\boldsymbol{A}'\boldsymbol{f}||^2/||\boldsymbol{f}||^2. \end{aligned}$$

Lemma 5.1 indicates that $\boldsymbol{f}$ maximizing the equation above is obtained by solving

$$\boldsymbol{A}\boldsymbol{A}'\boldsymbol{f} = \lambda \boldsymbol{f}. \tag{6.120}$$

This implies that the maximum value of s is given by the maximum eigenvalue of $\boldsymbol{A}\boldsymbol{A}'$ (or of $\boldsymbol{A}'\boldsymbol{A}$). Substituting $\boldsymbol{f} = \boldsymbol{A}\boldsymbol{w}$ into the equation above, and premultiplying both sides by $\boldsymbol{A}'$, we obtain

$$(\boldsymbol{A}'\boldsymbol{A})^2 \boldsymbol{w} = \lambda (\boldsymbol{A}'\boldsymbol{A}) \boldsymbol{w}. \tag{6.121}$$

If $\boldsymbol{A}'\boldsymbol{A}$ is nonsingular, we further obtain

$$(\boldsymbol{A}'\boldsymbol{A}) \boldsymbol{w} = \lambda \boldsymbol{w}. \tag{6.122}$$

If we substitute $\boldsymbol{f} = \boldsymbol{A}\boldsymbol{w}$ into the equation above, we obtain

$$\boldsymbol{A}'\boldsymbol{f} = \lambda \boldsymbol{w}. \tag{6.123}$$

Let $\mu_1 > \mu_2 > \cdots > \mu_p$ denote the singular values of $\boldsymbol{A}$. (It is assumed that they are distinct.) Let $\lambda_1 > \lambda_2 > \cdots > \lambda_p$ ($\lambda_j = \mu_j^2$) denote the eigenvalues of $\boldsymbol{A}'\boldsymbol{A}$, and let $\boldsymbol{w}_1, \boldsymbol{w}_2, \cdots, \boldsymbol{w}_p$ denote the corresponding normalized eigenvectors of $\boldsymbol{A}'\boldsymbol{A}$. Then the p linear combinations

$$\begin{aligned}
\boldsymbol{f}_1 &= \boldsymbol{A}\boldsymbol{w}_1 = w_{11}\boldsymbol{a}_1 + w_{12}\boldsymbol{a}_2 + \cdots + w_{1p}\boldsymbol{a}_p \\
\boldsymbol{f}_2 &= \boldsymbol{A}\boldsymbol{w}_2 = w_{21}\boldsymbol{a}_1 + w_{22}\boldsymbol{a}_2 + \cdots + w_{2p}\boldsymbol{a}_p \\
&\vdots \\
\boldsymbol{f}_p &= \boldsymbol{A}\boldsymbol{w}_p = w_{p1}\boldsymbol{a}_1 + w_{p2}\boldsymbol{a}_2 + \cdots + w_{pp}\boldsymbol{a}_p
\end{aligned}$$

are respectively called the first principal component, the second principal component, and so on.

The norm of each vector is given by

$$||\boldsymbol{f}_j|| = \sqrt{\boldsymbol{w}_j'\boldsymbol{A}'\boldsymbol{A}\boldsymbol{w}_j} = \mu_j, \quad (j = 1, \cdots, p), \tag{6.124}$$

which is equal to the corresponding singular value. The sum of squares of $||\boldsymbol{f}_j||$ is

$$||\boldsymbol{f}_1||^2 + ||\boldsymbol{f}_2||^2 + \cdots + ||\boldsymbol{f}_p||^2 = \lambda_1 + \lambda_2 + \cdots + \lambda_p = \mathrm{tr}(\boldsymbol{A}'\boldsymbol{A}).$$

Let $\tilde{\boldsymbol{f}}_j = \boldsymbol{f}_j/||\boldsymbol{f}_j||$. Then $\tilde{\boldsymbol{f}}_j$ is a vector of length one, and the SVD of $\boldsymbol{A}$ is, by (5.18) and (5.19), given by

$$\boldsymbol{A} = \mu_1\tilde{\boldsymbol{f}}_1\boldsymbol{w}_1' + \mu_2\tilde{\boldsymbol{f}}_2\boldsymbol{w}_2' + \cdots + \mu_p\tilde{\boldsymbol{f}}_p\boldsymbol{w}_p' \tag{6.125}$$

from the viewpoint of PCA. Noting that $\boldsymbol{f}_j = \mu_j\tilde{\boldsymbol{f}}_j$ ($j = 1, \cdots, p$), the equation above can be rewritten as

$$\boldsymbol{A} = \boldsymbol{f}_1\boldsymbol{w}_1' + \boldsymbol{f}_2\boldsymbol{w}_2' + \cdots + \boldsymbol{f}_p\boldsymbol{w}_p'. \tag{6.126}$$

Let

$$\boldsymbol{b} = \boldsymbol{A}'\boldsymbol{f} = \boldsymbol{A}'\boldsymbol{A}\boldsymbol{w},$$

where $\boldsymbol{A}'\boldsymbol{A}$ is assumed singular. From (6.121), we have

$$(\boldsymbol{A}'\boldsymbol{A})\boldsymbol{b} = \lambda\boldsymbol{b}.$$

If we normalize the principal component vector $\boldsymbol{f}_j$, the SVD of $\boldsymbol{A}$ is given by

$$\boldsymbol{A} = \boldsymbol{f}_1\boldsymbol{b}_1' + \boldsymbol{f}_2\boldsymbol{b}_2' + \cdots + \boldsymbol{f}_r\boldsymbol{b}_r', \tag{6.127}$$

where $r = \text{rank}(\boldsymbol{A})$, and $\boldsymbol{b}_j = \boldsymbol{A}'\boldsymbol{f}_j$ since $||\boldsymbol{b}|| = \sqrt{\boldsymbol{f}'\boldsymbol{A}'\boldsymbol{A}\boldsymbol{f}} = \sqrt{\lambda} = \mu$.

Note The method presented above concerns a general theory of PCA. In practice, we take $\boldsymbol{A} = [\boldsymbol{a}_1, \boldsymbol{a}_2, \cdots, \boldsymbol{a}_p]$ as the matrix of mean centered scores. We then calculate the covariance matrix $\boldsymbol{S} = \boldsymbol{A}'\boldsymbol{A}/n$ between p variables and solve the eigenequation

$$\boldsymbol{S}\boldsymbol{w} = \lambda\boldsymbol{w}. \tag{6.128}$$

Hence, the variance ($s^2_{f_j}$) of principal component scores $\boldsymbol{f}_j$ is equal to the eigenvalue λ_j, and the standard deviation (s_{f_j}) is equal to the singular value μ_j. If the scores are standardized, the variance-covariance matrix $\boldsymbol{S}$ is replaced by the correlation matrix $\boldsymbol{R}$.

Note Equations (6.119) and (6.123) can be rewritten as

$$\mu_j\tilde{\boldsymbol{f}}_j = \boldsymbol{A}\boldsymbol{w}_j \text{ and } \boldsymbol{A}'\tilde{\boldsymbol{f}}_j = \mu_j\boldsymbol{w}_j.$$

They correspond to the basic equations of the SVD of $\boldsymbol{A}$ in (5.18) (or (5.19)) and (5.24), and are derived from maximizing $(\tilde{\boldsymbol{f}}, \boldsymbol{A}\boldsymbol{w})$ subject to $||\tilde{\boldsymbol{f}}||^2 = 1$ and $||\boldsymbol{w}||^2 = 1$.

Let $\boldsymbol{A}$ denote an n by m matrix whose element a_{ij} indicates the joint frequency of category i and category j of two categorical variables, X and Y. Let x_i and y_j denote the weights assigned to the categories. The correlation between X and Y can be expressed as

$$r_{XY} = \frac{\sum_i \sum_j a_{ij}x_i y_j - n\bar{x}\bar{y}}{\sqrt{\sum_i a_{i.}x_i^2 - n\bar{x}^2}\sqrt{\sum_j a_{.j}y_j^2 - n\bar{y}^2}},$$

where $\bar{x} = \sum_i a_{i.}x_i/n$ and $\bar{y} = \sum_j a_{.j}y_j/n$ are the means of X and Y. Let us obtain $\boldsymbol{x} = (x_1, x_2, \cdots, x_n)'$ and $\boldsymbol{y} = (y_1, y_2, \cdots, y_m)'$ that maximize r_{XY} subject to the constraints that the means are $\bar{x} = \bar{y} = 0$ and the variances are $\sum_i a_{i.}x_i^2/n = 1$ and $\sum_j a_{.j}y_j^2/n = 1$. Define the diagonal matrices $\boldsymbol{D}_X$ and $\boldsymbol{D}_Y$ of orders n and m, respectively, as

$$\boldsymbol{D}_X = \begin{bmatrix} a_{1.} & 0 & \cdots & 0 \\ 0 & a_{2.} & \cdots & 0 \\ \vdots & \vdots & \ddots & \vdots \\ 0 & 0 & \cdots & a_{n.} \end{bmatrix} \text{ and } \boldsymbol{D}_Y = \begin{bmatrix} a_{.1} & 0 & \cdots & 0 \\ 0 & a_{.2} & \cdots & 0 \\ \vdots & \vdots & \ddots & \vdots \\ 0 & 0 & \cdots & a_{.m} \end{bmatrix},$$

where $a_{i.} = \sum_j a_{ij}$ and $a_{.j} = \sum_i a_{ij}$. The problem reduces to that of maximizing $\boldsymbol{x}'\boldsymbol{A}\boldsymbol{y}$ subject to the constraints

$$\boldsymbol{x}'\boldsymbol{D}_X\boldsymbol{x} = \boldsymbol{y}'\boldsymbol{D}_Y\boldsymbol{y} = 1.$$

Differentiating

$$f(\boldsymbol{x}, \boldsymbol{y}) = \boldsymbol{x}'\boldsymbol{A}\boldsymbol{y} - \frac{\lambda}{2}(\boldsymbol{x}'\boldsymbol{D}_X\boldsymbol{x} - 1) - \frac{\mu}{2}(\boldsymbol{y}'\boldsymbol{D}_Y\boldsymbol{y} - 1)$$

with respect to $\boldsymbol{x}$ and $\boldsymbol{y}$ and setting the results equal to zero, we obtain

$$\boldsymbol{A}\boldsymbol{y} = \lambda\boldsymbol{D}_X\boldsymbol{x} \text{ and } \boldsymbol{A}'\boldsymbol{x} = \mu\boldsymbol{D}_Y\boldsymbol{y}. \tag{6.129}$$

(It can be easily verified that $\lambda = \mu$, so μ is used for λ hereafter.) Let

$$\boldsymbol{D}_X^{-1/2} = \begin{bmatrix} 1/\sqrt{a_{1.}} & 0 & \cdots & 0 \\ 0 & 1/\sqrt{a_{2.}} & \cdots & 0 \\ \vdots & \vdots & \ddots & \vdots \\ 0 & 0 & \cdots & 1/\sqrt{a_{n.}} \end{bmatrix}$$

and

$$\boldsymbol{D}_Y^{-1/2} = \begin{bmatrix} 1/\sqrt{a_{.1}} & 0 & \cdots & 0 \\ 0 & 1/\sqrt{a_{.2}} & \cdots & 0 \\ \vdots & \vdots & \ddots & \vdots \\ 0 & 0 & \cdots & 1/\sqrt{a_{.m}} \end{bmatrix}.$$

Let

$$\tilde{\boldsymbol{A}} = \boldsymbol{D}_X^{-1/2}\boldsymbol{A}\boldsymbol{D}_Y^{-1/2},$$

and let $\tilde{\boldsymbol{x}}$ and $\tilde{\boldsymbol{y}}$ be such that $\boldsymbol{x} = \boldsymbol{D}_X^{-1/2}\tilde{\boldsymbol{x}}$ and $\boldsymbol{y} = \boldsymbol{D}_Y^{-1/2}\tilde{\boldsymbol{y}}$. Then, (6.129) can be rewritten as

$$\tilde{\boldsymbol{A}}\tilde{\boldsymbol{y}} = \mu\tilde{\boldsymbol{x}} \text{ and } \tilde{\boldsymbol{A}}'\tilde{\boldsymbol{x}} = \mu\tilde{\boldsymbol{y}}, \tag{6.130}$$

and the SVD of $\tilde{\boldsymbol{A}}$ can be written as

$$\tilde{\boldsymbol{A}} = \mu_1\tilde{\boldsymbol{x}}_1\tilde{\boldsymbol{y}}_1' + \mu_2\tilde{\boldsymbol{x}}_2\tilde{\boldsymbol{y}}_2' + \cdots + \mu_r\tilde{\boldsymbol{x}}_r\tilde{\boldsymbol{y}}_r', \tag{6.131}$$

where $r = \min(n, m)$ and where $\mu_1 = 1$, $\boldsymbol{x}_1 = \boldsymbol{1}_n$, and $\boldsymbol{y}_1 = \boldsymbol{1}_m$.

The method described above is a multivariate data analysis technique called optimal scaling or dual scaling (Nishisato, 1980).

Let us obtain $\boldsymbol{F} = [\boldsymbol{f}_1, \boldsymbol{f}_2, \cdots, \boldsymbol{f}_r]$, where $r = \text{rank}(\boldsymbol{A})$, that maximizes

$$s = \sum_{j=1}^{p} ||\boldsymbol{P}_F\boldsymbol{a}_j||^2, \tag{6.132}$$

where $\boldsymbol{P}_F$ is the orthogonal projector onto $\text{Sp}(\boldsymbol{F})$ and $\boldsymbol{a}_j$ is the jth column vector of $\boldsymbol{A} = [\boldsymbol{a}_1, \boldsymbol{a}_2, \cdots, \boldsymbol{a}_p]$. The criterion above can be rewritten as

$$s = \text{tr}(\boldsymbol{A}'\boldsymbol{P}_F\boldsymbol{A}) = \text{tr}\{(\boldsymbol{F}'\boldsymbol{F})^{-1}\boldsymbol{F}'\boldsymbol{A}\boldsymbol{A}'\boldsymbol{F}\},$$

and so, for maximizing this under the restriction that $\boldsymbol{F}'\boldsymbol{F} = \boldsymbol{I}_r$, we introduce

$$f(\boldsymbol{F}, \boldsymbol{L}) = \text{tr}(\boldsymbol{F}'\boldsymbol{A}\boldsymbol{A}'\boldsymbol{F}) - \text{tr}\{(\boldsymbol{F}'\boldsymbol{F} - \boldsymbol{I}_r)\boldsymbol{L}\},$$

where $\boldsymbol{L}$ is a symmetric matrix of Lagrangean multipliers. Differentiating $f(\boldsymbol{F}, \boldsymbol{L})$ with respect to $\boldsymbol{F}$ and setting the results equal to zero, we obtain

$$\boldsymbol{A}\boldsymbol{A}'\boldsymbol{F} = \boldsymbol{F}\boldsymbol{L}. \tag{6.133}$$

Since $\boldsymbol{L}$ is symmetric, it can be decomposed as $\boldsymbol{L} = \boldsymbol{V}\boldsymbol{\Delta}_r^2\boldsymbol{V}'$, where $r = \text{rank}(\boldsymbol{A}'\boldsymbol{A})$, by spectral decomposition. Substituting this into (6.133), we obtain

$$\boldsymbol{A}\boldsymbol{A}'\boldsymbol{F} = \boldsymbol{F}\boldsymbol{V}\boldsymbol{\Delta}_r^2\boldsymbol{V}' \Rightarrow \boldsymbol{A}\boldsymbol{A}'(\boldsymbol{F}\boldsymbol{V}) = (\boldsymbol{F}\boldsymbol{V})\boldsymbol{\Delta}_r^2.$$

Since $\boldsymbol{F}\boldsymbol{V}$ is columnwise orthogonal, we let $\tilde{\boldsymbol{F}} = \boldsymbol{F}\boldsymbol{V}$. $\tilde{\boldsymbol{F}}$ is the matrix of eigenvectors of $\boldsymbol{A}\boldsymbol{A}'$ corresponding to the r largest eigenvalues, so the maximum of s is given by

$$\begin{aligned}\text{tr}(\boldsymbol{F}'\boldsymbol{A}\boldsymbol{A}'\boldsymbol{F}) &= \text{tr}(\boldsymbol{F}'\boldsymbol{A}\boldsymbol{A}'\boldsymbol{F}\boldsymbol{V}\boldsymbol{V}') \\ &= \text{tr}(\boldsymbol{V}'\boldsymbol{F}'\boldsymbol{A}\boldsymbol{A}'\boldsymbol{F}\boldsymbol{V}) = \text{tr}(\boldsymbol{V}'\boldsymbol{F}'\boldsymbol{F}\boldsymbol{V}\boldsymbol{\Delta}_r^2) \\ &= \text{tr}(\boldsymbol{V}'\boldsymbol{V}\boldsymbol{\Delta}_r^2) = \text{tr}(\boldsymbol{\Delta}_r^2) = \lambda_1 + \lambda_2 + \cdots + \lambda_r. \end{aligned} \tag{6.134}$$

Hence, the r principal component vectors $\boldsymbol{F} = \tilde{\boldsymbol{F}}\boldsymbol{V}'$ are not the set of eigenvectors corresponding to the r largest eigenvalues of the symmetric matrix $\boldsymbol{A}\boldsymbol{A}'$ but a linear combination of those eigenvectors. That is, $\text{Sp}(\boldsymbol{F})$ is the subspace spanned by the r principal components.

In practice, it is advisable to compute $\boldsymbol{F}$ by solving

$$\boldsymbol{A}'\boldsymbol{A}(\boldsymbol{A}'\tilde{\boldsymbol{F}}) = (\boldsymbol{A}'\tilde{\boldsymbol{F}})\boldsymbol{\Delta}_r^2, \tag{6.135}$$

obtained by pre- and postmultiplying (6.133) by $\boldsymbol{A}'$ and $\boldsymbol{V}$, respectively.

Note that s in (6.132) is equal to the sum of squared norms of the projection of $\boldsymbol{a}_j$ onto $\text{Sp}(\boldsymbol{F})$, as depicted in Figure 6.4(a). The sum of squared lengths of the perpendicular line from the head of the vector $\boldsymbol{a}_j$ to its projection onto $\text{Sp}(\boldsymbol{F})$,

$$\tilde{s} = \sum_{j=1}^{p} ||\boldsymbol{Q}_F\boldsymbol{a}_j||^2,$$

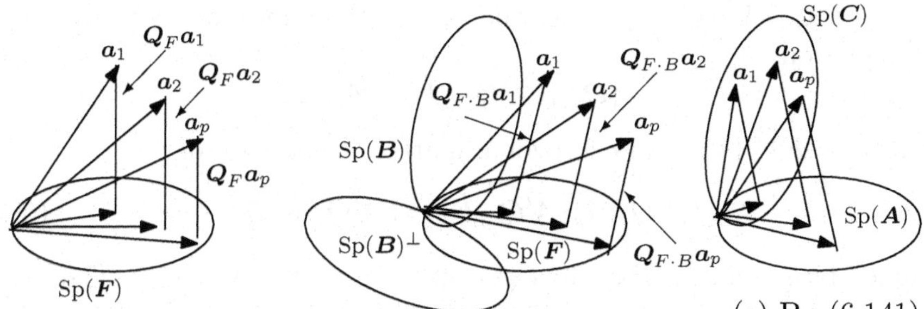

(a) General case by (6.135)

(b) By (6.137)

(c) By (6.141)

Figure 6.4: Three methods of PCA.

where $\boldsymbol{Q}_f = \boldsymbol{I}_n - \boldsymbol{P}_F$, is equal to

$$\begin{aligned}\tilde{s} &= \operatorname{tr}(\boldsymbol{A}'\boldsymbol{Q}_F\boldsymbol{A}) = \operatorname{tr}(\boldsymbol{A} - \boldsymbol{P}_F\boldsymbol{A})'(\boldsymbol{A} - \boldsymbol{P}_F\boldsymbol{A}) \\ &= \operatorname{tr}(\boldsymbol{A} - \boldsymbol{F}\boldsymbol{F}'\boldsymbol{A})'(\boldsymbol{A} - \boldsymbol{F}\boldsymbol{F}'\boldsymbol{A}) = \operatorname{tr}(\boldsymbol{A}'\boldsymbol{A}) - s,\end{aligned}$$

where s is as given in (6.134), due to the constraint that $\boldsymbol{F}'\boldsymbol{F} = \boldsymbol{I}_r$. Hence, maximizing s in (6.132) is equivalent to minimizing $\tilde{s}$, and the minimum of $\tilde{s}$ is given by $\lambda_{r+1} + \lambda_{r+2} + \cdots + \lambda_p$.

Let us now extend the PCA in two ways. First of all, suppose that Sp($\boldsymbol{B}$) is given, which is not necessarily orthogonal to Sp($\boldsymbol{A}$) but disjoint with it, as illustrated in Figure 6.4(b). We express the projection of $\boldsymbol{a}_j$ onto Sp($\boldsymbol{F}$) (Sp($\boldsymbol{F}$) $\subset$ Sp($\boldsymbol{A}$)) as $\boldsymbol{P}_{F\cdot B}\boldsymbol{a}_j$, where

$$\boldsymbol{P}_{F\cdot B} = \boldsymbol{F}(\boldsymbol{F}'\boldsymbol{Q}_B\boldsymbol{F})^-\boldsymbol{F}'\boldsymbol{Q}_B$$

is the projector onto Sp($\boldsymbol{F}$) along Sp($\boldsymbol{B}$) (see (4.9)). The residual vector is obtained by $\boldsymbol{a}_j - \boldsymbol{P}_{F\cdot B}\boldsymbol{a}_j = \boldsymbol{Q}_{F\cdot B}\boldsymbol{a}_j$. (This is the vector connecting the tip of the vector $\boldsymbol{P}_{F\cdot B}\boldsymbol{a}_j$ to the tip of the vector $\boldsymbol{a}_j$.) Since

$$\begin{aligned}\sum_{j=1}^{p}||\boldsymbol{Q}_{F\cdot B}\boldsymbol{a}_j||^2_{Q_B} &= \operatorname{tr}(\boldsymbol{A}'\boldsymbol{Q}_B\boldsymbol{Q}'_{F\cdot B}\boldsymbol{Q}_{F\cdot B}\boldsymbol{Q}_B\boldsymbol{A}) \\ &= \operatorname{tr}(\boldsymbol{A}'\boldsymbol{Q}_B\boldsymbol{A}) - \operatorname{tr}(\boldsymbol{A}'\boldsymbol{P}_{F[B]}\boldsymbol{A}), \qquad (6.136)\end{aligned}$$

we obtain $\boldsymbol{F}$ that maximizes

$$\tilde{s}_2 = \operatorname{tr}(\boldsymbol{A}'\boldsymbol{P}_{F[B]}\boldsymbol{A}) = \operatorname{tr}(\boldsymbol{A}'\boldsymbol{Q}_B\boldsymbol{F}(\boldsymbol{F}'\boldsymbol{Q}_B\boldsymbol{F})^-\boldsymbol{F}'\boldsymbol{Q}_B\boldsymbol{A})$$

under the restriction that $\boldsymbol{F}'\boldsymbol{Q}_B\boldsymbol{F} = \boldsymbol{I}_r$. Maximizing $\tilde{s}_2 = \text{tr}(\boldsymbol{A}'\boldsymbol{Q}_B\boldsymbol{F}\boldsymbol{F}'\boldsymbol{Q}_B \boldsymbol{A}) = \text{tr}(\boldsymbol{F}'\boldsymbol{Q}_B\boldsymbol{A}\boldsymbol{A}'\boldsymbol{Q}_B\boldsymbol{F})$ under the same restriction reduces to solving the eigenequation

$$(\boldsymbol{Q}_B\boldsymbol{A}\boldsymbol{A}'\boldsymbol{Q}_B)\tilde{\boldsymbol{F}} = \tilde{\boldsymbol{F}}\boldsymbol{\Delta}_r^2,$$

where $\tilde{\boldsymbol{F}} = \boldsymbol{F}\boldsymbol{V}$ ($\boldsymbol{V}$ is an orthogonal matrix of order r), or

$$(\boldsymbol{A}'Q_B\boldsymbol{A})(\boldsymbol{A}'\boldsymbol{Q}_B\tilde{\boldsymbol{F}}) = (\boldsymbol{A}'\boldsymbol{Q}_B\tilde{\boldsymbol{F}})\boldsymbol{\Delta}_r^2, \tag{6.137}$$

obtained by premultiplying the eigenequation above by $\boldsymbol{A}'\boldsymbol{Q}_B$. The derived $\tilde{\boldsymbol{F}}$ represents the principal components of $\boldsymbol{A}$ eliminating the effects of $\boldsymbol{B}$.

Let $\boldsymbol{W} = \boldsymbol{A}'\boldsymbol{Q}_B\tilde{\boldsymbol{F}}$. Let the normalized vectors of $\boldsymbol{W}$ and $\tilde{\boldsymbol{F}}$ be denoted by $\boldsymbol{w}_1, \boldsymbol{w}_2, \cdots, \boldsymbol{w}_r$ and $\tilde{\boldsymbol{f}}_1, \tilde{\boldsymbol{f}}_2, \cdots, \tilde{\boldsymbol{f}}_r$, and let the diagonal elements of $\boldsymbol{\Delta}_r^2$ be denoted by $\mu_1^2, \mu_2^2, \cdots, \mu_r^2$. Then,

$$\boldsymbol{Q}_B\boldsymbol{A} = \mu_1\tilde{\boldsymbol{f}}_1\boldsymbol{w}_1' + \mu_2\tilde{\boldsymbol{f}}_2\boldsymbol{w}_2' + \cdots + \mu_r\tilde{\boldsymbol{f}}_r\boldsymbol{w}_r', \tag{6.138}$$

where μ_j ($j = 1, \cdots, r$) is the positive square root of μ_j^2.

The other method involves the projection of vectors $\boldsymbol{C} = [\boldsymbol{c}_1, \boldsymbol{c}_2, \cdots, \boldsymbol{c}_s]$ in $\text{Sp}(\boldsymbol{C})$, not necessarily contained in $\text{Sp}(\boldsymbol{A})$, onto $\text{Sp}(\boldsymbol{F})(\subset \text{Sp}(\boldsymbol{A}))$ spanned by the principal components. We minimize

$$s_2 = \sum_{j=1}^{s} ||\boldsymbol{Q}_F\boldsymbol{c}_j||^2 = \text{tr}(\boldsymbol{C}'\boldsymbol{Q}_F\boldsymbol{C}) = \text{tr}(\boldsymbol{C}'\boldsymbol{C}) - \text{tr}(\boldsymbol{C}'\boldsymbol{P}_F\boldsymbol{C}) \tag{6.139}$$

with respect to $\boldsymbol{F}$, but minimizing the criterion above is obviously equivalent to maximizing

$$\tilde{s}_2 = \text{tr}(\boldsymbol{C}'\boldsymbol{P}_F\boldsymbol{C}) = \text{tr}(\boldsymbol{C}'\boldsymbol{F}(\boldsymbol{F}'\boldsymbol{F})^{-1}\boldsymbol{F}'\boldsymbol{C}). \tag{6.140}$$

Let $\boldsymbol{F} = \boldsymbol{A}\boldsymbol{W}$, where $\boldsymbol{W}$ is an n by r matrix of weights. Then, (6.140) can be rewritten as

$$\begin{aligned}\tilde{s}_2 &= \text{tr}(\boldsymbol{C}'\boldsymbol{A}\boldsymbol{W}(\boldsymbol{W}'\boldsymbol{A}'\boldsymbol{A}\boldsymbol{W})^{-1}\boldsymbol{W}'\boldsymbol{A}'\boldsymbol{C}) \\ &= \text{tr}(\boldsymbol{W}'\boldsymbol{A}'\boldsymbol{C}\boldsymbol{C}'\boldsymbol{A}\boldsymbol{W}(\boldsymbol{W}'\boldsymbol{A}'\boldsymbol{A}\boldsymbol{W})^{-1}),\end{aligned}$$

which is to be maximized with respect to $\boldsymbol{W}$ subject to the restriction that $\boldsymbol{W}'\boldsymbol{A}'\boldsymbol{A}\boldsymbol{W} = \boldsymbol{I}_r$. This leads to the following generalized eigenequation to be solved.

$$(\boldsymbol{A}'\boldsymbol{C}\boldsymbol{C}\boldsymbol{A})\boldsymbol{W}\boldsymbol{T} = \boldsymbol{A}'\boldsymbol{A}\boldsymbol{W}\boldsymbol{T}\boldsymbol{\Delta}_r^2.$$

Premultiplying both sides of the equation above by $\boldsymbol{C}'\boldsymbol{A}(\boldsymbol{A}'\boldsymbol{A})^-$, we can reduce the generalized eigenproblem to an ordinary one:

$$(\boldsymbol{C}'\boldsymbol{P}_A\boldsymbol{C})(\boldsymbol{C}'\boldsymbol{A}\boldsymbol{W}\boldsymbol{T}) = (\boldsymbol{C}'\boldsymbol{A}\boldsymbol{W}\boldsymbol{T})\boldsymbol{\Delta}_r^2. \tag{6.141}$$

The eigenvectors $\boldsymbol{C}'\boldsymbol{AWT}$ of $\boldsymbol{C}'\boldsymbol{P}_A\boldsymbol{C}$ are equal to the product of $\boldsymbol{C}'$ and the principal components $\boldsymbol{F} = \boldsymbol{AWT}$. The PCA by (6.137) and (6.140) is sometimes called redundancy analysis (RA; Van den Wollenberg, 1977) or PCA of instrumental variables (Rao, 1964). Takane and his collaborators (Takane and Shibayama, 1991; Takane and Hunter, 2001) developed a comprehensive method called CPCA (constrained PCA), which subsumes a number of representative techniques in multivariate analysis discussed in this book, including RA as a special case.

6.3.4 Distance and projection matrices

In this subsection, we represent distances in the n-dimensional Euclidean space from a variety of angles using projection matrices.

Lemma 6.7 *Let $\boldsymbol{e}_j$ denote an n-component vector in which only the jth element is unity and all other elements are zero. Then,*

$$\frac{1}{2n}\sum_{i=1}^{n}\sum_{j=1}^{n}(\boldsymbol{e}_i - \boldsymbol{e}_j)(\boldsymbol{e}_i - \boldsymbol{e}_j)' = \boldsymbol{Q}_M. \tag{6.142}$$

Proof.

$$\sum_{i=1}^{n}\sum_{j=1}^{n}(\boldsymbol{e}_i - \boldsymbol{e}_j)(\boldsymbol{e}_i - \boldsymbol{e}_j)'$$

$$= n\sum_{i=1}^{n}\boldsymbol{e}_i\boldsymbol{e}_i' + n\sum_{j=1}^{n}\boldsymbol{e}_j\boldsymbol{e}_j' - 2\sum_{i=1}^{n}\boldsymbol{e}_i\left(\sum_{j=1}^{n}\boldsymbol{e}_j\right)'$$

$$= 2n\boldsymbol{I}_n - 2\boldsymbol{1}_n\boldsymbol{1}_n' = 2n\left(\boldsymbol{I}_n - \frac{1}{n}\boldsymbol{1}_n\boldsymbol{1}_n'\right) = 2n\boldsymbol{Q}_M.$$

Q.E.D.

Example 6.2 That $\frac{1}{n}\sum_{i<j}(x_i - x_j)^2 = \sum_{i=1}^{n}(x_i - \bar{x})^2$ can be shown as follows using the result given above.

Let $\boldsymbol{x}_R = (x_1, x_2, \cdots, x_n)'$. Then, $x_j = (\boldsymbol{x}_R, \boldsymbol{e}_j)$, and so

$$\begin{aligned}\sum_{i<j}(x_i - x_j)^2 &= \frac{1}{2}\sum_{i}\sum_{j}\boldsymbol{x}_R'(\boldsymbol{e}_i - \boldsymbol{e}_j)(\boldsymbol{e}_i - \boldsymbol{e}_j)'\boldsymbol{x}_R \\ &= \frac{1}{2}\boldsymbol{x}_R'\left(\sum_{i}\sum_{j}(\boldsymbol{e}_i - \boldsymbol{e}_j)(\boldsymbol{e}_i - \boldsymbol{e}_j)'\right)\boldsymbol{x}_R = n\boldsymbol{x}_R'\boldsymbol{Q}_M\boldsymbol{x}_R\end{aligned}$$

$$= n\boldsymbol{x}'\boldsymbol{x} = n||\boldsymbol{x}||^2 = n\sum_{i=1}^{n}(x_i - \bar{x})^2.$$

We next consider the situation in which a matrix of raw scores on p variables is given:

$$\boldsymbol{X}_R = \begin{bmatrix} x_{11} & x_{12} & \cdots & x_{1p} \\ x_{21} & x_{22} & \cdots & x_{2p} \\ \vdots & \vdots & \ddots & \vdots \\ x_{n1} & x_{n2} & \cdots & x_{np} \end{bmatrix}.$$

Let

$$\tilde{\boldsymbol{x}}_j = (x_{j1}, x_{j2}, \cdots, x_{jp})'$$

denote the p-component vector pertaining to the jth subject's scores. Then,

$$\boldsymbol{x}_j = \boldsymbol{X}'_R\boldsymbol{e}_j. \tag{6.143}$$

Hence, the squared Euclidean distance between subjects i and j can be expressed as

$$\begin{aligned} d^2_{X_R}(\boldsymbol{e}_i, \boldsymbol{e}_j) &= \sum_{k=1}^{p}(x_{ik} - x_{jk})^2 \\ &= ||\tilde{\boldsymbol{x}}_i - \tilde{\boldsymbol{x}}_j||^2 = (\boldsymbol{e}_i - \boldsymbol{e}_j)'\boldsymbol{X}_R\boldsymbol{X}'_R(\boldsymbol{e}_i - \boldsymbol{e}_j). \end{aligned} \tag{6.144}$$

Let $\boldsymbol{X} = \boldsymbol{Q}_M\boldsymbol{X}_R$ represent the transformation that turns the matrix of raw scores $\boldsymbol{X}_R$ into the matrix $\boldsymbol{X}$ of mean deviation scores. We have

$$(\boldsymbol{e}_i - \boldsymbol{e}_j)'\boldsymbol{X} = (\boldsymbol{e}_i - \boldsymbol{e}_j)'\boldsymbol{Q}_M\boldsymbol{X}_R = (\boldsymbol{e}_i - \boldsymbol{e}_j)'\boldsymbol{X}_R,$$

and so

$$d^2_{X_R}(\boldsymbol{e}_i, \boldsymbol{e}_j) = d^2_X(\boldsymbol{e}_i, \boldsymbol{e}_j) = (\boldsymbol{e}_i - \boldsymbol{e}_j)'\boldsymbol{X}\boldsymbol{X}'(\boldsymbol{e}_i - \boldsymbol{e}_j), \tag{6.145}$$

from which the following theorem can be derived.

Theorem 6.13

$$\sum_{i=1}^{n}\sum_{j=1}^{n} d^2_{X_R}(\boldsymbol{e}_i, \boldsymbol{e}_j) = n\mathrm{tr}(\boldsymbol{X}'\boldsymbol{X}). \tag{6.146}$$

Proof. Use the fact that

$$\sum_{i=1}^{n}\sum_{j=1}^{n} d^2_{X_R}(\boldsymbol{e}_i, \boldsymbol{e}_j)$$
$$= \frac{1}{2}\mathrm{tr}\left\{(\boldsymbol{X}\boldsymbol{X}')\sum_i\sum_j(\boldsymbol{e}_i - \boldsymbol{e}_j)(\boldsymbol{e}_i - \boldsymbol{e}_j)'\right\}$$
$$= n\mathrm{tr}(\boldsymbol{X}\boldsymbol{X}'\boldsymbol{Q}_M) = n\mathrm{tr}(\boldsymbol{Q}_M\boldsymbol{X}\boldsymbol{X}') = n\mathrm{tr}(\boldsymbol{X}\boldsymbol{X}').$$

Q.E.D.

Corollary *Let* $\boldsymbol{f} = \boldsymbol{x}_1 a_1 + \boldsymbol{x}_2 a_2 + \cdots + \boldsymbol{x}_p a_p = \boldsymbol{X}\boldsymbol{a}$. *Then,*

$$\sum_{i<j} d^2_f(\boldsymbol{e}_i, \boldsymbol{e}_j) = n\mathrm{tr}(\boldsymbol{f}\boldsymbol{f}') = n\mathrm{tr}(\boldsymbol{a}'\boldsymbol{X}'\boldsymbol{X}\boldsymbol{a}). \tag{6.147}$$

(Proof omitted.)

Let $\boldsymbol{D}^{(2)} = [d^2_{ij}]$, where $d^2_{ij} = d^2_{X_R}(\boldsymbol{e}_i, \boldsymbol{e}_j)$ as defined in (6.145). Then, $\boldsymbol{e}_i'\boldsymbol{X}\boldsymbol{X}'\boldsymbol{e}_i$ represents the ith diagonal element of the matrix $\boldsymbol{X}\boldsymbol{X}'$ and $\boldsymbol{e}_i'\boldsymbol{X}\boldsymbol{X}' \times \boldsymbol{e}_j$ represents its (i, j)th element. Hence,

$$\boldsymbol{D}^{(2)} = \mathrm{diag}(\boldsymbol{X}\boldsymbol{X}')\boldsymbol{1}_n\boldsymbol{1}_n' - 2\boldsymbol{X}\boldsymbol{X}' + \boldsymbol{1}_n\boldsymbol{1}_n'\mathrm{diag}(\boldsymbol{X}\boldsymbol{X}'), \tag{6.148}$$

where diag($\boldsymbol{A}$) indicates the diagonal matrix with the diagonal elements of $\boldsymbol{A}$ as its diagonal entries. Pre- and postmultiplying the formula above by $\boldsymbol{Q}_M = \boldsymbol{I}_n - \frac{1}{n}\boldsymbol{1}_n\boldsymbol{1}_n'$, we obtain

$$\boldsymbol{S} = -\frac{1}{2}\boldsymbol{Q}_M\boldsymbol{D}^{(2)}\boldsymbol{Q}_M = \boldsymbol{X}\boldsymbol{X}' \geq \boldsymbol{O} \tag{6.149}$$

since $\boldsymbol{Q}_M\boldsymbol{1}_n = \boldsymbol{0}$. (6.149) indicates that $\boldsymbol{S}$ is *nnd*.

Note Let $\boldsymbol{D}^{(2)} = [d^2_{ij}]$ and $\boldsymbol{S} = [s_{ij}]$. Then,

$$s_{ij} = -\frac{1}{2}(d^2_{ij} - \bar{d}^2_{i.} - \bar{d}^2_{.j} + \bar{d}^2_{..}),$$

where $\bar{d}^2_{i.} = \frac{1}{n}\sum_j d^2_{ij}$, $\bar{d}^2_{.j} = \frac{1}{n}\sum_i d^2_{ij}$, and $\bar{d}^2_{..} = \frac{1}{n^2}\sum_{i,j} d^2_{ij}$.

The transformation (6.149) that turns $\boldsymbol{D}^{(2)}$ into $\boldsymbol{S}$ is called the Young-Householder transformation. It indicates that the n points corresponding to the n rows and columns of $\boldsymbol{S}$ can be embedded in a Euclidean space of dimensionality rank($\boldsymbol{S}$), which is equal to the number of positive eigenvalues of $\boldsymbol{S}$. This method of embedding points in a Euclidean space is called metric multidimensional scaling (MDS) (Torgerson, 1958).

We now consider the situation in which n subjects are classified into m groups. Each group has n_j subjects with $\sum_j n_j = n$. Denote the matrix of dummy variables defined in (6.46) by

$$\boldsymbol{G} = [\boldsymbol{g}_1, \boldsymbol{g}_2, \cdots, \boldsymbol{g}_m], \tag{6.150}$$

where $\boldsymbol{g}_j$ is an n-component vector of ones and zeroes. Assume that

$$||\boldsymbol{g}_j||^2 = n_j \text{ and } (\boldsymbol{g}_i, \boldsymbol{g}_j) = 0 \ \ (i \neq j).$$

Let

$$\boldsymbol{h}_j = \boldsymbol{g}_j(\boldsymbol{g}_j'\boldsymbol{g}_j)^{-1}.$$

Then the vector of group means of the jth group,

$$\boldsymbol{m}_j = (\bar{x}_{j1}, \bar{x}_{j2}, \cdots, \bar{x}_{jp})',$$

on p variables can be expressed as

$$\boldsymbol{m}_j = \boldsymbol{X}_R'\boldsymbol{g}_j(\boldsymbol{g}_j'\boldsymbol{g}_j)^{-1} = \boldsymbol{X}_R'\boldsymbol{h}_j. \tag{6.151}$$

Thus, the squared Euclidean distance between means of groups i and j is given by

$$d_X^2(\boldsymbol{g}_i, \boldsymbol{g}_j) = (\boldsymbol{h}_i - \boldsymbol{h}_j)'\boldsymbol{X}\boldsymbol{X}'(\boldsymbol{h}_i - \boldsymbol{h}_j). \tag{6.152}$$

Hence, the following lemma is obtained.

Lemma 6.8

$$\frac{1}{2n}\sum_{i,j} n_i n_j (\boldsymbol{h}_i - \boldsymbol{h}_j)(\boldsymbol{h}_i - \boldsymbol{h}_j)' = \boldsymbol{P}_G - \boldsymbol{P}_M, \tag{6.153}$$

where $\boldsymbol{P}_G$ *is the orthogonal projector onto* Sp($\boldsymbol{G}$).

Proof. Use the definition of the vector $\boldsymbol{h}_j$, $n_j = \boldsymbol{g}_j'\boldsymbol{g}_j$, and the fact that $\boldsymbol{P}_G = \boldsymbol{P}_{g_1} + \boldsymbol{P}_{g_2} + \cdots + \boldsymbol{P}_{g_m}$. Q.E.D.

Theorem 6.14

$$\frac{1}{n}\sum_{i<j} n_i n_j d_X^2(\boldsymbol{g}_i, \boldsymbol{g}_j) = \mathrm{tr}(\boldsymbol{X}'\boldsymbol{P}_G\boldsymbol{X}). \tag{6.154}$$

(Proof omitted.)

Note Dividing (6.146) by n, we obtain the trace of the variance-covariance matrix $\boldsymbol{C}$, which is equal to the sum of variances of the p variables, and by dividing (6.154) by n, we obtain the trace of the between-group covariance matrix $\boldsymbol{C}_A$, which is equal to the sum of the between-group variances of the p variables.

In general, even if $\boldsymbol{X}$ is columnwise standardized, correlations among the p variables in $\boldsymbol{X}$ have a grave impact on distances among the n subjects. To adjust for the effects of correlations, it is often useful to introduce a generalized distance between subjects i and j defined by

$$\tilde{d}_X^2(\boldsymbol{e}_i, \boldsymbol{e}_j) = (\boldsymbol{e}_i - \boldsymbol{e}_j)'\boldsymbol{P}_X(\boldsymbol{e}_i - \boldsymbol{e}_j) \tag{6.155}$$

(Takeuchi, Yanai, and Mukherjee, 1982, pp. 389–391). Note that the p columns of $\boldsymbol{X}$ are not necessarily linearly independent. By Lemma 6.7, we have

$$\frac{1}{n}\sum_{i<j} \tilde{d}_X^2(\boldsymbol{e}_i, \boldsymbol{e}_j) = \mathrm{tr}(\boldsymbol{P}_X). \tag{6.156}$$

Furthermore, from (6.153), the generalized distance between the means of groups i and j, namely

$$\begin{aligned}\tilde{d}_X^2(\boldsymbol{g}_i, \boldsymbol{g}_j) &= (\boldsymbol{h}_i - \boldsymbol{h}_j)'\boldsymbol{P}_X(\boldsymbol{h}_i - \boldsymbol{h}_j)\\ &= \frac{1}{n}(\boldsymbol{m}_i - \boldsymbol{m}_j)'\boldsymbol{C}_{XX}^-(\boldsymbol{m}_i - \boldsymbol{m}_j),\end{aligned}$$

satisfies

$$\sum_{i<j} \tilde{d}_X^2(\boldsymbol{g}_i, \boldsymbol{g}_j) = \mathrm{tr}(\boldsymbol{P}_X\boldsymbol{P}_G) = \mathrm{tr}(\boldsymbol{C}_{XX}^-\boldsymbol{C}_A).$$

Let $\boldsymbol{A} = [\boldsymbol{a}_1, \boldsymbol{a}_2, \cdots, \boldsymbol{a}_{m-1}]$ denote the matrix of eigenvectors corresponding to the positive eigenvalues in the matrix equation (6.113) for canonical discriminant analysis. We assume that $\boldsymbol{a}_j'\boldsymbol{X}'\boldsymbol{X}\boldsymbol{a}_j = 1$ and $\boldsymbol{a}_j'\boldsymbol{X}'\boldsymbol{X}\boldsymbol{a}_i = 0$ $(j \neq i)$, that is, $\boldsymbol{A}'\boldsymbol{X}'\boldsymbol{X}\boldsymbol{A} = \boldsymbol{I}_{m-1}$. Then the following relation holds.

Lemma 6.9

$$\boldsymbol{P}_{XA}\boldsymbol{P}_G = \boldsymbol{P}_X\boldsymbol{P}_G. \tag{6.157}$$

Proof. Since canonical discriminant analysis is equivalent to canonical correlation analysis between $\tilde{\boldsymbol{G}} = \boldsymbol{Q}_M\boldsymbol{G}$ and $\boldsymbol{X}$, it follows from Theorem 6.11 that $\boldsymbol{P}_{XA}\boldsymbol{P}_{\tilde{G}} = \boldsymbol{P}_X\boldsymbol{P}_{\tilde{G}}$. It also holds that $\boldsymbol{P}_{\tilde{G}} = \boldsymbol{Q}_M\boldsymbol{P}_G$, and $\boldsymbol{X}'\boldsymbol{Q}_M = (\boldsymbol{Q}_M\boldsymbol{X})' = \boldsymbol{X}'$, from which the proposition in the lemma follows immediately. Q.E.D.

The following theorem can be derived from the result given above (Yanai, 1981).

Theorem 6.15

$$(\boldsymbol{X}'\boldsymbol{X})\boldsymbol{A}\boldsymbol{A}'(\boldsymbol{m}_i - \boldsymbol{m}_j) = \boldsymbol{m}_i - \boldsymbol{m}_j, \tag{6.158}$$

where $\boldsymbol{m}_j$ is the group mean vector, as defined in (6.151).

Proof. Postmultiplying both sides of $\boldsymbol{P}_{XA}\boldsymbol{P}_G = \boldsymbol{P}_X\boldsymbol{P}_G$ by $\boldsymbol{h}_i - \boldsymbol{h}_j$, we obtain $\boldsymbol{P}_{XA}\boldsymbol{P}_G(\boldsymbol{h}_i - \boldsymbol{h}_j) = \boldsymbol{P}_X\boldsymbol{P}_G(\boldsymbol{h}_i - \boldsymbol{h}_j)$. Since $\text{Sp}(\boldsymbol{G}) \supset \text{Sp}(\boldsymbol{g}_i)$, $\boldsymbol{P}_G\boldsymbol{g}_i = \boldsymbol{g}_i$ implies $\boldsymbol{P}_G\boldsymbol{h}_i = \boldsymbol{h}_i$, which in turn implies

$$\boldsymbol{P}_{XA}(\boldsymbol{h}_i - \boldsymbol{h}_j) = \boldsymbol{P}_X(\boldsymbol{h}_i - \boldsymbol{h}_j).$$

Premultiplying the equation above by $\boldsymbol{X}'$, we obtain (6.158) by noting that $\boldsymbol{A}'\boldsymbol{X}'\boldsymbol{X}\boldsymbol{A} = \boldsymbol{I}_r$ and (6.151). Q.E.D.

Corollary

$$(\boldsymbol{m}_i - \boldsymbol{m}_j)'\boldsymbol{A}\boldsymbol{A}'(\boldsymbol{m}_i - \boldsymbol{m}_j) = (\boldsymbol{m}_i - \boldsymbol{m}_j)'(\boldsymbol{X}'\boldsymbol{X})^-(\boldsymbol{m}_i - \boldsymbol{m}_j). \tag{6.159}$$

Proof. Premultiply (6.158) by $(\boldsymbol{h}_i - \boldsymbol{h}_j)'\boldsymbol{X}(\boldsymbol{X}'\boldsymbol{X})^- = (\boldsymbol{m}_i - \boldsymbol{m}_j)'(\boldsymbol{X}'\boldsymbol{X})^-$. Q.E.D.

The left-hand side of (6.159) is equal to $d^2_{XA}(\boldsymbol{g}_i, \boldsymbol{g}_j)$, and the right-hand side is equal to $d^2_X(\boldsymbol{g}_i, \boldsymbol{g}_j)$. Hence, in general, it holds that

$$d^2_{XA}(\boldsymbol{g}_i, \boldsymbol{g}_j) = \tilde{d}^2_X(\boldsymbol{g}_i, \boldsymbol{g}_j).$$

That is, between-group distances defined on the canonical variates $\boldsymbol{XA}$ obtained by canonical discriminant analysis coincide with generalized distances based on the matrix $\boldsymbol{X}$ of mean deviation scores.

Assume that the second set of variables exists in the form of $\boldsymbol{Z}$. Let $\boldsymbol{X}_{Z^\perp} = \boldsymbol{Q}_Z\boldsymbol{X}$, where $\boldsymbol{Q}_Z = \boldsymbol{I}_r - \boldsymbol{Z}(\boldsymbol{Z}'\boldsymbol{Z})^-\boldsymbol{Z}'$, denote the matrix of predictor variables from which the effects of $\boldsymbol{Z}$ are eliminated. Let $\boldsymbol{X}\tilde{\boldsymbol{A}}$ denote the matrix of discriminant scores obtained, using $\boldsymbol{X}_{Z^\perp}$ as the predictor variables. The relations

$$(\boldsymbol{X}'\boldsymbol{Q}_Z\boldsymbol{X})\tilde{\boldsymbol{A}}\tilde{\boldsymbol{A}}'(\tilde{\boldsymbol{m}}_i - \tilde{\boldsymbol{m}}_j) = \tilde{\boldsymbol{m}}_i - \tilde{\boldsymbol{m}}_j$$

and

$$(\tilde{\boldsymbol{m}}_i - \tilde{\boldsymbol{m}}_j)'\tilde{\boldsymbol{A}}\tilde{\boldsymbol{A}}'(\tilde{\boldsymbol{m}}_i - \tilde{\boldsymbol{m}}_j) = (\tilde{\boldsymbol{m}}_i - \tilde{\boldsymbol{m}}_j)'(\boldsymbol{X}'\boldsymbol{Q}_Z\boldsymbol{X})^-(\tilde{\boldsymbol{m}}_i - \tilde{\boldsymbol{m}}_j)$$

hold, where $\tilde{\boldsymbol{m}}_i = \boldsymbol{m}_{i\cdot X} - \boldsymbol{X}'\boldsymbol{Z}(\boldsymbol{Z}'\boldsymbol{Z})^-\boldsymbol{m}_{i\cdot Z}$ ($\boldsymbol{m}_{i\cdot X}$ and $\boldsymbol{m}_{i\cdot Z}$ are vectors of group means of $\boldsymbol{X}$ and $\boldsymbol{Z}$, respectively).

6.4 Linear Simultaneous Equations

As a method to obtain the solution vector $\boldsymbol{x}$ for a linear simultaneous equation $\boldsymbol{A}\boldsymbol{x} = \boldsymbol{b}$ or for a normal equation $\boldsymbol{A}'\boldsymbol{A}\boldsymbol{x} = \boldsymbol{A}'\boldsymbol{b}$ derived in the context of multiple regression analysis, a sweep-out method called the Gauss-Doolittle method is well known. In this section, we discuss other methods for solving linear simultaneous equations based on the QR decomposition of $\boldsymbol{A}$.

6.4.1 QR decomposition by the Gram-Schmidt orthogonalization method

Assume that m linearly independent vectors, $\boldsymbol{a}_1, \boldsymbol{a}_2, \cdots, \boldsymbol{a}_m$, in E^n are given (these vectors are collected to form a matrix $\boldsymbol{A}$), and let $\boldsymbol{P}_{[j]}$ denote the orthogonal projector onto $\text{Sp}([\boldsymbol{a}_1, \boldsymbol{a}_2, \cdots, \boldsymbol{a}_j]) = \text{Sp}(\boldsymbol{a}_1) \oplus \text{Sp}(\boldsymbol{a}_2) \oplus \cdots \oplus \text{Sp}(\boldsymbol{a}_j)$. Construct a sequence of vectors as follows:

$$\begin{aligned}
\boldsymbol{t}_1 &= \boldsymbol{a}_1/||\boldsymbol{a}_1|| \\
\boldsymbol{t}_2 &= (\boldsymbol{a}_2 - \boldsymbol{P}_{[1]}\boldsymbol{a}_2)/||\boldsymbol{a}_2 - \boldsymbol{P}_{[1]}\boldsymbol{a}_2|| \\
\boldsymbol{t}_3 &= (\boldsymbol{a}_3 - \boldsymbol{P}_{[2]}\boldsymbol{a}_3)/||\boldsymbol{a}_3 - \boldsymbol{P}_{[2]}\boldsymbol{a}_3|| \\
&\vdots \\
\boldsymbol{t}_j &= (\boldsymbol{a}_j - \boldsymbol{P}_{[j-1]}\boldsymbol{a}_j)/||\boldsymbol{a}_j - \boldsymbol{P}_{[j-1]}\boldsymbol{a}_j|| \\
&\vdots \\
\boldsymbol{t}_m &= (\boldsymbol{a}_m - \boldsymbol{P}_{[m-1]}\boldsymbol{a}_m)/||\boldsymbol{a}_m - \boldsymbol{P}_{[m-1]}\boldsymbol{a}_m||.
\end{aligned} \tag{6.160}$$

This way of generating orthonormal basis vectors is called the Gram-Schmidt orthogonalization method.

Let $i > j$. From Theorem 2.11, it holds that $\boldsymbol{P}_{[i]}\boldsymbol{P}_{[j]} = \boldsymbol{P}_{[j]}$. Hence, we have

$$\begin{aligned}(\boldsymbol{t}_i, \boldsymbol{t}_j) &= (\boldsymbol{a}_i - \boldsymbol{P}_{[i-1]}\boldsymbol{a}_i)'(\boldsymbol{a}_j - \boldsymbol{P}_{[j-1]}\boldsymbol{a}_j) \\ &= \boldsymbol{a}_i'\boldsymbol{a}_j - \boldsymbol{a}_i'\boldsymbol{P}_{[j-1]}\boldsymbol{a}_j - \boldsymbol{a}_i'\boldsymbol{P}_{[i-1]}\boldsymbol{a}_j + \boldsymbol{a}_i'\boldsymbol{P}_{[i-1]}\boldsymbol{P}_{[j-1]}\boldsymbol{a}_j \\ &= \boldsymbol{a}_i'\boldsymbol{a}_j - \boldsymbol{a}_i'\boldsymbol{a}_j = 0.\end{aligned}$$

Furthermore, it is clear that $||\boldsymbol{t}_j|| = 1$, so we obtain a set of orthonormal basis vectors.

Let $\boldsymbol{P}_{t_j}$ denote the orthogonal projector onto $\text{Sp}(\boldsymbol{t}_j)$. Since $\text{Sp}(\boldsymbol{A}) = \text{Sp}([\boldsymbol{a}_1, \boldsymbol{a}_2, \cdots, \boldsymbol{a}_m]) = \text{Sp}(\boldsymbol{t}_1) \dot{\oplus} \text{Sp}(\boldsymbol{t}_2) \dot{\oplus} \cdots \dot{\oplus} \text{Sp}(\boldsymbol{t}_m)$,

$$\boldsymbol{P}_{[j]} = \boldsymbol{P}_{t_1} + \boldsymbol{P}_{t_2} + \cdots + \boldsymbol{P}_{t_j} = \boldsymbol{t}_1\boldsymbol{t}_1' + \boldsymbol{t}_2\boldsymbol{t}_2' + \cdots + \boldsymbol{t}_j\boldsymbol{t}_j'.$$

Substituting this into (6.160), we obtain

$$\boldsymbol{t}_j = (\boldsymbol{a}_j - (\boldsymbol{a}_j, \boldsymbol{t}_1)\boldsymbol{t}_1 - (\boldsymbol{a}_j, \boldsymbol{t}_2)\boldsymbol{t}_2 - \cdots - (\boldsymbol{a}_j, \boldsymbol{t}_{j-1})\boldsymbol{t}_{j-1})/R_{jj}, \tag{6.161}$$

where $R_{jj} = ||\boldsymbol{a}_j - (\boldsymbol{a}_j, \boldsymbol{t}_1)\boldsymbol{t}_1 - (\boldsymbol{a}_j, \boldsymbol{t}_2)\boldsymbol{t}_2 - \cdots - (\boldsymbol{a}_j, \boldsymbol{t}_{j-1})\boldsymbol{t}_{j-1}||$. Let $\boldsymbol{R}_{ji} = (\boldsymbol{a}_i, \boldsymbol{t}_j)$. Then,

$$\boldsymbol{a}_j = R_{1j}\boldsymbol{t}_1 + R_{2j}\boldsymbol{t}_2 + \cdots + R_{j-1}\boldsymbol{t}_{j-1} + R_{jj}\boldsymbol{t}_j$$

for $j = 1, \cdots, m$. Let $\boldsymbol{Q} = [\boldsymbol{t}_1, \boldsymbol{t}_2, \cdots, \boldsymbol{t}_m]$ and

$$\boldsymbol{R} = \begin{bmatrix} R_{11} & R_{12} & \cdots & R_{1m} \\ 0 & R_{22} & \cdots & R_{2m} \\ \vdots & \vdots & \ddots & \vdots \\ 0 & 0 & \cdots & R_{mm} \end{bmatrix}.$$

Then $\boldsymbol{Q}$ is an n by m matrix such that $\boldsymbol{Q}'\boldsymbol{Q} = \boldsymbol{I}_m$, $\boldsymbol{R}$ is an upper triangular matrix of order m, and $\boldsymbol{A}$ is decomposed as

$$\boldsymbol{A} = [\boldsymbol{a}_1, \boldsymbol{a}_2, \cdots, \boldsymbol{a}_m] = \boldsymbol{Q}\boldsymbol{R}. \tag{6.162}$$

The factorization above is called the (compact) QR decomposition by the Gram-Schmidt orthogonalization. It follows that

$$\boldsymbol{A}^+ = \boldsymbol{R}^{-1}\boldsymbol{Q}'. \tag{6.163}$$

6.4.2 QR decomposition by the Householder transformation

Lemma 6.10 *Let $\boldsymbol{t}_1$ be a vector of unit length. Then, $\boldsymbol{Q}_1 = (\boldsymbol{I}_n - 2\boldsymbol{t}_1\boldsymbol{t}_1')$ is an orthogonal matrix.*

Proof. $\boldsymbol{Q}_1^2 = (\boldsymbol{I}_n - 2\boldsymbol{t}_1\boldsymbol{t}_1')^2 = \boldsymbol{I}_n - 2\boldsymbol{t}_1\boldsymbol{t}_1' - 2\boldsymbol{t}_1\boldsymbol{t}_1' + 4\boldsymbol{t}_1\boldsymbol{t}_1'\boldsymbol{t}_1\boldsymbol{t}_1' = \boldsymbol{I}_n$. Since $\boldsymbol{Q}_1$ is symmetric, $\boldsymbol{Q}_1'\boldsymbol{Q}_1 = \boldsymbol{Q}_1^2 = \boldsymbol{I}_n$. Q.E.D.

Let
$$\tilde{\boldsymbol{Q}}_2 = \boldsymbol{I}_{n-1} - 2\boldsymbol{t}_2\boldsymbol{t}_2',$$
where $\boldsymbol{t}_2$ is an $(n-1)$-component vector of unit length. It follows that the square matrix of order n
$$\boldsymbol{Q}_2 = \begin{bmatrix} 1 & \mathbf{0}' \\ \mathbf{0} & \tilde{\boldsymbol{Q}}_2 \end{bmatrix}$$
is orthogonal (i.e., $\boldsymbol{Q}_2^2 = \boldsymbol{Q}_2'\boldsymbol{Q}_2 = \boldsymbol{I}_n$). More generally, define
$$\tilde{\boldsymbol{Q}}_j = \boldsymbol{I}_{n-j+1} - 2\boldsymbol{t}_j\boldsymbol{t}_j',$$
where $\boldsymbol{t}_j$ is an $(n-j+1)$-component vector of unit length. Then the square matrix of order n defined by
$$\boldsymbol{Q}_j = \begin{bmatrix} \boldsymbol{I}_{j-1} & \boldsymbol{O} \\ \boldsymbol{O} & \tilde{\boldsymbol{Q}}_j \end{bmatrix}, \quad j = 2, \cdots, n,$$
is an orthogonal matrix. Hence, it holds that
$$\boldsymbol{Q}_1'\boldsymbol{Q}_2' \cdots \boldsymbol{Q}_{p-1}'\boldsymbol{Q}_p'\boldsymbol{Q}_p\boldsymbol{Q}_{p-1} \cdots \boldsymbol{Q}_2\boldsymbol{Q}_1 = \boldsymbol{I}_n. \tag{6.164}$$
Let
$$\boldsymbol{A}_j = \boldsymbol{Q}_j\boldsymbol{Q}_{j-1} \cdots \boldsymbol{Q}_2\boldsymbol{Q}_1\boldsymbol{A}, \tag{6.165}$$
and determine $\boldsymbol{t}_1, \boldsymbol{t}_2, \cdots, \boldsymbol{t}_j$ in such a way that
$$\boldsymbol{A}_j = \begin{bmatrix} a_{1.1(j)} & a_{1.2(j)} & \cdots & a_{1.j(j)} & a_{1.j+1(j)} & \cdots & a_{1.m(j)} \\ 0 & a_{2.2(j)} & \cdots & a_{2.j(j)} & a_{2.j+1(j)} & \cdots & a_{2.m(j)} \\ \vdots & \vdots & \ddots & \vdots & \vdots & \ddots & \vdots \\ 0 & 0 & \cdots & a_{j.j(j)} & a_{j.j+1(j)} & \cdots & a_{j.m(j)} \\ 0 & 0 & \cdots & 0 & a_{j+1.j+1(j)} & \cdots & a_{j+1.m(j)} \\ \vdots & \vdots & \ddots & \vdots & \vdots & \ddots & \vdots \\ 0 & 0 & \cdots & 0 & a_{n.j+1(j)} & \cdots & a_{n.m(j)} \end{bmatrix}.$$

First, let $\boldsymbol{A} = [\boldsymbol{a}_1, \boldsymbol{a}_2, \cdots, \boldsymbol{a}_m]$ and $\boldsymbol{A}_{(1)} = \boldsymbol{Q}_1\boldsymbol{A} = [\boldsymbol{a}_{1(1)}, \boldsymbol{a}_{2(1)}, \cdots, \boldsymbol{a}_{m(1)}]$. Let us determine $\boldsymbol{Q}_1$ so that $\boldsymbol{a}_{1(1)} = \boldsymbol{Q}_1\boldsymbol{a}_1$ has a nonzero element only in the first element. (All other elements are zero.) Let $\boldsymbol{b}_1 = \boldsymbol{a}_{1(1)}$. We have

$$\boldsymbol{Q}_1\boldsymbol{a}_1 = \boldsymbol{b}_1 \Rightarrow (\boldsymbol{I}_n - 2\boldsymbol{t}_1\boldsymbol{t}_1')\boldsymbol{a}_1 = \boldsymbol{b}_1.$$

Hence, $\boldsymbol{a}_1 - \boldsymbol{b}_1 = 2\boldsymbol{t}_1 k_1$, where $k_1 = \boldsymbol{t}_1'\boldsymbol{a}_1$. Since $\boldsymbol{Q}_1$ is orthogonal, $||\boldsymbol{a}_1|| = ||\boldsymbol{b}_1||$. Hence, $\boldsymbol{b}_1 = (a_{1\cdot 1(1)}, 0, 0, \cdots, 0)'$, where $a_{1\cdot 1(1)} = ||\boldsymbol{a}_1||$ (assuming that $a_{1\cdot 1(1)} > 0$). Also, since $||\boldsymbol{a}_1 - \boldsymbol{b}_1||^2 = 4k_1^2||\boldsymbol{t}_1||^2 = 4k_1^2$, it follows that $k_1 = \sqrt{||\boldsymbol{a}_1||(||\boldsymbol{a}_1|| - a_{1\cdot 1(1)})/2}$, and so

$$\boldsymbol{t}_1 = (a_{11} - ||\boldsymbol{a}_1||, a_{21}, \cdots, a_{n1})'/(2k_1). \tag{6.166}$$

To obtain $\boldsymbol{t}_j$ for $j \geq 2$, let $\boldsymbol{a}_{(j)} = (a_{j\cdot j(j-1)}, a_{j+1\cdot j(j-1)}, \cdots, a_{n\cdot j(j-1)})'$ be the $(n-j+1)$-component vector obtained by eliminating the first $j-1$ elements from the jth column vector $\boldsymbol{a}_{j(j-1)}$ in the n by m matrix $\boldsymbol{A}_{(j-1)}$. Using a similar procedure to obtain $\boldsymbol{t}_1$ in (6.166), we obtain

$$\boldsymbol{t}_j = (a_{j\cdot j(j-1)} - ||\boldsymbol{b}_1||, a_{j+1\cdot j(j-1)}, \cdots, a_{n\cdot j(j-1)})'/(2k_j), \tag{6.167}$$

where $k_j = \sqrt{||\boldsymbol{a}_{(j)}||(||\boldsymbol{a}_{(j)}|| - a_{j\cdot j(j-1)})/2}$.

Construct $\tilde{\boldsymbol{Q}}_j$ and $\boldsymbol{Q}_j$ using $\boldsymbol{t}_1, \boldsymbol{t}_2, \cdots, \boldsymbol{t}_m$, and obtain $\boldsymbol{Q} = \boldsymbol{Q}_1\boldsymbol{Q}_2\cdots\boldsymbol{Q}_m$. Then $\boldsymbol{Q}'\boldsymbol{A}$ is an upper triangular matrix $\boldsymbol{R}$. Premultiplying by $\boldsymbol{Q}$, we obtain $\boldsymbol{A} = \boldsymbol{Q}\boldsymbol{R}$, which is the QR decomposition of $\boldsymbol{A}$.

Note Let $\boldsymbol{a}$ and $\boldsymbol{b}$ be two n-component vectors having the same norm, and let

$$\boldsymbol{t} = (\boldsymbol{b} - \boldsymbol{a})/||\boldsymbol{b} - \boldsymbol{a}||$$

and

$$\boldsymbol{S} = \boldsymbol{I}_n - 2\boldsymbol{t}\boldsymbol{t}'. \tag{6.168}$$

It can be easily shown that the symmetric matrix $\boldsymbol{S}$ satisfies

$$\boldsymbol{S}\boldsymbol{a} = \boldsymbol{b} \text{ and } \boldsymbol{S}\boldsymbol{b} = \boldsymbol{a}. \tag{6.169}$$

This type of transformation is called the Householder transformation (or reflection).

Example 6.3 Apply the QR decomposition to the matrix

$$\boldsymbol{A} = \begin{bmatrix} 1 & 1 & 1 & 1 \\ 1 & -3 & 2 & 4 \\ 1 & -2 & -3 & 7 \\ 1 & -2 & -4 & 10 \end{bmatrix}.$$

Since $\boldsymbol{a}_1 = (1,1,1,1)'$, we have $\boldsymbol{t}_1 = (-1,1,1,1)'/2$, and it follows that

$$\boldsymbol{Q}_1 = \frac{1}{2}\begin{bmatrix} 1 & 1 & 1 & 1 \\ 1 & 1 & -1 & -1 \\ 1 & -1 & 1 & -1 \\ 1 & -1 & -1 & -1 \end{bmatrix} \text{ and } \boldsymbol{Q}_1\boldsymbol{A} = \begin{bmatrix} 2 & -3 & -2 & 11 \\ 0 & 1 & 5 & -6 \\ 0 & 2 & 0 & -3 \\ 0 & 2 & 1 & 0 \end{bmatrix}.$$

Next, since $\boldsymbol{a}_{(2)} = (1,2,2)'$, we obtain $\boldsymbol{t}_2 = (-1,1,1)'/\sqrt{3}$. Hence,

$$\tilde{\boldsymbol{Q}}_2 = \frac{1}{3}\begin{bmatrix} 1 & 2 & 2 \\ 2 & 1 & -2 \\ 2 & -2 & 1 \end{bmatrix} \text{ and } \boldsymbol{Q}_2 = \begin{bmatrix} 1 & 0\ 0\ 0 \\ 0 & \\ 0 & \tilde{\boldsymbol{Q}}_2 \\ 0 & \end{bmatrix},$$

and so

$$\boldsymbol{Q}_2\boldsymbol{Q}_1\boldsymbol{A} = \begin{bmatrix} 2 & -3 & -2 & 11 \\ 0 & 3 & 1 & 4 \\ 0 & 0 & 4 & -5 \\ 0 & 0 & 3 & -2 \end{bmatrix}.$$

Next, since $\boldsymbol{a}_{(3)} = (4,3)'$, we obtain $\boldsymbol{t}_3 = (-1,3)'/\sqrt{10}$. Hence,

$$\tilde{\boldsymbol{Q}}_3 = \frac{1}{5}\begin{bmatrix} 4 & 3 \\ 3 & -4 \end{bmatrix} \text{ and } \tilde{\boldsymbol{Q}}_3\begin{bmatrix} 4 & -5 \\ 3 & -2 \end{bmatrix} = \begin{bmatrix} 5 & -5.2 \\ 0 & -1.4 \end{bmatrix}.$$

Putting this all together, we obtain

$$\boldsymbol{Q} = \boldsymbol{Q}_1\boldsymbol{Q}_2\boldsymbol{Q}_3 = \frac{1}{30}\begin{bmatrix} 15 & 25 & 7 & -1 \\ 15 & -15 & 21 & -3 \\ 15 & -5 & -11 & 23 \\ 15 & -5 & -17 & -19 \end{bmatrix}$$

and

$$\boldsymbol{R} = \begin{bmatrix} 2 & -3 & -2 & 11 \\ 0 & 3 & 1 & 4 \\ 0 & 0 & 5 & -5.2 \\ 0 & 0 & 0 & -1.4 \end{bmatrix}.$$

It can be confirmed that $\boldsymbol{A} = \boldsymbol{QR}$, and $\boldsymbol{Q}$ is orthogonal.

Note To get the inverse of $\boldsymbol{A}$, we obtain

$$\boldsymbol{R}^{-1} = \begin{bmatrix} .5 & .5 & 1/10 & -2.129 \\ 0 & 1/3 & -1/20 & 0.705 \\ 0 & 0 & 1/5 & 0.743 \\ 0 & 0 & 0 & 0.714 \end{bmatrix}.$$

Since $\boldsymbol{A}^{-1} = \boldsymbol{R}^{-1}\boldsymbol{Q}'$, we obtain

$$\boldsymbol{A}^{-1} = \begin{bmatrix} 0.619 & -0.143 & 1.762 & -1.228 \\ 0.286 & -0.143 & -0.571 & 0.429 \\ 0.071 & 0.214 & -0.643 & 0.357 \\ 0.024 & 0.071 & -0.548 & 0.452 \end{bmatrix}.$$

Note The description above assumed that $\boldsymbol{A}$ is square and nonsingular. When $\boldsymbol{A}$ is a tall matrix, the QR decomposition takes the form of

$$\boldsymbol{A} = \begin{bmatrix} \boldsymbol{Q} & \boldsymbol{Q}_0 \end{bmatrix} \begin{bmatrix} \boldsymbol{R} \\ \boldsymbol{O} \end{bmatrix} = \boldsymbol{Q}^*\boldsymbol{R}^* = \boldsymbol{Q}\boldsymbol{R},$$

where $\boldsymbol{Q}^* = \begin{bmatrix} \boldsymbol{Q} & \boldsymbol{Q}_0 \end{bmatrix}$, $\boldsymbol{R}^* = \begin{bmatrix} \boldsymbol{R} \\ \boldsymbol{O} \end{bmatrix}$, and $\boldsymbol{Q}_0$ is the matrix of orthogonal basis vectors spanning $\text{Ker}(\boldsymbol{A}')$. (The matrix $\boldsymbol{Q}_0$ usually is not unique.) The $\boldsymbol{Q}^*\boldsymbol{R}^*$ is called sometimes the complete QR decomposition of $\boldsymbol{A}$, and $\boldsymbol{Q}\boldsymbol{R}$ is called the compact (or incomplete) QR decomposition. When $\boldsymbol{A}$ is singular, $\boldsymbol{R}$ is truncated at the bottom to form an upper echelon matrix.

6.4.3 Decomposition by projectors

A simultaneous linear equation $\boldsymbol{A}\boldsymbol{x} = \boldsymbol{b}$, where $\boldsymbol{A}$ is an n by m matrix, has a solution if $\boldsymbol{b} \in \text{Sp}(\boldsymbol{A})$. If we decompose $\boldsymbol{A}$ using QR decomposition described in the previous subsection, we obtain

$$\boldsymbol{Q}\boldsymbol{R}\boldsymbol{x} = \boldsymbol{b} \Rightarrow \boldsymbol{x} = \boldsymbol{R}^{-1}\boldsymbol{Q}'\boldsymbol{b}.$$

The QR decomposition can be interpreted geometrically as obtaining a set of basis vectors $\boldsymbol{Q} = [\boldsymbol{q}_1, \boldsymbol{q}_2, \cdots, \boldsymbol{q}_m]$ in the subspace $\text{Sp}(\boldsymbol{A})$ in such a way that the coefficient matrix $\boldsymbol{R}$ is upper triangular. However, this is not an absolute requirement for solving the equation. It is possible to define a set of arbitrary orthonormal basis vectors, $\boldsymbol{f}_1 = \boldsymbol{A}\boldsymbol{w}_1, \boldsymbol{f}_2 = \boldsymbol{A}\boldsymbol{w}_2, \cdots, \boldsymbol{f}_m = \boldsymbol{A}\boldsymbol{w}_m$, directly on $\text{Sp}(\boldsymbol{A})$. Since these vectors are orthogonal, the orthogonal projector $\boldsymbol{P}_A$ onto $\text{Sp}(\boldsymbol{A})$ can be expressed as

$$\boldsymbol{P}_A = \boldsymbol{P}_{f_1} + \boldsymbol{P}_{f_2} + \cdots + \boldsymbol{P}_{f_m}. \tag{6.170}$$

Pre- and postmultiplying the equation above by $\boldsymbol{A}'$ and $\boldsymbol{A}\boldsymbol{x} = \boldsymbol{b}$, respectively, we obtain

$$\boldsymbol{A}'\boldsymbol{A}\boldsymbol{x} = \boldsymbol{A}'(\boldsymbol{P}_{f_1} + \boldsymbol{P}_{f_2} + \cdots + \boldsymbol{P}_{f_m})\boldsymbol{b}$$

since $\boldsymbol{A}'\boldsymbol{P}_A = \boldsymbol{A}'$. If $\boldsymbol{A}'\boldsymbol{A}$ is nonsingular, the equation above can be rewritten as

$$\boldsymbol{x} = \boldsymbol{w}_1(\boldsymbol{f}_1'\boldsymbol{f}_1)^{-1}\boldsymbol{f}_1'\boldsymbol{b} + \boldsymbol{w}_2(\boldsymbol{f}_2'\boldsymbol{f}_2)^{-1}\boldsymbol{f}_2'\boldsymbol{b} + \cdots + \boldsymbol{w}_m(\boldsymbol{f}_m'\boldsymbol{f}_m)^{-1}\boldsymbol{f}_m'\boldsymbol{b}. \quad (6.171)$$

The equation above can further be rewritten as

$$\boldsymbol{x} = \boldsymbol{w}_1\boldsymbol{f}_1'\boldsymbol{b} + \boldsymbol{w}_2\boldsymbol{f}_2'\boldsymbol{b} + \cdots + \boldsymbol{w}_m\boldsymbol{f}_m'\boldsymbol{b} = \boldsymbol{W}\boldsymbol{F}'\boldsymbol{b}, \quad (6.172)$$

where $\boldsymbol{F} = [\boldsymbol{f}_1, \boldsymbol{f}_2, \cdots, \boldsymbol{f}_m]$, since $\boldsymbol{f}_i'\boldsymbol{f}_i = 1$ $(i = 1, \cdots, m)$, assuming that the $\boldsymbol{f}_j$'s constitute a set of orthonormal basis vectors.

One way of obtaining $\boldsymbol{f}_1, \boldsymbol{f}_2, \cdots, \boldsymbol{f}_m$ is by the Gram-Schmidt method as described above. In this case, $\boldsymbol{F} = \boldsymbol{A}\boldsymbol{W} \Rightarrow \boldsymbol{A} = \boldsymbol{F}\boldsymbol{W}^{-1}$, so that $\boldsymbol{F} = \boldsymbol{Q}$ and $\boldsymbol{W}^{-1} = \boldsymbol{R}$ in (6.172).

Another way of obtaining a set of orthonormal basis vectors is via singular value decomposition (SVD). Let $\mu_1, \mu_2, \cdots, \mu_m$ denote the positive singular values of $\boldsymbol{A}$, where the SVD of $\boldsymbol{A}$ is obtained by (5.18). Then, $\boldsymbol{w}_j = \mu_j\boldsymbol{v}_j$ and $\boldsymbol{f}_j = \boldsymbol{u}_j$, so that the solution vector in (6.171) can be expressed as

$$\boldsymbol{x} = \frac{1}{\mu_1}\boldsymbol{v}_1\boldsymbol{u}_1'\boldsymbol{b} + \frac{1}{\mu_2}\boldsymbol{v}_2\boldsymbol{u}_2'\boldsymbol{b} + \cdots + \frac{1}{\mu_m}\boldsymbol{v}_m\boldsymbol{u}_m'\boldsymbol{b}. \quad (6.173)$$

Let $\boldsymbol{A} = \boldsymbol{Q}\boldsymbol{R}$ be the QR decomposition of $\boldsymbol{A}$, and let $\boldsymbol{B} = \boldsymbol{A}'\boldsymbol{A}$. We have

$$\boldsymbol{B} = \boldsymbol{R}'\boldsymbol{Q}'\boldsymbol{Q}\boldsymbol{R} = \boldsymbol{R}'\boldsymbol{R}.$$

This is called the Cholesky decomposition of $\boldsymbol{B}$. Let $\boldsymbol{B} = [b_{ij}]$ and $\boldsymbol{R} = [r_{ij}]$. Since $b_{ij} = \sum_{k=1}^{i} r_{ki}r_{kj}$, we have

$$\begin{aligned} r_{11} &= \sqrt{b_{11}},\ \ r_{1j} = b_{1j}/r_{11},\ \ (j = 2, \cdots, m), \\ r_{jj} &= \left(b_{jj} - \sum_{k=1}^{j-1} r_{kj}^2\right)^{1/2},\ \ (j = 2, \cdots, m), \\ r_{ij} &= \left(b_{ij} - \sum_{k=1}^{j-1} r_{ki}r_{kj}\right)/r_{jj},\ \ (i < j). \end{aligned}$$

6.5 Exercises for Chapter 6

1. Show that $R^2_{X\cdot y} = R^2_{\tilde{X}\cdot y}$ if $\mathrm{Sp}(\boldsymbol{X}) = \mathrm{Sp}(\tilde{\boldsymbol{X}})$.

2. Show that $1 - R^2_{X\cdot y} = (1 - r^2_{x_1y})(1 - r_{x_2y|x_1})^2 \cdots (1 - r^2_{x_py|x_1x_2\cdots x_{p-1}})$, where $r_{x_jy|x_1x_2\cdots x_{j-1}}$ is the correlation between x_j and y eliminating the effects due to $x_1, x_2, \cdots, x_{j-1}$.

3. Show that the necessary and sufficient condition for $\boldsymbol{Ly}$ to be the BLUE of $E(\boldsymbol{L}'\boldsymbol{y})$ in the Gauss-Markov model $(\boldsymbol{y}, \boldsymbol{X\beta}, \sigma^2\boldsymbol{G})$ is

$$\boldsymbol{GL} \in \mathrm{Sp}(\boldsymbol{X}).$$

4. Show that the BLUE of $\boldsymbol{e}'\boldsymbol{\beta}$ in the Gauss-Markov model $(\boldsymbol{y}, \boldsymbol{X\beta}, \sigma^2\boldsymbol{G})$ is $\boldsymbol{e}'\hat{\boldsymbol{\beta}}$, where $\hat{\boldsymbol{\beta}}$ is an unbiased estimator of $\boldsymbol{\beta}$.

5. Show that, in the Gauss-Markov model above, an estimator for $f\sigma^2$, where $f = \mathrm{rank}(\boldsymbol{X}, \boldsymbol{G}) - \mathrm{rank}(\boldsymbol{X})$, is given by one of the following:
(i) $\boldsymbol{y}'\boldsymbol{Z}(\boldsymbol{ZGZ})^-\boldsymbol{Zy}$.
(ii) $\boldsymbol{y}'T^-(\boldsymbol{I}_n - \boldsymbol{P}_{X/T^-})\boldsymbol{y}$, where $\boldsymbol{T} = \boldsymbol{G} + \boldsymbol{XUX}'$ and $\mathrm{rank}(\boldsymbol{T}) = \mathrm{rank}([\boldsymbol{G}, \boldsymbol{X}])$.

6. For $\boldsymbol{G} = [\boldsymbol{g}_1, \boldsymbol{g}_2, \cdots, \boldsymbol{g}_m]$ given in (6.46):
(i) Show that $\boldsymbol{Q}_M\boldsymbol{G}(\boldsymbol{G}'\boldsymbol{Q}_M\boldsymbol{G})^-\boldsymbol{G}'\boldsymbol{Q}_M = \boldsymbol{Q}_M\tilde{\boldsymbol{G}}(\tilde{\boldsymbol{G}}'\boldsymbol{Q}_M\tilde{\boldsymbol{G}})^{-1}\tilde{\boldsymbol{G}}\boldsymbol{Q}_M$, where $\tilde{\boldsymbol{G}}$ is a matrix obtained by eliminating an arbitrary column from $\boldsymbol{G}$.
(ii) Show that $\min_\alpha ||\boldsymbol{y} - \boldsymbol{G}^*\boldsymbol{\alpha}||^2 = \boldsymbol{y}'(\boldsymbol{I}_n - \tilde{\boldsymbol{G}}(\tilde{\boldsymbol{G}}'\boldsymbol{Q}_M\tilde{\boldsymbol{G}})^{-1}\tilde{\boldsymbol{G}}')\boldsymbol{y}$, where $\boldsymbol{G}^* = [\boldsymbol{G}, \boldsymbol{1}_n]$, $\boldsymbol{\alpha}$ is an $(m+1)$-component vector of weights, and $\boldsymbol{y}$ is an n-component vector with zero mean.

7. Define the projectors

$$\boldsymbol{P}_{x[G]} = \boldsymbol{Q}_G\boldsymbol{x}(\boldsymbol{x}'\boldsymbol{Q}_G\boldsymbol{x})^{-1}\boldsymbol{x}'\boldsymbol{Q}_G$$

and

$$\boldsymbol{P}_{D_x[G]} = \boldsymbol{Q}_G\boldsymbol{D}_x(\boldsymbol{D}_x'\boldsymbol{Q}_G\boldsymbol{D}_x)^{-1}\boldsymbol{D}_x'\boldsymbol{Q}_G$$

using $\boldsymbol{x} = \begin{pmatrix} x_1 \\ x_2 \\ \vdots \\ x_m \end{pmatrix}$, $\boldsymbol{D}_x = \begin{bmatrix} \boldsymbol{x}_1 & \boldsymbol{0} & \cdots & \boldsymbol{0} \\ \boldsymbol{0} & \boldsymbol{x}_2 & \cdots & \boldsymbol{0} \\ \vdots & \vdots & \ddots & \vdots \\ \boldsymbol{0} & \boldsymbol{0} & \cdots & \boldsymbol{x}_m \end{bmatrix}$, $\boldsymbol{y} = \begin{pmatrix} y_1 \\ y_2 \\ \vdots \\ y_m \end{pmatrix}$, and the matrix of dummy variables $\boldsymbol{G}$ given in (6.46). Assume that $\boldsymbol{x}_j$ and $\boldsymbol{y}_j$ have the same size n_j. Show that the following relations hold:
(i) $\boldsymbol{P}_{x[G]}\boldsymbol{P}_{D_x[G]} = \boldsymbol{P}_{x[G]}$.
(ii) $\boldsymbol{P}_x\boldsymbol{P}_{D_x[G]} = \boldsymbol{P}_x\boldsymbol{P}_{x[G]}$.
(iii) $\min_b ||\boldsymbol{y} - b\boldsymbol{x}||^2_{Q_G} = ||\boldsymbol{y} - \boldsymbol{P}_{x[G]}\boldsymbol{y}||^2_{Q_G}$.
(iv) $\min_b ||\boldsymbol{y} - \boldsymbol{D}_x\boldsymbol{b}||^2_{Q_G} = ||\boldsymbol{y} - \boldsymbol{P}_{D_x[G]}\boldsymbol{y}||^2_{Q_G}$.
(v) Show that $\hat{\beta}_i\boldsymbol{x}_i = \boldsymbol{P}_{D_x[G]}\boldsymbol{y}$ and $\hat{\beta}\boldsymbol{x}_i = \boldsymbol{P}_{x[G]}\boldsymbol{y}$, where $\beta = \beta_1 = \beta_2 = \cdots = \beta_m$ in the least squares estimation in the linear model $y_{ij} = \alpha_i + \beta_i x_{ij} + \epsilon_{ij}$, where $1 \geq i \geq m$ and $1 \geq j \geq n_i$.

8. Let $\boldsymbol{X} = \boldsymbol{U}_X\boldsymbol{\Delta}_X\boldsymbol{V}'_X$ and $\boldsymbol{Y} = \boldsymbol{U}_Y\boldsymbol{\Delta}_Y\boldsymbol{V}'_Y$ represent the SVDs of $\boldsymbol{X}$ and $\boldsymbol{Y}$. Show that the singular values of the matrix $S = \boldsymbol{\Delta}_X^{-1}\boldsymbol{U}_X\boldsymbol{C}_{XY}\boldsymbol{U}'_Y\boldsymbol{\Delta}_Y^{-1}$ are equal to the canonical correlations between $\boldsymbol{X}$ and $\boldsymbol{Y}$.

9. Let $\boldsymbol{Q}_Z\boldsymbol{X}\boldsymbol{A}$ and $\boldsymbol{Q}_Z\boldsymbol{Y}\boldsymbol{B}$ denote the canonical variates corresponding to $\boldsymbol{Q}_Z\boldsymbol{X}$ and $\boldsymbol{Q}_Z\boldsymbol{Y}$. Show that (Yanai, 1980):
(i) $\boldsymbol{P}_{XA\cdot Z} = (\boldsymbol{P}_{X\cdot Z}\boldsymbol{P}_{Y\cdot Z})(\boldsymbol{P}_{X\cdot Z}\boldsymbol{P}_{Y\cdot Z})^-_{\ell(Z)}$.
(ii) $\boldsymbol{P}_{YB\cdot Z} = (\boldsymbol{P}_{Y\cdot Z}\boldsymbol{P}_{X\cdot Z})(\boldsymbol{P}_{Y\cdot Z}\boldsymbol{P}_{X\cdot Z})^-_{\ell(Z)}$.
(iii) $\boldsymbol{P}_{XA\cdot Z}\boldsymbol{P}_{YB\cdot Z} = \boldsymbol{P}_{XA\cdot Z}\boldsymbol{P}_{Y\cdot Z} = \boldsymbol{P}_{X\cdot Z}\boldsymbol{P}_{YB\cdot Z} = \boldsymbol{P}_{X\cdot Z}\boldsymbol{P}_{Y\cdot Z}$.

10. Let $\boldsymbol{X}$ and $\boldsymbol{Y}$ be n by p and n by q matrices, respectively, and let

$$\boldsymbol{R} = \begin{bmatrix} \boldsymbol{R}_{XX} & \boldsymbol{R}_{XY} \\ \boldsymbol{R}_{YX} & \boldsymbol{R}_{YY} \end{bmatrix} \text{ and } \boldsymbol{R}\boldsymbol{R}^- = \begin{bmatrix} \boldsymbol{S}_{11} & \boldsymbol{S}_{12} \\ \boldsymbol{S}_{21} & \boldsymbol{S}_{22} \end{bmatrix}.$$

Show the following:
(i) $\mathrm{Sp}(\boldsymbol{I}_p - \boldsymbol{R}\boldsymbol{R}^-) = \mathrm{Ker}([\boldsymbol{X}, \boldsymbol{Y}])$.
(ii) $(\boldsymbol{I}_p - \boldsymbol{S}_{11})\boldsymbol{X}'\boldsymbol{Q}_Y = \boldsymbol{O}$, and $(\boldsymbol{I}_q - \boldsymbol{S}_{22})\boldsymbol{Y}'\boldsymbol{Q}_X = \boldsymbol{O}$.
(iii) If $\mathrm{Sp}(\boldsymbol{X})$ and $\mathrm{Sp}(\boldsymbol{Y})$ are disjoint, $\boldsymbol{S}_{11}\boldsymbol{X}' = \boldsymbol{X}'$, $\boldsymbol{S}_{12}\boldsymbol{Y}' = \boldsymbol{O}$, $\boldsymbol{S}_{21}\boldsymbol{X}' = \boldsymbol{O}$, and $\boldsymbol{S}_{22}\boldsymbol{Y}' = \boldsymbol{Y}'$.

11. Let $\boldsymbol{Z} = [\boldsymbol{z}_1, \boldsymbol{z}_2, \cdots, \boldsymbol{z}_p]$ denote the matrix of columnwise standardized scores, and let $\boldsymbol{F} = [\boldsymbol{f}_1, \boldsymbol{f}_2, \cdots, \boldsymbol{f}_r]$ denote the matrix of common factors in the factor analysis model ($r < p$). Show the following:
(i) $\frac{1}{n}||\boldsymbol{P}_F\boldsymbol{z}_j||^2 = h_j^2$, where h_j^2 is called the communality of the variable j.
(ii) $\mathrm{tr}(\boldsymbol{P}_F\boldsymbol{P}_Z) \le r$.
(iii) $h_j^2 \ge ||\boldsymbol{P}_{Z_{(j)}}\boldsymbol{z}_j||^2$, where $\boldsymbol{Z}_{(j)} = [\boldsymbol{z}_1, \cdots, \boldsymbol{z}_{j-1}, \boldsymbol{z}_{j+1}, \cdots, \boldsymbol{z}_p]$.

12. Show that $\lim_{k\to\infty}(\boldsymbol{P}_X\boldsymbol{P}_Y)^k = \boldsymbol{P}_Z$ if $\mathrm{Sp}(\boldsymbol{X}) \cap \mathrm{Sp}(\boldsymbol{Y}) = \mathrm{Sp}(\boldsymbol{Z})$.

13. Consider the perturbations $\Delta\boldsymbol{x}$ and $\Delta\boldsymbol{b}$ of $\boldsymbol{X}$ and $\boldsymbol{b}$ in the linear equation $\boldsymbol{A}\boldsymbol{x} = \boldsymbol{b}$, that is, $\boldsymbol{A}(\boldsymbol{x} + \Delta\boldsymbol{x}) = \boldsymbol{b} + \Delta\boldsymbol{b}$. Show that

$$\frac{||\Delta\boldsymbol{x}||}{||\boldsymbol{x}||} \le \mathrm{Cond}(\boldsymbol{A})\frac{||\Delta\boldsymbol{b}||}{||\boldsymbol{b}||},$$

where $\mathrm{Cond}(\boldsymbol{A})$ indicates the ratio of the largest singular value $\mu_{\max}(\boldsymbol{A})$ of $\boldsymbol{A}$ to the smallest singular value $\mu_{\min}(\boldsymbol{A})$ of $\boldsymbol{A}$ and is called the condition number.

Chapter 7

Answers to Exercises

7.1 Chapter 1

1. (a) Premultiplying the right-hand side by $\boldsymbol{A} + \boldsymbol{BCB}'$, we obtain

$$\begin{aligned}
&(\boldsymbol{A} + \boldsymbol{BCB}')[\boldsymbol{A}^{-1} - \boldsymbol{A}^{-1}\boldsymbol{B}(\boldsymbol{B}'\boldsymbol{A}^{-1}\boldsymbol{B} + \boldsymbol{C}^{-1})^{-1}\boldsymbol{B}'\boldsymbol{A}^{-1}] \\
&\quad = \boldsymbol{I} - \boldsymbol{B}(\boldsymbol{B}'\boldsymbol{A}^{-1}\boldsymbol{B} + \boldsymbol{C}^{-1})^{-1}\boldsymbol{B}'\boldsymbol{A}^{-1} + \boldsymbol{BCB}'\boldsymbol{A}^{-1} \\
&\qquad\qquad - \boldsymbol{BCB}'\boldsymbol{A}^{-1}\boldsymbol{B}(\boldsymbol{B}'\boldsymbol{A}^{-1}\boldsymbol{B} + \boldsymbol{C}^{-1})^{-1}\boldsymbol{B}'\boldsymbol{A}^{-1} \\
&\quad = \boldsymbol{I} + \boldsymbol{B}[\boldsymbol{C} - (\boldsymbol{I} + \boldsymbol{CB}'\boldsymbol{A}^{-1}\boldsymbol{B})(\boldsymbol{B}'\boldsymbol{A}^{-1}\boldsymbol{B} + \boldsymbol{C}^{-1})^{-1}]\boldsymbol{B}'\boldsymbol{A}^{-1} \\
&\quad = \boldsymbol{I} + \boldsymbol{B}[\boldsymbol{C} - \boldsymbol{C}(\boldsymbol{C}^{-1} + \boldsymbol{B}'\boldsymbol{A}^{-1}\boldsymbol{B})(\boldsymbol{B}'\boldsymbol{A}^{-1}\boldsymbol{B} + \boldsymbol{C}^{-1})^{-1}]\boldsymbol{B}'\boldsymbol{A}^{-1} \\
&\quad = \boldsymbol{I}.
\end{aligned}$$

(b) In (a) above, set $\boldsymbol{C} = \boldsymbol{I}$ and $\boldsymbol{B} = \boldsymbol{c}$.

2. To obtain $\boldsymbol{x}_1 = (x_1, x_2)'$ and $\boldsymbol{x}_2 = (x_3, x_4)'$ that satisfy $\boldsymbol{Ax}_1 = \boldsymbol{Bx}_2$, we solve

$$\begin{aligned}
x_1 + 2x_2 - 3x_3 + 2x_4 &= 0, \\
2x_1 + x_2 - x_3 - 3x_4 &= 0, \\
3x_1 + 3x_2 - 2x_3 - 5x_4 &= 0.
\end{aligned}$$

Then, $x_1 = 2x_4$, $x_2 = \boldsymbol{x}_4$, and $x_3 = 2x_4$. Hence, $\boldsymbol{Ax}_1 = \boldsymbol{Bx}_2 = (4x_4, 5x_4, 9x_4)' = x_4(4, 5, 9)'$. Let $\boldsymbol{d} = (4, 5, 9)'$. We have $\mathrm{Sp}(\boldsymbol{A}) \cap \mathrm{Sp}(\boldsymbol{B}) = \{\boldsymbol{x}|\boldsymbol{x} = \alpha\boldsymbol{d}\}$, where α is an arbitrary nonzero real number.

3. Since $\boldsymbol{M}$ is a *pd* matrix, we have $\boldsymbol{M} = \boldsymbol{T\Delta}^2\boldsymbol{T}' = (\boldsymbol{T\Delta})(\boldsymbol{T\Delta})' = \boldsymbol{SS}'$, where $\boldsymbol{S}$ is a nonsingular matrix. Let $\tilde{\boldsymbol{A}} = \boldsymbol{S}'\boldsymbol{A}$ and $\tilde{\boldsymbol{B}} = \boldsymbol{S}^{-1}\boldsymbol{B}$. From (1.19),

$$[\mathrm{tr}(\tilde{\boldsymbol{A}}'\tilde{\boldsymbol{B}})]^2 \le \mathrm{tr}(\tilde{\boldsymbol{A}}'\tilde{\boldsymbol{A}})\mathrm{tr}(\tilde{\boldsymbol{B}}'\tilde{\boldsymbol{B}}).$$

On the other hand, $\tilde{\boldsymbol{A}}'\tilde{\boldsymbol{B}} = \boldsymbol{A}'\boldsymbol{SS}^{-1}\boldsymbol{B} = \boldsymbol{A}'\boldsymbol{B}$, $\tilde{\boldsymbol{A}}'\tilde{\boldsymbol{A}} = \boldsymbol{A}'\boldsymbol{SS}'\boldsymbol{A} = \boldsymbol{A}'\boldsymbol{MA}$, and $\tilde{\boldsymbol{B}}'\tilde{\boldsymbol{B}} = \boldsymbol{B}'(\boldsymbol{S}')^{-1}\boldsymbol{S}^{-1}\boldsymbol{B} = \boldsymbol{B}'(\boldsymbol{SS}')^{-1}\boldsymbol{B} = \boldsymbol{B}'\boldsymbol{M}^{-1}\boldsymbol{B}$, leading to the given formula.

4. (a) Correct.

(b) Incorrect. Let $\boldsymbol{x} \in E^n$. Then $\boldsymbol{x}$ can be decomposed as $\boldsymbol{x} = \boldsymbol{x}_1 + \boldsymbol{x}_2$, where

$\boldsymbol{x}_1 \in V$ and $\boldsymbol{x}_2 \in W$. That is, $\boldsymbol{x}$ is necessarily contained in neither V nor W. Even if $\boldsymbol{x} \notin V$, $\boldsymbol{x} \in W$ is not necessarily true. In general, $\boldsymbol{x} \in V \oplus W$. Try, for example, $V = \left\{\begin{pmatrix} 1 \\ 0 \end{pmatrix}\right\}$, $W = \left\{\begin{pmatrix} 0 \\ 1 \end{pmatrix}\right\}$, and $\boldsymbol{x} = \begin{pmatrix} 1 \\ 1 \end{pmatrix}$.
(c) Incorrect. Even if $\boldsymbol{x} \in V$, it is possible that $\boldsymbol{x} = \boldsymbol{x}_1 + \boldsymbol{x}_2$, where $\boldsymbol{x}_1 \in \tilde{V}$ and $\boldsymbol{x}_2 \in \tilde{W}$, and $E^n = \tilde{V} \oplus \tilde{W}$ is an arbitrary decomposition of E^n.
(d) Incorrect. $V \cap \mathrm{Ker}(\boldsymbol{A}) = \{\boldsymbol{0}\}$ is equivalent to $\mathrm{rank}(\boldsymbol{A}) = \mathrm{rank}(\boldsymbol{A}^2)$. For example, for $\boldsymbol{A} = \begin{bmatrix} 0 & 1 \\ 0 & 0 \end{bmatrix}$, $\mathrm{Sp}(\boldsymbol{A}) = \mathrm{Ker}(\boldsymbol{A}) = \mathrm{Sp}\left\{\begin{pmatrix} 1 \\ 0 \end{pmatrix}\right\}$.
5. $\dim(V_1+V_2) = \dim(V_1)+\dim(V_2)-\dim(V_1\cap V_2)$ and $\dim(W_1+W_2) = \dim(W_1)+\dim(W_2) - \dim(W_1 \cap W_2)$. On the other hand, $\dim(V_1) + \dim(W_1) = \dim(V_2) + \dim(W_2) = n$, from which (1.87) follows.
6. (a) ($\Rightarrow$): Let $\boldsymbol{y} \in \mathrm{Ker}(\boldsymbol{A})$ and $\boldsymbol{Bx} = \boldsymbol{y} = \boldsymbol{0}$. From $\boldsymbol{ABx} = \boldsymbol{Ay} = \boldsymbol{0}$, we obtain $\boldsymbol{Ay} = \boldsymbol{0}$, which implies $\boldsymbol{ABx} = \boldsymbol{0}$. On the other hand, from $\mathrm{Ker}(\boldsymbol{AB}) = \mathrm{Ker}(\boldsymbol{B})$, we have $\boldsymbol{ABx} = \boldsymbol{0}$, which implies $\boldsymbol{Bx} = \boldsymbol{0}$. Hence, we have $\mathrm{Sp}(\boldsymbol{B}) \cap \mathrm{Ker}(\boldsymbol{A}) = \{\boldsymbol{0}\}$ by Theorem 1.4.

($\Leftarrow$): $\boldsymbol{ABx} = \boldsymbol{0}$ implies $\boldsymbol{Bx} \in \mathrm{Ker}(\boldsymbol{A})$. On the other hand, $\boldsymbol{Bx} = \boldsymbol{0}$ from $\mathrm{Sp}(\boldsymbol{B}) \cap \mathrm{Ker}(\boldsymbol{A}) = \{\boldsymbol{0}\}$. Thus, $\mathrm{Ker}(\boldsymbol{AB}) \subset \mathrm{Ker}(\boldsymbol{B})$. Clearly, $\mathrm{Ker}(\boldsymbol{AB}) \supset \mathrm{Ker}(\boldsymbol{B})$, so that $\mathrm{Ker}(\boldsymbol{AB}) = \mathrm{Ker}(\boldsymbol{B})$.
(b) Setting $\boldsymbol{B} = \boldsymbol{A}$ in (a) above, we obtain

$$\mathrm{Ker}(\boldsymbol{A}) \cap \mathrm{Sp}(\boldsymbol{A}) = \{\boldsymbol{0}\} \Leftrightarrow \mathrm{Ker}(\boldsymbol{A}) = \mathrm{Ker}(\boldsymbol{A}^2).$$

On the other hand, we must have $\mathrm{rank}(\boldsymbol{A}) = \mathrm{rank}(\boldsymbol{A}^2)$ from $\dim(\mathrm{Ker}(\boldsymbol{A})) = n - \mathrm{rank}(\boldsymbol{A})$, from which the given formula follows.
7. (a) The given equation follows from $\begin{bmatrix} \boldsymbol{I}_m & \boldsymbol{O} \\ -\boldsymbol{C} & \boldsymbol{I}_p \end{bmatrix} \begin{bmatrix} \boldsymbol{A} & \boldsymbol{AB} \\ \boldsymbol{CA} & \boldsymbol{O} \end{bmatrix} \begin{bmatrix} \boldsymbol{I}_n & -\boldsymbol{B} \\ \boldsymbol{O} & \boldsymbol{I}_m \end{bmatrix}$ $= \begin{bmatrix} \boldsymbol{A} & \boldsymbol{O} \\ \boldsymbol{O} & -\boldsymbol{CAB} \end{bmatrix}$.
(b) Let $\boldsymbol{E} = \begin{bmatrix} \boldsymbol{I}_n & \boldsymbol{I}_n - \boldsymbol{BA} \\ \boldsymbol{A} & \boldsymbol{O} \end{bmatrix}$. From (a) above, it follows that

$$\begin{bmatrix} \boldsymbol{I}_n & \boldsymbol{O} \\ -\boldsymbol{A} & \boldsymbol{I}_m \end{bmatrix} \boldsymbol{E} \begin{bmatrix} \boldsymbol{I}_n & -(\boldsymbol{I}_n - \boldsymbol{BA}) \\ \boldsymbol{O} & \boldsymbol{I}_n \end{bmatrix} = \begin{bmatrix} \boldsymbol{I}_n & \boldsymbol{O} \\ \boldsymbol{O} & -\boldsymbol{A}(\boldsymbol{I}_n - \boldsymbol{BA}) \end{bmatrix}.$$

Thus, $\mathrm{rank}(\boldsymbol{E}) = n + \mathrm{rank}(\boldsymbol{A} - \boldsymbol{ABA})$.

On the other hand,

$$\begin{aligned} \mathrm{rank}(\boldsymbol{E}) &= \mathrm{rank}\left\{\begin{bmatrix} \boldsymbol{I}_n & -\boldsymbol{B} \\ \boldsymbol{O} & \boldsymbol{I}_m \end{bmatrix} \begin{bmatrix} \boldsymbol{O} & \boldsymbol{I}_n - \boldsymbol{BA} \\ \boldsymbol{A} & \boldsymbol{O} \end{bmatrix} \begin{bmatrix} \boldsymbol{I}_n & \boldsymbol{O} \\ -\boldsymbol{I}_n & \boldsymbol{I}_n \end{bmatrix}\right\} \\ &= \mathrm{rank}\begin{bmatrix} \boldsymbol{O} & \boldsymbol{I}_n - \boldsymbol{BA} \\ \boldsymbol{A} & \boldsymbol{O} \end{bmatrix} = \mathrm{rank}(\boldsymbol{A}) + \mathrm{rank}(\boldsymbol{I}_n - \boldsymbol{BA}). \end{aligned}$$

Hence, $\mathrm{rank}(\boldsymbol{A} - \boldsymbol{ABA}) = \mathrm{rank}(\boldsymbol{A}) + \mathrm{rank}(\boldsymbol{I}_n - \boldsymbol{BA}) - n$ is established. The other formula can be derived similarly. This method of proof is called the matrix rank method, which was used by Guttman (1944) and Khatri (1961), but it was later greatly amplified by Tian and his collaborators (e.g., Tian, 1998, 2002; Tian and Styan, 2009).

8. (a) Assume that the basis vectors $[\boldsymbol{e}_1, \cdots, \boldsymbol{e}_p, \boldsymbol{e}_{p+1}, \cdots, \boldsymbol{e}_q]$ for $\text{Sp}(\boldsymbol{B})$ are obtained by expanding the basis vectors $[\boldsymbol{e}_1, \cdots, \boldsymbol{e}_p]$ for W_1. We are to prove that $[\boldsymbol{A}\boldsymbol{e}_{p+1}, \cdots, \boldsymbol{A}\boldsymbol{e}_q]$ are basis vectors for $W_2 = \text{Sp}(\boldsymbol{AB})$.

For $\boldsymbol{y} \in W_2$, there exists $\boldsymbol{x} \in \text{Sp}(\boldsymbol{B})$ such that $\boldsymbol{y} = \boldsymbol{Ax}$. Let $\boldsymbol{x} = c_1\boldsymbol{e}_1 + \cdots + c_q\boldsymbol{e}_q$. Since $\boldsymbol{A}\boldsymbol{e}_i = \boldsymbol{0}$ for $i = 1, \cdots, p$, we have $\boldsymbol{y} = \boldsymbol{Ax} = c_{p+1}\boldsymbol{A}\boldsymbol{e}_{p+1} + \cdots + c_q\boldsymbol{A}\boldsymbol{e}_q$. That is, an arbitrary $\boldsymbol{y} \in W_2$ can be expressed as a sum of $\boldsymbol{A}\boldsymbol{e}_i$ $(i = p+1, \cdots, q)$. On the other hand, let $c_{p+1}\boldsymbol{A}\boldsymbol{e}_{p+1} + \cdots + c_q\boldsymbol{A}\boldsymbol{e}_q = \boldsymbol{0}$. Then $\boldsymbol{A}(c_{p+1}\boldsymbol{e}_{p+1} + \cdots + c_q\boldsymbol{e}_q) = \boldsymbol{0}$ implies $c_{p+1}\boldsymbol{e}_{p+1} + \cdots c_q\boldsymbol{e}_q \in W_1$. Hence, $b_1\boldsymbol{e}_1 + \cdots + b_p\boldsymbol{e}_p + c_{p+1}\boldsymbol{e}_{p+1} + \cdots + c_q\boldsymbol{e}_q = \boldsymbol{0}$. Since $\boldsymbol{e}_1, \cdots \boldsymbol{e}_q$ are linearly independent, we must have $b_1 = \cdots = b_p = c_{p+1} = \cdots = c_q = 0$. That is, $c_{p+1}\boldsymbol{A}\boldsymbol{e}_{p+1} + \cdots + c_q\boldsymbol{A}\boldsymbol{e}_q = \boldsymbol{0}$ implies $c_{p=1} = \cdots = c_q$, which in turn implies that $[\boldsymbol{A}\boldsymbol{e}_{p+1}, \cdots, \boldsymbol{A}\boldsymbol{e}_q]$ constitutes basis vectors for $\text{Sp}(\boldsymbol{AB})$.

(b) From (a) above, $\text{rank}(\boldsymbol{AB}) = \text{rank}(\boldsymbol{B}) - \dim[\text{Sp}(\boldsymbol{B}) \cap \text{Ker}(\boldsymbol{A})]$, and so

$$\begin{aligned}\text{rank}(\boldsymbol{AB}) &= \text{rank}(\boldsymbol{B}'\boldsymbol{A}') = \text{rank}(\boldsymbol{A}') - \dim\{\text{Sp}(\boldsymbol{A}') \cap \text{Ker}(\boldsymbol{B}')\} \\ &= \text{rank}(\boldsymbol{A}) - \dim\{\text{Sp}(\boldsymbol{A}') \cap \text{Sp}(\boldsymbol{B})^{\perp}\}.\end{aligned}$$

9. $(\boldsymbol{I} - \boldsymbol{A})(\boldsymbol{I} + \boldsymbol{A} + \boldsymbol{A}^2 + \cdots + \boldsymbol{A}^{n-1}) = \boldsymbol{I} - \boldsymbol{A}^n$. Since $\boldsymbol{Ax} = \lambda\boldsymbol{x}$ does not have $\lambda = 1$ as a solution, $\boldsymbol{I} - \boldsymbol{A}$ is nonsingular, from which it follows that

$$(\boldsymbol{I} - \boldsymbol{A})^{-1}(\boldsymbol{I} - \boldsymbol{A}^n) = \boldsymbol{I} + \boldsymbol{A} + \boldsymbol{A}^2 + \cdots + \boldsymbol{A}^{n-1}.$$

Let $\boldsymbol{A} = \boldsymbol{T}_1\boldsymbol{\Delta}\boldsymbol{T}_2'$ be the spectral decomposition of $\boldsymbol{A}$, where $\boldsymbol{T}_1$ and $\boldsymbol{T}_2$ are orthogonal matrices and $\boldsymbol{\Delta}$ is a diagonal matrix with λ_j $(0 < \lambda_j < 1)$ as the jth diagonal element. Then, $\boldsymbol{A}^n = \boldsymbol{T}_1\boldsymbol{\Delta}^n\boldsymbol{T}_2'$, which goes to $\boldsymbol{O}$ as $n \to \infty$, from which the given formula follows immediately.

(b) Let $\boldsymbol{A} = \begin{bmatrix} 0 & 1 & 0 & 0 & 0 \\ 0 & 0 & 1 & 0 & 0 \\ 0 & 0 & 0 & 1 & 0 \\ 0 & 0 & 0 & 0 & 1 \\ 0 & 0 & 0 & 0 & 0 \end{bmatrix}$. Then, $\boldsymbol{A}^2 = \begin{bmatrix} 0 & 0 & 1 & 0 & 0 \\ 0 & 0 & 0 & 1 & 0 \\ 0 & 0 & 0 & 0 & 1 \\ 0 & 0 & 0 & 0 & 0 \\ 0 & 0 & 0 & 0 & 0 \end{bmatrix}$,

$\boldsymbol{A}^3 = \begin{bmatrix} 0 & 0 & 0 & 1 & 0 \\ 0 & 0 & 0 & 0 & 1 \\ 0 & 0 & 0 & 0 & 0 \\ 0 & 0 & 0 & 0 & 0 \\ 0 & 0 & 0 & 0 & 0 \end{bmatrix}$, $\boldsymbol{A}^4 = \begin{bmatrix} 0 & 0 & 0 & 0 & 1 \\ 0 & 0 & 0 & 0 & 0 \\ 0 & 0 & 0 & 0 & 0 \\ 0 & 0 & 0 & 0 & 0 \\ 0 & 0 & 0 & 0 & 0 \end{bmatrix}$, and $\boldsymbol{A}^5 = \boldsymbol{O}$. That is, the eigenvalues of $\boldsymbol{A}$ are all zero, and so

$$\boldsymbol{B} = \boldsymbol{I}_5 + \boldsymbol{A} + \boldsymbol{A}^2 + \boldsymbol{A}^3 + \boldsymbol{A}^4 + \boldsymbol{A}^5 = (\boldsymbol{I}_5 - \boldsymbol{A})^{-1}.$$

Hence,

$$\boldsymbol{B}^{-1} = \boldsymbol{I}_5 - \boldsymbol{A} = \begin{bmatrix} 1 & -1 & 0 & 0 & 0 \\ 0 & 1 & -1 & 0 & 0 \\ 0 & 0 & 1 & -1 & 0 \\ 0 & 0 & 0 & 1 & -1 \\ 0 & 0 & 0 & 0 & 1 \end{bmatrix}.$$

Note that if we let $\boldsymbol{x} = (x_1, x_2, x_3, x_4, x_5)'$, then

$$\boldsymbol{B}\boldsymbol{x} = \begin{pmatrix} x_1 + x_2 + x_3 + x_4 + x_5 \\ x_2 + x_3 + x_4 + x_5 \\ x_3 + x_4 + x_5 \\ x_4 + x_5 \\ x_5 \end{pmatrix} \text{ and } \boldsymbol{B}^{-1}\boldsymbol{x} = \begin{pmatrix} x_1 - x_2 \\ x_2 - x_3 \\ x_3 - x_4 \\ x_4 - x_5 \\ x_5 \end{pmatrix}.$$

This indicates that $\boldsymbol{B}\boldsymbol{x}$ is analogous to integration (summation) and $\boldsymbol{B}^{-1}\boldsymbol{x}$ is analogous to differentiation (taking differences).
10. Choose $\boldsymbol{M}$ as constituting a set of basis vectors for $\text{Sp}(\boldsymbol{A})$.
11. From $\boldsymbol{U}\boldsymbol{A}\boldsymbol{V}' = \tilde{\boldsymbol{U}}\boldsymbol{T}_1^{-1}\boldsymbol{A}(\boldsymbol{T}_2^{-1})'\tilde{\boldsymbol{V}}'$, we obtain $\tilde{\boldsymbol{A}} = \boldsymbol{T}_1^{-1}\boldsymbol{A}(\boldsymbol{T}_2^{-1})'$.
12. Assume $\boldsymbol{\beta} \notin \text{Sp}(X')$. Then $\boldsymbol{\beta}$ can be decomposed into $\boldsymbol{\beta} = \boldsymbol{\beta}_0 + \boldsymbol{\beta}_1$, where $\boldsymbol{\beta}_0 \in \text{Ker}(\boldsymbol{X})$ and $\boldsymbol{\beta}_1 \in \text{Sp}(\boldsymbol{X}')$. Hence, $\boldsymbol{X}\boldsymbol{\beta} = \boldsymbol{X}\boldsymbol{\beta}_0 + \boldsymbol{X}\boldsymbol{\beta}_1 = \boldsymbol{X}\boldsymbol{\beta}_1$. We may set $\boldsymbol{\beta} = \boldsymbol{\beta}_1$ without loss of generality.

7.2 Chapter 2

1. $\text{Sp}(\tilde{\boldsymbol{A}}) = \text{Sp}\begin{bmatrix} \boldsymbol{A}_1 & \boldsymbol{O} \\ \boldsymbol{O} & \boldsymbol{A}_2 \end{bmatrix} = \text{Sp}\begin{bmatrix} \boldsymbol{A}_1 \\ \boldsymbol{O} \end{bmatrix} \dot{\oplus} \text{Sp}\begin{bmatrix} \boldsymbol{O} \\ \boldsymbol{A}_2 \end{bmatrix} \supset \text{Sp}\begin{bmatrix} \boldsymbol{A}_1 \\ \boldsymbol{A}_2 \end{bmatrix}$. Hence $\boldsymbol{P}_{\tilde{A}}\boldsymbol{P}_A = \boldsymbol{P}_A$.
2. (Sufficiency) $\boldsymbol{P}_A\boldsymbol{P}_B = \boldsymbol{P}_B\boldsymbol{P}_A$ implies $\boldsymbol{P}_A(\boldsymbol{I} - \boldsymbol{P}_B) = (\boldsymbol{I} - \boldsymbol{P}_B)\boldsymbol{P}_A$. Hence, $\boldsymbol{P}_A\boldsymbol{P}_B$ and $\boldsymbol{P}_A(\boldsymbol{I} - \boldsymbol{P}_B)$ are the orthogonal projectors onto $\text{Sp}(\boldsymbol{A}) \cap \text{Sp}(\boldsymbol{B})$ and $\text{Sp}(\boldsymbol{A}) \cap \text{Sp}(\boldsymbol{B})^\perp$, respectively. Furthermore, since $\boldsymbol{P}_A\boldsymbol{P}_B\boldsymbol{P}_A(\boldsymbol{I} - \boldsymbol{P}_B) = \boldsymbol{P}_A(\boldsymbol{I} - \boldsymbol{P}_B)\boldsymbol{P}_A\boldsymbol{P}_B = \boldsymbol{O}$, the distributive law between subspaces holds, and

$$(\text{Sp}(\boldsymbol{A}) \cap \text{Sp}(\boldsymbol{B})) \dot{\oplus} (\text{Sp}(\boldsymbol{A}) \cap \text{Sp}(\boldsymbol{B})^\perp) = \text{Sp}(\boldsymbol{A}) \cap (\text{Sp}(\boldsymbol{B}) \dot{\oplus} \text{Sp}(\boldsymbol{B})^\perp) = \text{Sp}(\boldsymbol{A}).$$

(Necessity) $\boldsymbol{P}_A = \boldsymbol{P}_A\boldsymbol{P}_B + \boldsymbol{P}_A(\boldsymbol{I} - \boldsymbol{P}_B)$, and note that $\boldsymbol{P}_A\boldsymbol{P}_B = \boldsymbol{P}_B\boldsymbol{P}_A$ is the necessary and sufficient condition for $\boldsymbol{P}_A\boldsymbol{P}_B$ to be the orthogonal projector onto $\text{Sp}(\boldsymbol{A}) \cap \text{Sp}(\boldsymbol{B})$ and for $\boldsymbol{P}_A(\boldsymbol{I} - \boldsymbol{P}_B)$ to be the orthogonal projector onto $\text{Sp}(\boldsymbol{A}) \cap \text{Sp}(\boldsymbol{B})^\perp$.
3. (i) Let $\boldsymbol{x} \in (\text{Ker}(\boldsymbol{P}))^\perp$. Then $\boldsymbol{x}$ is decomposed as $\boldsymbol{x} = \boldsymbol{P}\boldsymbol{x} + (\boldsymbol{I} - \boldsymbol{P})\boldsymbol{x} = \boldsymbol{x}_1 + \boldsymbol{x}_2$, where $\boldsymbol{x}_2 \in \text{Ker}(\boldsymbol{P})$. Since $\boldsymbol{P}\boldsymbol{x} = \boldsymbol{x} - (\boldsymbol{I} - \boldsymbol{P})\boldsymbol{x}$ and $(\boldsymbol{x}, (\boldsymbol{I} - \boldsymbol{P})\boldsymbol{x}) = 0$, we obtain

$$||\boldsymbol{x}||^2 \geq ||\boldsymbol{P}\boldsymbol{x}||^2 = ||\boldsymbol{x}||^2 + ||(\boldsymbol{I} - \boldsymbol{P})\boldsymbol{x}||^2 \geq ||\boldsymbol{x}||^2.$$

Hence, $||\boldsymbol{P}\boldsymbol{x}||^2 = ||\boldsymbol{x}||^2 \Rightarrow (\boldsymbol{x} - \boldsymbol{P}\boldsymbol{x})'(\boldsymbol{x} - \boldsymbol{P}\boldsymbol{x}) = 0 \Rightarrow \boldsymbol{x} = \boldsymbol{P}\boldsymbol{x}$.

(ii) From (i) above, $\text{Ker}(\boldsymbol{P})^\perp \subset \text{Sp}(\boldsymbol{P})$. On the other hand, let $\boldsymbol{x} \in \text{Sp}(\boldsymbol{P})$, and let $\boldsymbol{x} = \boldsymbol{x}_1 + \boldsymbol{x}_2$, where $\boldsymbol{x}_1 \in \text{Ker}(\boldsymbol{P})^\perp$ and $\boldsymbol{x}_2 \in \text{Ker}(\boldsymbol{P})$. Then, $\boldsymbol{x} = \boldsymbol{P}\boldsymbol{x} = \boldsymbol{P}\boldsymbol{x}_1 + \boldsymbol{P}\boldsymbol{x}_2 = \boldsymbol{P}\boldsymbol{x}_1 = \boldsymbol{x}_1$. Hence,

$$\text{Sp}(\boldsymbol{P}) \subset \text{Ker}(\boldsymbol{P})^\perp \Rightarrow \text{Sp}(\boldsymbol{P}) = \text{Ker}(\boldsymbol{P})^\perp \Rightarrow \text{Sp}(\boldsymbol{P})^\perp = \text{Ker}(\boldsymbol{P}).$$

That is, $\boldsymbol{P}$ is the projector onto $\mathrm{Sp}(\boldsymbol{P})$ along $\mathrm{Sp}(\boldsymbol{P})$, and so $\boldsymbol{P}' = \boldsymbol{P}$. (This proof follows Yoshida (1981, p. 84).)

4. (i)

$$\begin{aligned} ||\boldsymbol{x}||^2 = ||\boldsymbol{P}_A\boldsymbol{x} + (\boldsymbol{I} - \boldsymbol{P}_A)\boldsymbol{x}||^2 \geq ||\boldsymbol{P}_A\boldsymbol{x}||^2 &= ||\boldsymbol{P}_1\boldsymbol{x} + \cdots + \boldsymbol{P}_m\boldsymbol{x}||^2 \\ &= ||\boldsymbol{P}_1\boldsymbol{x}||^2 + \cdots + ||\boldsymbol{P}_m\boldsymbol{x}||^2. \end{aligned}$$

The equality holds when $\boldsymbol{I} - \boldsymbol{P}_A = \boldsymbol{O} \Rightarrow \boldsymbol{P}_A = \boldsymbol{I}$, i.e., when $\mathrm{Sp}(\boldsymbol{A}) = E^n$.

(ii) Let $\boldsymbol{x}_j \in \mathrm{Sp}(\boldsymbol{A}_j)$. Then, $\boldsymbol{P}_j\boldsymbol{x}_j = \boldsymbol{x}_j$. From (2.84), $||\boldsymbol{P}_1\boldsymbol{x}_j||^2 + \cdots + ||\boldsymbol{P}_{j-1}\boldsymbol{x}_j||^2 + ||\boldsymbol{P}_{j+1}\boldsymbol{x}_j||^2 + \cdots + ||\boldsymbol{P}_m\boldsymbol{x}_j||^2 = 0 \Rightarrow ||\boldsymbol{P}_j\boldsymbol{x}_i|| = 0 \Rightarrow \boldsymbol{P}_j\boldsymbol{x}_i = \boldsymbol{0} \Rightarrow (\boldsymbol{P}_j)'\boldsymbol{x}_i = \boldsymbol{0}$ for $i \neq j$, which implies that $\mathrm{Sp}(\boldsymbol{A}_i)$ and $\mathrm{Sp}(\boldsymbol{A}_j)$ are orthogonal.

(iii) From $\boldsymbol{P}_j(\boldsymbol{P}_1 + \boldsymbol{P}_2 + \cdots \boldsymbol{P}_{j-1}) = \boldsymbol{0}$, we have $||\boldsymbol{P}_{(j)}\boldsymbol{x}||^2 = ||\boldsymbol{P}_{(j-1)}\boldsymbol{x} + \boldsymbol{P}_j\boldsymbol{x}||^2 = ||\boldsymbol{P}_{(j-1)}\boldsymbol{x}||^2 + ||\boldsymbol{P}_j\boldsymbol{x}||^2$, which implies $||\boldsymbol{P}_{(j)}\boldsymbol{x}|| \geq ||\boldsymbol{P}_{(j-1)}\boldsymbol{x}||$ for $j = 2, \cdots, m$.

5. (i) By Theorem 2.8, $\boldsymbol{P}_1 + \boldsymbol{P}_2$ is the projector onto $V_1 + V_2$ along $W_1 \cap W_2$. On the other hand, since $\boldsymbol{P}_3(\boldsymbol{P}_1 + \boldsymbol{P}_2) = \boldsymbol{O}$ and $(\boldsymbol{P}_1 + \boldsymbol{P}_2)\boldsymbol{P}_3 = \boldsymbol{O}$, $(\boldsymbol{P}_1 + \boldsymbol{P}_2) + \boldsymbol{P}_3$ is the projector onto $V_1 + V_2 + V_3$ along $W_1 \cap W_2 \cap W_3$, again by Theorem 2.8.

(ii) $\boldsymbol{P}_1\boldsymbol{P}_2$ is the projector onto $V_1 \cap V_2$ along $W_1 + W_2$. On the other hand, since $(\boldsymbol{P}_1\boldsymbol{P}_2)\boldsymbol{P}_3 = \boldsymbol{P}_3(\boldsymbol{P}_1\boldsymbol{P}_2)$, $\boldsymbol{P}_1\boldsymbol{P}_2\boldsymbol{P}_3$ is the projector onto $V_1 \cap V_2 \cap V_3$ along $W_1 + W_2 + W_3$. (Note, however, that $\boldsymbol{P}_1\boldsymbol{P}_2 = \boldsymbol{P}_2\boldsymbol{P}_1$, $\boldsymbol{P}_1\boldsymbol{P}_3 = \boldsymbol{P}_3\boldsymbol{P}_1$, or $\boldsymbol{P}_2\boldsymbol{P}_3 = \boldsymbol{P}_3\boldsymbol{P}_2$ may not hold even if $\boldsymbol{P}_1\boldsymbol{P}_2\boldsymbol{P}_3$ is a projector.)

(iii) $\boldsymbol{I} - \boldsymbol{P}_{1+2+3}$ is the projector onto $W_1 \cap W_2 \cap W_3$ along $V_1 + V_2 + V_3$. On the other hand, since $\boldsymbol{I} - \boldsymbol{P}_j$ $(j = 1, 2, 3)$ is the projector onto W_j along V_j, we obtain $\boldsymbol{I} - \boldsymbol{P}_{1+2+3} = (\boldsymbol{I} - \boldsymbol{P}_1)(\boldsymbol{I} - \boldsymbol{P}_2)(\boldsymbol{I} - \boldsymbol{P}_3)$ from (ii) above, leading to the equation to be shown.

6. $\boldsymbol{Q}_{[A,B]} = \boldsymbol{I} - \boldsymbol{P}_A - \boldsymbol{P}_{Q_AB} = \boldsymbol{Q}_A - \boldsymbol{P}_{Q_AB} = \boldsymbol{Q}_A - Q_A\boldsymbol{P}_{Q_AB} = \boldsymbol{Q}_A\boldsymbol{Q}_{Q_AB}$.

7. (a) It is clear that $\boldsymbol{X}\boldsymbol{A}$ and $\boldsymbol{X}(\boldsymbol{X}'\boldsymbol{X})^{-1}\boldsymbol{B}$ are orthogonal to each other (i.e., $\boldsymbol{A}'\boldsymbol{X}'\boldsymbol{X}(\boldsymbol{X}'\boldsymbol{X})^{-1}\boldsymbol{B} = \boldsymbol{O}$) and that they jointly span $\mathrm{Sp}(\boldsymbol{X})$. (Note that when $\boldsymbol{X}'\boldsymbol{X}$ is singular, $(\boldsymbol{X}'\boldsymbol{X})^{-1}$ can be replaced by a generalized inverse of $\boldsymbol{X}'\boldsymbol{X}$, provided that $\boldsymbol{B} \in \mathrm{Sp}(\boldsymbol{X}')$. See Takane and Yanai (1999) for more details.)

(b) Set $\boldsymbol{A}$ and $\boldsymbol{B}$ equal to selection matrices such that $\boldsymbol{X}\boldsymbol{A} = \boldsymbol{X}_1$ and $\boldsymbol{X}\boldsymbol{B} = \boldsymbol{X}_2$. Then, $\boldsymbol{X}(\boldsymbol{X}'\boldsymbol{X})^{-1}\boldsymbol{B} = \boldsymbol{Q}_{X_2}\boldsymbol{X}_1$.

8. (a) Note first that (i) $(\boldsymbol{P}_1\boldsymbol{P}_2)^2 = \boldsymbol{P}_1\boldsymbol{P}_2$ is equivalent to (ii) $\boldsymbol{P}_1\boldsymbol{Q}_2\boldsymbol{P}_1\boldsymbol{P}_2 = \boldsymbol{O}$, (iii) $\boldsymbol{P}_1\boldsymbol{Q}_2\boldsymbol{Q}_1\boldsymbol{P}_2 = \boldsymbol{O}$, and (iv) $\boldsymbol{P}_1\boldsymbol{P}_2\boldsymbol{Q}_1\boldsymbol{P}_2 = \boldsymbol{O}$, where $\boldsymbol{Q}_1 = \boldsymbol{I} - \boldsymbol{P}_1$ and $\boldsymbol{Q}_2 = \boldsymbol{I} - P_2$. The (ii) indicates that $(\boldsymbol{P}_1\boldsymbol{P}_2)^2 = \boldsymbol{P}_1\boldsymbol{P}_2$ holds if and only if $\mathrm{Sp}(\boldsymbol{Q}_2\boldsymbol{P}_1\boldsymbol{P}_2) \subset W_1 \cap W_2$.

($\Leftarrow$) That $V_{12} \in V_2 \oplus (W_1 \cap W_2)$ implies $\mathrm{Sp}(\boldsymbol{Q}_2\boldsymbol{P}_1\boldsymbol{P}_2) \in W_1 \cap W_2$ is trivial. (Obviously, it is not in V_2.)

($\Rightarrow$) Conversely, assume that $\mathrm{Sp}(\boldsymbol{Q}_2\boldsymbol{P}_1\boldsymbol{P}_2) \in W_1 \cap W_2$, and let $\boldsymbol{y} \in V_{12}$. Then, $\boldsymbol{y} = \boldsymbol{P}_1\boldsymbol{P}_2\boldsymbol{y} = \boldsymbol{P}_2\boldsymbol{P}_1\boldsymbol{P}_2\boldsymbol{y} + \boldsymbol{Q}_2\boldsymbol{P}_1\boldsymbol{P}_2\boldsymbol{y} = \boldsymbol{P}_2\boldsymbol{y} + \boldsymbol{Q}_2\boldsymbol{P}_1\boldsymbol{P}_2\boldsymbol{y} \in V_2 \oplus (W_1 \cap W_2)$. (See Groß and Trenkler (1998).)

(b) Let $\boldsymbol{y} \in V_2$. Then, $\boldsymbol{P}_2\boldsymbol{y} = \boldsymbol{y}$ and $\boldsymbol{y} = \boldsymbol{P}_1\boldsymbol{y} + \boldsymbol{P}_2\boldsymbol{Q}_1\boldsymbol{y} + \boldsymbol{Q}_2\boldsymbol{Q}_1\boldsymbol{y} = \boldsymbol{P}_1\boldsymbol{y} + \boldsymbol{P}_2\boldsymbol{Q}_1\boldsymbol{P}_2\boldsymbol{y} + \boldsymbol{Q}_2\boldsymbol{Q}_1\boldsymbol{P}_2\boldsymbol{y}$. However, $\boldsymbol{P}_1\boldsymbol{y} \in V_1$, $\boldsymbol{P}_2\boldsymbol{Q}_1\boldsymbol{P}_2\boldsymbol{y} \in W_1 \cap V_2$ because of (iv) in (a), and $\boldsymbol{Q}_2\boldsymbol{Q}_1\boldsymbol{P}_2\boldsymbol{y} \in W_1 \cap W_2$ because of (iii) in (a), implying that $V_2 \in V_1 \oplus (W_1 \cap V_2) \oplus (W_1 \cap W_2)$.

Conversely, let $\boldsymbol{y} \in E^n$. Then, $\boldsymbol{P}_2\boldsymbol{y} \in V_2$. Let $\boldsymbol{P}_2\boldsymbol{y} = \boldsymbol{y}_1 + \boldsymbol{y}_2 + \boldsymbol{y}_3$, where $\boldsymbol{y}_1 \in V_1$, $\boldsymbol{y}_2 \in W_1 \cap V_2$, and $\boldsymbol{y}_3 \in W_1 \cap W_2$. We have $(\boldsymbol{P}_1\boldsymbol{P}_2\boldsymbol{P}_1)\boldsymbol{P}_2\boldsymbol{y} = \boldsymbol{P}_1\boldsymbol{P}_2\boldsymbol{y}_1 = \boldsymbol{P}_1\boldsymbol{P}_2(\boldsymbol{y}_1+\boldsymbol{y}_2+\boldsymbol{y}_3) = \boldsymbol{P}_1\boldsymbol{P}_2\boldsymbol{y}$, implying (i) in (a). (See Takane and Yanai (1999).)

9. (1) → (2): Pre- and postmultiplying both sides of (1) by $\boldsymbol{A}$ and $\boldsymbol{B}$, respectively, yields (2).

(2) → (3): Pre- and postmultiplying both sides of (2) by $\boldsymbol{A}(\boldsymbol{A}'\boldsymbol{A})^-$ and $(\boldsymbol{B}'\boldsymbol{B})^- \times \boldsymbol{B}'$, respectively, yields (3).

(3) → (2): Pre- and postmultiplying both sides of (3) by $\boldsymbol{A}'$ and $\boldsymbol{B}$, respectively, yields (2).

(1) → (4): Observe that (1) implies that $\boldsymbol{P}_A\boldsymbol{P}_B$ is the orthogonal projector onto $\mathrm{Sp}(\boldsymbol{A}) \cap \mathrm{Sp}(\boldsymbol{B})$, and $\boldsymbol{Q}_A\boldsymbol{Q}_B = (\boldsymbol{I}-\boldsymbol{P}_A)(\boldsymbol{I}-\boldsymbol{P}_B) = \boldsymbol{I}-\boldsymbol{P}_A-\boldsymbol{P}_B+\boldsymbol{P}_A\boldsymbol{P}_B = \boldsymbol{I}-\boldsymbol{P}_A-\boldsymbol{P}_B+\boldsymbol{P}_B\boldsymbol{P}_A = \boldsymbol{Q}_B\boldsymbol{Q}_A$ is the orthogonal projector onto $\mathrm{Sp}(\boldsymbol{A})^\perp \cap \mathrm{Sp}(\boldsymbol{B})^\perp = (\mathrm{Sp}(\boldsymbol{A}) \cup \mathrm{Sp}(\boldsymbol{B}))^\perp$, showing that $\boldsymbol{I} - \boldsymbol{P}_{[A,B]} = (\boldsymbol{I}-\boldsymbol{P}_A)(\boldsymbol{I}-\boldsymbol{P}_B) = \boldsymbol{I}-\boldsymbol{P}_A-\boldsymbol{P}_B+\boldsymbol{P}_A\boldsymbol{P}_B$, from which (4) follows immediately.

(4) → (1): Since $\boldsymbol{P}_A$, $\boldsymbol{P}_B$, and $\boldsymbol{P}_{[A,B]}$ are all symmetric, (1) follows immediately.

(3) → (5): Pre- and postmultiplying (3) by $\boldsymbol{B}'$ and $\boldsymbol{B}$, respectively, yields $\boldsymbol{B}'\boldsymbol{P}_A\boldsymbol{B} = \boldsymbol{B}'\boldsymbol{P}_A\boldsymbol{P}_B\boldsymbol{P}_A\boldsymbol{B}$. Substituting $\boldsymbol{P}_A = \boldsymbol{I} - \boldsymbol{Q}_A$ and $\boldsymbol{P}_B = \boldsymbol{I} - \boldsymbol{Q}_B$ into this yields $\boldsymbol{B}'\boldsymbol{Q}_A\boldsymbol{Q}_B\boldsymbol{Q}_A\boldsymbol{B} = \boldsymbol{O}$, which implies $\boldsymbol{Q}_B\boldsymbol{Q}_A\boldsymbol{B} = \boldsymbol{O}$, which in turn implies $\boldsymbol{A}'\boldsymbol{Q}_B\boldsymbol{Q}_A\boldsymbol{B} = \boldsymbol{O}$.

(5) → (6): $0 = \mathrm{rank}(\boldsymbol{A}'\boldsymbol{Q}_B\boldsymbol{Q}_A\boldsymbol{B}) = \mathrm{rank}(\boldsymbol{Q}_B\boldsymbol{Q}_A\boldsymbol{B}) = \mathrm{rank}(\boldsymbol{Q}_B\boldsymbol{P}_A\boldsymbol{B}) = \mathrm{rank}([\boldsymbol{B},\boldsymbol{P}_A\boldsymbol{B}]) - \mathrm{rank}(\boldsymbol{B}) = \mathrm{rank}(\boldsymbol{P}_A\boldsymbol{B}) + \mathrm{rank}(\boldsymbol{Q}_{P_AB}\boldsymbol{B}) - \mathrm{rank}(\boldsymbol{B}) = \mathrm{rank}(\boldsymbol{A}'\boldsymbol{B}) + \mathrm{rank}(\boldsymbol{Q}_A\boldsymbol{B}) - \mathrm{rank}(\boldsymbol{B})$, establishing (6). Note that we used $\mathrm{rank}([\boldsymbol{X},\boldsymbol{Y}]) = \mathrm{rank}(\boldsymbol{X}) + \mathrm{rank}(\boldsymbol{Q}_X\boldsymbol{Y})$ to establish the fourth and fifth equalities, and that we used $\boldsymbol{Q}_{P_AB}\boldsymbol{B} = (\boldsymbol{I}-\boldsymbol{P}_{P_AB})\boldsymbol{B} = \boldsymbol{B} - \boldsymbol{P}_A\boldsymbol{B}(\boldsymbol{B}'\boldsymbol{P}_A\boldsymbol{B})^-\boldsymbol{B}'\boldsymbol{P}_A\boldsymbol{B} = \boldsymbol{Q}_A\boldsymbol{B}$ to establish the sixth equality.

(6) → (1): We first note that (6) is equivalent to $\mathrm{rank}(\boldsymbol{A}'\boldsymbol{B}) = \mathrm{rank}(\boldsymbol{A}) + \mathrm{rank}(\boldsymbol{B}) - \mathrm{rank}([\boldsymbol{A},\boldsymbol{B}])$, which implies $0 = \mathrm{rank}(\boldsymbol{A}'\boldsymbol{B}) - \mathrm{rank}(\boldsymbol{A}) - \mathrm{rank}(\boldsymbol{B}) + \mathrm{rank}([\boldsymbol{A},\boldsymbol{B}])$, which in turn implies (5). (The second equality is due to Baksalary and Styan (1990).) Furthermore, (5) implies (2) since $\boldsymbol{O} = \boldsymbol{A}'\boldsymbol{Q}_B\boldsymbol{Q}_A\boldsymbol{B} = \boldsymbol{A}'\boldsymbol{P}_B\boldsymbol{P}_A\boldsymbol{B} - \boldsymbol{A}'\boldsymbol{B}$. Combined with the previous result that (2) implies (3), we know that (5) also implies (3). That is, $\boldsymbol{P}_A\boldsymbol{P}_B$ and $\boldsymbol{P}_B\boldsymbol{P}_A$ are both idempotent. Now consider $\mathrm{tr}((\boldsymbol{P}_A\boldsymbol{P}_B - \boldsymbol{P}_B\boldsymbol{P}_A)'(\boldsymbol{P}_A\boldsymbol{P}_B - \boldsymbol{P}_A\boldsymbol{P}_B))$, which is equal to 0, thus implying $\boldsymbol{P}_A\boldsymbol{P}_B = \boldsymbol{P}_B\boldsymbol{P}_A$.

There are many other equivalent conditions for the commutativity of two orthogonal projectors. See Baksalary (1987) for some of them.

7.3 Chapter 3

1. (a) $(\boldsymbol{A}_{mr}^-)' = \frac{1}{12}\begin{bmatrix} -2 & 1 & 4 \\ 4 & 1 & -2 \end{bmatrix}$. (Use $\boldsymbol{A}_{mr}^- = (\boldsymbol{A}\boldsymbol{A}')^-\boldsymbol{A}$.)

(b) $\boldsymbol{A}_{\ell r}^- = \frac{1}{11}\begin{bmatrix} -4 & 7 & 1 \\ 7 & -4 & 1 \end{bmatrix}$. (Use $\boldsymbol{A}_{\ell r}^- = (\boldsymbol{A}'\boldsymbol{A})^-\boldsymbol{A}'$.)

(c) $A^+ = \frac{1}{9}\begin{bmatrix} 2 & -1 & -1 \\ -1 & 2 & -1 \\ -1 & -1 & 2 \end{bmatrix}$.

2. ($\Leftarrow$): From $P^2 = P$, we have $E^n = \text{Sp}(P) \oplus \text{Sp}(I-P)$. We also have $\text{Ker}(P) = \text{Sp}(I-P)$ and $\text{Ker}(I-P) = \text{Sp}(P)$. Hence, $E^n = \text{Ker}(P) \oplus \text{Ker}(I-P)$.

($\Rightarrow$): Let $\text{rank}(P) = r$. Then, $\dim(\text{Ker}(P)) = n - r$, and $\dim(\text{Ker}(I-P)) = r$. Let $x \in \text{Ker}(I-P)$. Then, $(I-P)x = 0 \Rightarrow x = Px$. Hence, $\text{Sp}(P) \supset \text{Ker}(I-P)$. Also, $\dim(\text{Sp}(P)) = \dim(\text{Ker}(I-P)) = r$, which implies $\text{Sp}(P) = \text{Ker}(I-P)$, and so $(I-P)P = O \Rightarrow P^2 = P$.

3. (i) Since $(I_m - BA)(I_m - A^-A) = I_m - A^-A$, $\text{Ker}(A) = \text{Sp}(I_m - A^-A) = \text{Sp}\{(I_m - BA)(I_m - A^-A)\}$. Also, since $m = \text{rank}(A) + \dim(\text{Ker}(A))$, $\text{rank}(I_m - BA) = \dim(\text{Ker}(A)) = \text{rank}(I_m - A^-A)$. Hence, from $\text{Sp}(I_m - A^-A) = \text{Sp}\{(I_m - BA)(I_m - A^-A)\} \subset \text{Sp}(I_m - BA)$, we have $\text{Sp}(I_m - BA) = \text{Sp}(I_m - A^-A) \Rightarrow I_m - BA = (I_m - A^-A)W$. Premultiplying both sides by A, we obtain $A - ABA = O \Rightarrow A = ABA$, which indicates that $B = A^-$.

(Another proof) $\text{rank}(BA) \le \text{rank}(A) \Rightarrow \text{rank}(I_m - BA) \le m - \text{rank}(BA)$. Also, $\text{rank}(I_m - BA) + \text{rank}(BA) \ge m \Rightarrow \text{rank}(I_m - BA) + \text{rank}(BA) = m \Rightarrow \text{rank}(BA) = \text{rank}(A) \Rightarrow (BA)^2 = BA$. We then use (ii) below.

(ii) From $\text{rank}(BA) = \text{rank}(A)$, we have $\text{Sp}(A') = \text{Sp}(A'B')$. Hence, for some K we have $A = KBA$. Premultiplying $(BA)^2 = BABA = BA$ by K, we obtain $KBABA = KBA$, from which it follows that $ABA = A$.

(iii) From $\text{rank}(AB) = \text{rank}(A)$, we have $\text{Sp}(AB) = \text{Sp}(A)$. Hence, for some L, $A = ABL$. Postmultiplying both sides of $(AB)^2 = AB$ by L, we obtain $ABABL = ABL$, from which we obtain $ABA = A$.

4. (i) ($\Rightarrow$): From $\text{rank}(AB) = \text{rank}(A)$, $A = ABK$ for some K. Hence, $AB(AB)^-A = AB(AB)^-ABK = ABK = A$, which shows $B(AB)^- \in \{A^-\}$.

($\Leftarrow$): From $B(AB)^- \in \{A^-\}$, $AB(AB)^-A = A$, and $\text{rank}(AB(AB)^-A) \le \text{rank}(AB)$. On the other hand, $\text{rank}(AB(AB)^-A) \ge \text{rank}(AB(AB)^-AB) = \text{rank}(AB)$. Thus, $\text{rank}(AB(AB)^-A) = \text{rank}(AB)$.

(ii) ($\Rightarrow$): $\text{rank}(A) = \text{rank}(CAD) = \text{rank}\{(CAD)(CAD)^-\} = \text{rank}(AD(CA \times D)^-C)$. Hence, $AD(CAD)^-C = AK$ for some K, and so $AD(CAD)^-CAD \times (CAD)^-C = AD(CAD)^-CAK = AD(CAD)^-C$, from which it follows that $D(CAD)^-C \in \{A^-\}$. Finally, the given equation is obtained by noting $(CAD)(CAD)^-C = C \Rightarrow CAK = C$.

($\Leftarrow$): $\text{rank}(AA^-) = \text{rank}(AD(CAD)^-C) = \text{rank}(A)$. Let $H = AD(CAD)^- C$. Then, $H^2 = AD(CAD)^-CAD(CAD)^-C = AD(CAD)^-C = H$, which implies $\text{rank}(H) = \text{tr}(H)$. Hence, $\text{rank}(AD(CAD)^-C) = \text{tr}(AD(CAD)^-C) = \text{tr}(CAD(CAD)^-) = \text{rank}(CAD(CAD)^-) = \text{rank}(CAD)$, that is, $\text{rank}(A) = \text{rank}(CAD)$.

5. (i) (Necessity) $AB(B^-A^-)AB = AB$. Premultiplying and postmultiplying both sides by A^- and B^-, respectively, leads to $(A^-ABB^-)^2 = A^-ABB^-$.

(Sufficiency) Pre- and postmultiply both sides of $A^-ABB^-A^-ABB^- = A^-ABB^-$ by A and B, respectively.

(ii) $(A_m^-ABB')' = BB'A_m^-A = A_m^-ABB'$. That is, A_m^-A and BB' are commutative. Hence, $ABB_m^-A_m^-AB = ABB_m^-A_m^-ABB_m^-B = ABB_m^-A_m^-ABB' \times$

$(B_m^-)' = ABB_m^-BB'A_m^-A(B_m^-)' = ABB'A_m^-A(B_m^-)' = AA_m^-ABB'(B_m^-)' = AB$, and so (1) $B_m^-A_m^- \in \{(AB)^-\}$. Next, $(B_m^-A_m^-AB)' = B'A_m^-A(B_m^-)' = B_m^-BB'A_m^-A(B_m^-)' = B_m^-A_m^-ABB'(B_m^-)' = B_m^-A_m^-AB(B_m^-B)' = B_m^-A_m^-AB$ $B_m^-B = B_m^-A_m^-AB$, so that (2) $B_m^-A_m^-AB$ is symmetric. Combining (1) and (2) and considering the definition of a minimum norm g-inverse, we have $\{B_m^-A_m^-\} = \{(AB)_m^-\}$.

(iii) When $P_AP_B = P_BP_A$, $Q_AP_B = P_BQ_A$. In this case, $(Q_AB)'Q_ABB_\ell^- = B'Q_AP_B = B'P_BQ_A = B'Q_A$, and so $B_\ell^- \in \{(Q_AB)_\ell^-\}$. Hence, $(Q_AB)(Q_A\times B)_\ell^- = Q_AP_B = P_B - P_AP_B$.

6. (i) → (ii) From $A^2 = AA^-$, we have $\text{rank}(A^2) = \text{rank}(AA^-) = \text{rank}(A)$. Furthermore, $A^2 = AA^- \Rightarrow A^4 = (AA^-)^2 = AA^- = A^2$.

(ii) → (iii) From $\text{rank}(A) = \text{rank}(A^2)$, we have $A = A^2D$ for some D. Hence, $A = A^2D = A^4D = A^2(A^2D) = A^3$.

(iii) → (i) From $AAA = A$, $A \in \{A^-\}$. (The matrix A having this property is called a tripotent matrix, whose eigenvalues are either −1, 0, or 1. See Rao and Mitra (1971) for details.)

7. (i) Since $A = [A, B]\begin{bmatrix} I \\ O \end{bmatrix}$, $[A, B][A, B]^-A = [A, B][A, B]^-[A, B]\begin{bmatrix} I \\ O \end{bmatrix} = A$.

(ii) $AA' + BB' = FF'$, where $F = [A, B]$. Furthermore, since $A = [A, B]\times \begin{bmatrix} I \\ O \end{bmatrix} = F\begin{bmatrix} I \\ O \end{bmatrix}$, $(AA' + BB')(AA' + BB')^-A = FF'(FF')^-F\begin{bmatrix} I \\ O \end{bmatrix} = F\begin{bmatrix} I \\ O \end{bmatrix} = A$.

8. From $V = W_1A$, we have $V = VA^-A$ and from $U = AW_2$, we have $U = AA^-U$. It then follows that

$$\begin{aligned}
&(A + UV)\{A^- - A^-U(I + VA^-U)^-VA^-\}(A + UV) \\
&\quad = (A + UV)A^-(A + UV) - (AA^-U + UVA^-U)(I + VA^-U) \\
&\qquad\qquad (VA^-A + VA^-UV) \\
&\quad = A + 2UV + UVA^-UV - U(I + VA^-U)V \\
&\quad = A + UV.
\end{aligned}$$

9. $A = B^{-1}\begin{bmatrix} I_r & O \\ O & O \end{bmatrix}C^{-1}$, and $AGA = B^{-1}\begin{bmatrix} I_r & O \\ O & O \end{bmatrix}C^{-1}C\begin{bmatrix} I_r & O \\ O & E \end{bmatrix}B\times B^{-1}\begin{bmatrix} I_r & O \\ O & O \end{bmatrix}C^{-1} = B^{-1}\begin{bmatrix} I_r & O \\ O & O \end{bmatrix}C^{-1}$. Hence, $G \in \{A^-\}$. It is clear that $\text{rank}(G) = r + \text{rank}(E)$.

10. Let $Q_{A'}a$ denote an arbitrary vector in $\text{Sp}(Q_{A'}) = \text{Sp}(A')^\perp$. The vector $Q_{A'}a$ that minimizes $||x - Q_{A'}a||^2$ is given by the orthogonal projection of x onto $\text{Sp}(A')^\perp$, namely $Q_{A'}x$. In this case, the minimum attained is given by $||x - Q_{A'}x||^2 = ||(I - Q_{A'})x||^2 = ||P_{A'}x||^2 = x'P_{A'}x$. (This is equivalent to obtaining the minimum of $x'x$ subject to $Ax = b$, that is, obtaining a minimum norm g-inverse as a least squares g-inverse of $Q_{A'}$.)

11. (i) $\boldsymbol{ABA} = \boldsymbol{AA}_m^-\boldsymbol{AA}_\ell^-\boldsymbol{A} = \boldsymbol{A}$.
(ii) $\boldsymbol{BAB} = \boldsymbol{A}_m^-\boldsymbol{AA}_\ell^-\boldsymbol{AA}_m^-\boldsymbol{AA}_\ell^- = \boldsymbol{A}_m^-\boldsymbol{AA}_\ell^- = \boldsymbol{B}$.
(iii) $(\boldsymbol{BA})' = (\boldsymbol{A}_m^-\boldsymbol{AA}_\ell^-\boldsymbol{A})' = (\boldsymbol{A}_m^-\boldsymbol{A})' = \boldsymbol{A}_m^-\boldsymbol{A} = \boldsymbol{BA}$.
(iv) $(\boldsymbol{AB})' = (\boldsymbol{AA}_m^-\boldsymbol{AA}_\ell^-)' = (\boldsymbol{AA}_\ell^-)' = \boldsymbol{AA}_\ell^- = \boldsymbol{AB}$.
By (i) through (iv), $\boldsymbol{B} = \boldsymbol{A}_m^-\boldsymbol{AA}_\ell^-$ is the Moore-Penrose inverse of $\boldsymbol{A}$.
12. Let $\boldsymbol{P}_{1+2}$ denote the orthogonal projector onto $V_1 + V_2$. Since $V_1 + V_2 \supset V_2$,

$$(1)\ \ \boldsymbol{P}_{1+2}\boldsymbol{P}_2 = \boldsymbol{P}_2 = \boldsymbol{P}_2\boldsymbol{P}_{1+2}.$$

On the other hand, $\boldsymbol{P}_{1+2} = [\boldsymbol{P}_1, \boldsymbol{P}_2]\begin{bmatrix}\boldsymbol{P}_1\\ \boldsymbol{P}_2\end{bmatrix}\left[[\boldsymbol{P}_1, \boldsymbol{P}_2]\begin{bmatrix}\boldsymbol{P}_1\\ \boldsymbol{P}_2\end{bmatrix}\right]^+ = (\boldsymbol{P}_1+\boldsymbol{P}_2)(\boldsymbol{P}_1 + \boldsymbol{P}_2)^+$.

Similarly, we obtain

$$\boldsymbol{P}_{1+2} = (\boldsymbol{P}_1 + \boldsymbol{P}_2)^+(\boldsymbol{P}_1 + \boldsymbol{P}_2),$$

and so, by substituting this into (1),

$$(\boldsymbol{P}_1 + \boldsymbol{P}_2)(\boldsymbol{P}_1 + \boldsymbol{P}_2)^+\boldsymbol{P}_2 = \boldsymbol{P}_2 = \boldsymbol{P}_2(\boldsymbol{P}_1 + \boldsymbol{P}_2)^+(\boldsymbol{P}_1 + \boldsymbol{P}_2),$$

by which we have $2\boldsymbol{P}_1(\boldsymbol{P}_1 + \boldsymbol{P}_2)^+\boldsymbol{P}_2 = 2\boldsymbol{P}_2(\boldsymbol{P}_1 + \boldsymbol{P}_2)^+\boldsymbol{P}_1$ (which is set to $\boldsymbol{H}$). Clearly, $\text{Sp}(\boldsymbol{H}) \subset V_1 \cap V_2$. Hence,

$$\begin{aligned}\boldsymbol{H} = \boldsymbol{P}_{1\cap 2}\boldsymbol{H} &= \boldsymbol{P}_{1\cap 2}(\boldsymbol{P}_1(\boldsymbol{P}_1 + \boldsymbol{P}_2)^+\boldsymbol{P}_2 + \boldsymbol{P}_2(\boldsymbol{P}_1 + \boldsymbol{P}_2)^+\boldsymbol{P}_1)\\ &= \boldsymbol{P}_{1\cap 2}(\boldsymbol{P}_1 + \boldsymbol{P}_2)^+(\boldsymbol{P}_1 + \boldsymbol{P}_2) = \boldsymbol{P}_{1\cap 2}\boldsymbol{P}_{1+2} = \boldsymbol{P}_{1\cap 2}.\end{aligned}$$

Therefore,

$$\boldsymbol{P}_{1\cap 2} = 2\boldsymbol{P}_1(\boldsymbol{P}_1 + \boldsymbol{P}_2)^+\boldsymbol{P}_2 = 2\boldsymbol{P}_2(\boldsymbol{P}_1 + \boldsymbol{P}_2)^+\boldsymbol{P}_1.$$

(This proof is due to Ben-Israel and Greville (1974).)
13. (i): Trivial.

(ii): Let $\boldsymbol{v} \in V$ belong to both M and $\text{Ker}(\boldsymbol{A})$. It follows that $\boldsymbol{Ax} = \boldsymbol{0}$, and $\boldsymbol{x} = (\boldsymbol{G} - \boldsymbol{N})\boldsymbol{y}$ for some $\boldsymbol{y}$. Then, $\boldsymbol{A}(\boldsymbol{G} - \boldsymbol{N})\boldsymbol{y} = \boldsymbol{AGAGy} = \boldsymbol{AGy} = \boldsymbol{0}$. Premultiplying both sides by $\boldsymbol{G}'$, we obtain $\boldsymbol{0} = \boldsymbol{GAGy} = (\boldsymbol{G} - \boldsymbol{N})\boldsymbol{y} = \boldsymbol{x}$, indicating $M \cap \text{Ker}(\boldsymbol{A}) = \{\boldsymbol{0}\}$. Let $\boldsymbol{x} \in V$. It follows that $\boldsymbol{x} = \boldsymbol{GAx} + (\boldsymbol{I} - \boldsymbol{GA})\boldsymbol{x}$, where $(\boldsymbol{I} - \boldsymbol{GA})\boldsymbol{x} \in \text{Ker}(\boldsymbol{A})$, since $\boldsymbol{A}(\boldsymbol{I} - \boldsymbol{GA})\boldsymbol{x} = \boldsymbol{0}$ and $\boldsymbol{GAx} = (\boldsymbol{G} - \boldsymbol{A})\boldsymbol{x} \in \text{Sp}(\boldsymbol{G} - \boldsymbol{N})$. Hence, $M \oplus \text{Ker}(\boldsymbol{A}) = V$.

(iii): This can be proven in a manner similar to (2). Note that $\boldsymbol{G}$ satisfying (1) $\boldsymbol{N} = \boldsymbol{G} - \boldsymbol{GAG}$, (2) $M = \text{Sp}(\boldsymbol{G} - \boldsymbol{N})$, and (3) $L = \text{Ker}(\boldsymbol{G} - \boldsymbol{N})$ exists and is called the LMN-inverse or the Rao-Yanai inverse (Rao and Yanai, 1985).

The proofs given above are due to Rao and Rao (1998).
14. We first show a lemma by Mitra (1968; Theorem 2.1).

Lemma *Let $\boldsymbol{A}$, $\boldsymbol{M}$, and $\boldsymbol{B}$ be as introduced in Question 14. Then the following two statements are equivalent:*
(i) $\boldsymbol{AGA} = \boldsymbol{A}$, *where* $\boldsymbol{G} = \boldsymbol{L}(\boldsymbol{M}'\boldsymbol{AL})^-\boldsymbol{M}'$.
(ii) $\text{rank}(\boldsymbol{M}'\boldsymbol{AL}) = \text{rank}(\boldsymbol{A})$.

Proof. (i) $\Rightarrow$ (ii): $\boldsymbol{A} = \boldsymbol{AGA} = \boldsymbol{AGAGA}$. Hence, $\text{rank}(\boldsymbol{A}) = \text{rank}(\boldsymbol{AGAGA}) = \text{rank}(\boldsymbol{AL}(\boldsymbol{M}'\boldsymbol{AL})^{-}\boldsymbol{M}'\boldsymbol{AL}(\boldsymbol{M}'\boldsymbol{AL})^{-}\boldsymbol{M}'\boldsymbol{A})$, which implies $\text{rank}(\boldsymbol{M}'\boldsymbol{AL}) \geq \text{rank}(\boldsymbol{A})$. Trivially, $\text{rank}(\boldsymbol{A}) \geq \text{rank}(\boldsymbol{M}'\boldsymbol{AL})$, and so $\text{rank}(\boldsymbol{A}) = \text{rank}(\boldsymbol{M}'\boldsymbol{AL})$.

(ii) $\Rightarrow$ (i): Condition (ii) implies that $\text{rank}(\boldsymbol{A}) = \text{rank}(\boldsymbol{M}'\boldsymbol{A}) = \text{rank}(\boldsymbol{AL}) = \text{rank}(\boldsymbol{M}'\boldsymbol{AL})$. This in turn implies that $\boldsymbol{A}$ can be expressed as $\boldsymbol{A} = \boldsymbol{BM}'\boldsymbol{A} = \boldsymbol{ALC}$ for some $\boldsymbol{B}$ and $\boldsymbol{C}$. Thus, $\boldsymbol{AL}(\boldsymbol{M}'\boldsymbol{AL})^{-}\boldsymbol{M}'\boldsymbol{A} = \boldsymbol{BM}'\boldsymbol{AL}(\boldsymbol{M}'\boldsymbol{AL})^{-}\boldsymbol{M}'\boldsymbol{AL} \times \boldsymbol{C} = \boldsymbol{BM}'\boldsymbol{ALC} = \boldsymbol{A}$. Q.E.D.

We now prove the equivalence of the three conditions in Question 14.

(i) $\Leftrightarrow$ (ii): This follows from Mitra's lemma above by setting $\boldsymbol{L} = \boldsymbol{I}$.

(ii) $\Rightarrow$ (iii): Let $\boldsymbol{x} \in \text{Sp}(\boldsymbol{A}) \oplus \text{Ker}(\boldsymbol{H})$. Then, $\boldsymbol{Hx} = \boldsymbol{0}$ and $\boldsymbol{x} = \boldsymbol{Az}$ for some $\boldsymbol{z}$. Hence, $\boldsymbol{0} = \boldsymbol{HAz} = \boldsymbol{Az} = \boldsymbol{x}$, which implies $\text{Sp}(\boldsymbol{A})$ and $\text{Ker}(\boldsymbol{H})$ are disjoint. Condition (iii) immediately follows since $\text{rank}(\boldsymbol{H}) = \text{rank}(\boldsymbol{A})$.

(iii) $\Rightarrow$ (ii): It can be readily verified that $\boldsymbol{H}^2\boldsymbol{A} = \boldsymbol{HA}$. This implies $\boldsymbol{H}(\boldsymbol{I} - \boldsymbol{H})\boldsymbol{A} = \boldsymbol{O}$, which in turn implies $\text{Sp}((\boldsymbol{I} - \boldsymbol{H})\boldsymbol{A}) \subset \text{Ker}(\boldsymbol{H})$. Since $(\boldsymbol{I} - \boldsymbol{H})\boldsymbol{A} = \boldsymbol{A}(\boldsymbol{I} - \boldsymbol{L}(\boldsymbol{M}'\boldsymbol{AL})^{-}\boldsymbol{M}'\boldsymbol{A})$, $\text{Sp}((\boldsymbol{I} - \boldsymbol{H})\boldsymbol{A}$ is also a subset of $\text{Sp}(\boldsymbol{A})$. Since $\text{Ker}(\boldsymbol{H})$ and $\text{Sp}(\boldsymbol{A})$ are disjoint, this implies $(\boldsymbol{I} - \boldsymbol{H})\boldsymbol{A} = \boldsymbol{O}$, namely $\boldsymbol{HA} = \boldsymbol{A}$.

The propositions in this question are given as Theorem 2.1 in Yanai (1990). See also Theorems 3.1, 3.2, and 3.3 in the same article.

7.4 Chapter 4

1. We use (4.77). We have $\boldsymbol{Q}_{C'} = \boldsymbol{I}_3 - \frac{1}{3}\begin{pmatrix} 1 \\ 1 \\ 1 \end{pmatrix}(1,1,1) = \frac{1}{3}\begin{bmatrix} 2 & -1 & -1 \\ -1 & 2 & -1 \\ -1 & -1 & 2 \end{bmatrix}$,

$\boldsymbol{Q}_{C'}\boldsymbol{A}' = \frac{1}{3}\begin{bmatrix} 2 & -1 & -1 \\ -1 & 2 & -1 \\ -1 & -1 & 2 \end{bmatrix}\begin{bmatrix} 1 & 2 \\ 2 & 3 \\ 3 & 1 \end{bmatrix} = \frac{1}{3}\begin{bmatrix} -3 & 0 \\ 0 & 3 \\ 3 & -3 \end{bmatrix}$, and

$\boldsymbol{A}(\boldsymbol{Q}_{C'}\boldsymbol{A}') = \frac{1}{3}\begin{bmatrix} 1 & 2 & 3 \\ 2 & 3 & 1 \end{bmatrix}\begin{bmatrix} -3 & 0 \\ 0 & 3 \\ 3 & -3 \end{bmatrix} = \frac{1}{3}\begin{bmatrix} 6 & -3 \\ -3 & 6 \end{bmatrix} = \begin{bmatrix} 2 & -1 \\ -1 & 2 \end{bmatrix}$.

Hence,

$$\begin{aligned} A^{-}_{mr(C)} &= \boldsymbol{Q}_{C'}\boldsymbol{A}'(\boldsymbol{AQ}_{C'}\boldsymbol{A}')^{-1} \\ &= \frac{1}{3}\begin{bmatrix} -3 & 0 \\ 0 & 3 \\ 3 & -3 \end{bmatrix}\begin{bmatrix} 2 & -1 \\ -1 & 2 \end{bmatrix}^{-1} = \frac{1}{9}\begin{bmatrix} -3 & 0 \\ 0 & 3 \\ 3 & -3 \end{bmatrix}\begin{bmatrix} 2 & 1 \\ 1 & 2 \end{bmatrix} \\ &= \frac{1}{3}\begin{bmatrix} -2 & -1 \\ 1 & 2 \\ 1 & -1 \end{bmatrix}. \end{aligned}$$

2. We use (4.65).

(i) $\boldsymbol{Q}_B = \boldsymbol{I}_3 - \boldsymbol{P}_B = \boldsymbol{I}_3 - \frac{1}{3}\begin{bmatrix} 1 & 1 & 1 \\ 1 & 1 & 1 \\ 1 & 1 & 1 \end{bmatrix} = \frac{1}{3}\begin{bmatrix} 2 & -1 & -1 \\ -1 & 2 & -1 \\ -1 & -1 & 2 \end{bmatrix}$, and

$\boldsymbol{A}'\boldsymbol{Q}_B\boldsymbol{A} = \frac{1}{3}\begin{bmatrix} 1 & 2 & 1 \\ 2 & 1 & 1 \end{bmatrix}\begin{bmatrix} 2 & -1 & -1 \\ -1 & 2 & -1 \\ -1 & -1 & 2 \end{bmatrix}\begin{bmatrix} 1 & 2 \\ 2 & 1 \\ 1 & 1 \end{bmatrix} = \frac{1}{3}\begin{bmatrix} 2 & -1 \\ -1 & 2 \end{bmatrix}$.

Thus,

$$\begin{aligned} \boldsymbol{A}^-_{\ell r(B)} = (\boldsymbol{A}'\boldsymbol{Q}_B\boldsymbol{A})^{-1}\boldsymbol{A}'\boldsymbol{Q}_B &= 3\begin{bmatrix} 2 & -1 \\ -1 & 2 \end{bmatrix}^{-1} \times \frac{1}{3}\begin{bmatrix} -1 & 2 & -1 \\ 2 & -1 & -1 \end{bmatrix} \\ &= \frac{1}{3}\begin{bmatrix} 2 & 1 \\ 1 & 2 \end{bmatrix}\begin{bmatrix} -1 & 2 & -1 \\ 2 & -1 & -1 \end{bmatrix} \\ &= \begin{bmatrix} 0 & 1 & -1 \\ 1 & 0 & -1 \end{bmatrix}. \end{aligned}$$

(ii) We have

$$\begin{aligned} \boldsymbol{Q}_{\tilde{B}} = \boldsymbol{I}_3 - \boldsymbol{P}_{\tilde{B}} &= \boldsymbol{I}_3 - \frac{1}{1+a^2+b^2}\begin{bmatrix} 1 & a & b \\ a & a^2 & ab \\ b & ab & b^2 \end{bmatrix} \\ &= \frac{1}{1+a^2+b^2}\begin{bmatrix} a^2+b^2 & -a & -b \\ -a & 1+b^2 & -ab \\ -b & -ab & 1+a^2 \end{bmatrix}, \end{aligned}$$

from which the equation

$$\boldsymbol{A}'\boldsymbol{Q}_{\tilde{B}}\boldsymbol{A} = \frac{1}{1+a^2+b^2}\begin{bmatrix} f_1 & f_2 \\ f_2 & f_3 \end{bmatrix}$$

can be derived, where $f_1 = 2a^2 + 5b^2 - 4ab - 4a - 2b + 5$, $f_2 = 3a^2 + 4b^2 - 3ab - 5a - 3b + 3$, and $f_3 = 5a^2 + 5b^2 - 2ab - 4a - 4b + 2$. Hence,

$$\begin{aligned} \boldsymbol{Q}_{\tilde{B}} = \boldsymbol{I}_3 - \boldsymbol{P}_{\tilde{B}} &= \boldsymbol{I}_3 - \frac{1}{2+a^2}\begin{bmatrix} 1 & 1 & a \\ 1 & 1 & a \\ a & a & a^2 \end{bmatrix} \\ &= \frac{1}{2+a^2}\begin{bmatrix} 1+a^2 & -1 & -a \\ -1 & 1+a^2 & -a \\ -a & -a & 2 \end{bmatrix}, \end{aligned}$$

$$\boldsymbol{A}'\boldsymbol{Q}_{\tilde{B}}\boldsymbol{A} = \frac{1}{2+a^2}\begin{bmatrix} e_1 & e_2 \\ e_2 & e_1 \end{bmatrix}, \text{ and } \boldsymbol{A}'\boldsymbol{Q}_{\tilde{B}} = \frac{1}{2+a^2}\begin{bmatrix} g_1 & g_2 & g_3 \\ g_2 & g_1 & g_3 \end{bmatrix},$$

where $e_1 = 5a^2 - 6a + 3$, $e_2 = 4a^2 - 6a + 1$, $g_1 = a^2 - a - 1$, $g_2 = 2a^2 - a + 1$, and $g_3 = 2 - 3a$. Hence, when $a \neq \frac{2}{3}$,

$$\boldsymbol{A}^-_{\ell r(\tilde{B})} = (\boldsymbol{A}'\boldsymbol{Q}_{\tilde{B}}\boldsymbol{A})^{-1}\boldsymbol{A}'\boldsymbol{Q}_{\tilde{B}}$$

$$= \frac{1}{(2+a^2)(3a-2)^2} \begin{bmatrix} e_1 & -e_2 \\ -e_2 & e_1 \end{bmatrix} \begin{bmatrix} g_1 & g_2 & g_3 \\ g_2 & g_1 & g_3 \end{bmatrix}$$
$$= \frac{1}{(2+a^2)(3a-2)^2} \begin{bmatrix} h_1 & h_2 & h_3 \\ h_2 & h_1 & h_3 \end{bmatrix},$$

where $h_1 = -3a^4 + 5a^3 - 8a^2 + 10a - 4$, $h_2 = 6a^4 - 7a^3 + 14a^2 - 14a + 4$, and $h_3 = (2-3a)(a^2+2)$. Furthermore, when $a = -3$ in the equation above,

$$\boldsymbol{A}^-_{\ell r(\tilde{B})} = \frac{1}{11} \begin{bmatrix} -4 & 7 & 1 \\ 7 & -4 & 1 \end{bmatrix}.$$

Hence, by letting $\boldsymbol{E} = \boldsymbol{A}^-_{\ell r(\tilde{B})}$, we have $\boldsymbol{AEA} = \boldsymbol{A}$ and $(\boldsymbol{AE})' = \boldsymbol{AE}$, and so $\boldsymbol{A}^-_{\ell r(\tilde{B})} = \boldsymbol{A}^-_{\ell}$.

3. We use (4.101). We have

$$(\boldsymbol{A}'\boldsymbol{A} + \boldsymbol{C}'\boldsymbol{C})^{-1} = \frac{1}{432} \begin{bmatrix} 45 & 19 & 19 \\ 19 & 69 & 21 \\ 19 & 21 & 69 \end{bmatrix},$$

and

$$(\boldsymbol{A}\boldsymbol{A}' + \boldsymbol{B}\boldsymbol{B}')^{-1} = \frac{1}{432} \begin{bmatrix} 69 & 9 & 21 \\ 9 & 45 & 9 \\ 21 & 9 & 69 \end{bmatrix}.$$

Furthermore,

$$\boldsymbol{A}'\boldsymbol{A}\boldsymbol{A}' = 9 \begin{bmatrix} 2 & -1 & -1 \\ -1 & 2 & -1 \\ -1 & -1 & 2 \end{bmatrix},$$

so that

$$\boldsymbol{A}^+_{B\cdot C} = (\boldsymbol{A}'\boldsymbol{A} + \boldsymbol{C}'\boldsymbol{C})^{-1}\boldsymbol{A}'\boldsymbol{A}\boldsymbol{A}'(\boldsymbol{A}\boldsymbol{A}' + \boldsymbol{B}\boldsymbol{B}')^{-1}$$
$$= \begin{bmatrix} 12.75 & -8.25 & -7.5 \\ -11.25 & 24.75 & -4.5 \\ -14.25 & -8.25 & 19.5 \end{bmatrix}.$$

(The Moore-Penrose inverse of Question 1(c) in Chapter 3 can also be calculated using the same formula.)

4. (i) $(\boldsymbol{I} - \boldsymbol{P}_A\boldsymbol{P}_B)\boldsymbol{a} = \boldsymbol{0}$ implies $\boldsymbol{a} = \boldsymbol{P}_A\boldsymbol{P}_B\boldsymbol{a}$. On the other hand, from $||\boldsymbol{a}||^2 = ||\boldsymbol{P}_A\boldsymbol{P}_B\boldsymbol{a}||^2 \leq ||\boldsymbol{P}_B\boldsymbol{a}||^2 \leq ||\boldsymbol{a}||^2$, we have $||\boldsymbol{P}_B\boldsymbol{a}||^2 = ||\boldsymbol{a}||^2$, which implies $\boldsymbol{a}'\boldsymbol{a} = \boldsymbol{a}'\boldsymbol{P}_A\boldsymbol{a}$. Hence, $||\boldsymbol{a} - \boldsymbol{P}_B\boldsymbol{a}||^2 = \boldsymbol{a}'\boldsymbol{a} - \boldsymbol{a}'\boldsymbol{P}_B\boldsymbol{a} - \boldsymbol{a}'\boldsymbol{P}_B\boldsymbol{a} + \boldsymbol{a}'\boldsymbol{P}_B\boldsymbol{a} = \boldsymbol{a}'\boldsymbol{a} - \boldsymbol{a}'\boldsymbol{P}_B\boldsymbol{a} = 0 \rightarrow \boldsymbol{a} = \boldsymbol{P}_B\boldsymbol{a}$. That is, $\boldsymbol{a} = \boldsymbol{P}_B\boldsymbol{a} = \boldsymbol{P}_A\boldsymbol{a}$, and so $\boldsymbol{a} \in \text{Sp}(\boldsymbol{A}) \cap \text{Sp}(\boldsymbol{B}) = \{\boldsymbol{0}\} \Rightarrow \boldsymbol{a} = \boldsymbol{0}$. Hence, $\boldsymbol{I} - \boldsymbol{P}_A\boldsymbol{P}_B$ is nonsingular.

(ii) Clear from $\boldsymbol{P}_A(\boldsymbol{I} - \boldsymbol{P}_B\boldsymbol{P}_A) = (\boldsymbol{I} - \boldsymbol{P}_A\boldsymbol{P}_B)\boldsymbol{P}_A$.

(iii) $(\boldsymbol{I}-\boldsymbol{P}_A\boldsymbol{P}_B)^{-1}\boldsymbol{P}_A(\boldsymbol{I}-\boldsymbol{P}_A\boldsymbol{P}_B)\boldsymbol{P}_A = (\boldsymbol{I}-\boldsymbol{P}_A\boldsymbol{P}_B)^{-1}(\boldsymbol{I}-\boldsymbol{P}_A\boldsymbol{P}_B)\boldsymbol{P}_A = \boldsymbol{P}_A$ and $(\boldsymbol{I}-\boldsymbol{P}_A\boldsymbol{P}_B)^{-1}\boldsymbol{P}_A(\boldsymbol{I}-\boldsymbol{P}_A\boldsymbol{P}_B)\boldsymbol{P}_B = \boldsymbol{O}$. Hence, $(\boldsymbol{I}-\boldsymbol{P}_A\boldsymbol{P}_B)^{-1}\boldsymbol{P}_A(\boldsymbol{I}-\boldsymbol{P}_A\boldsymbol{P}_B)$ is the projector onto $\text{Sp}(\boldsymbol{A}) = \text{Sp}(\boldsymbol{P}_A)$ along $\text{Sp}(\boldsymbol{B}) = \text{Sp}(\boldsymbol{P}_B)$.

5. $\mathrm{Sp}(\boldsymbol{A}')\oplus\mathrm{Sp}(\boldsymbol{C}')\oplus\mathrm{Sp}(\boldsymbol{D}') = E^m$. Let $\boldsymbol{E}$ be such that $\mathrm{Sp}(\boldsymbol{E}') = \mathrm{Sp}(\boldsymbol{C}')\oplus\mathrm{Sp}(\boldsymbol{D}')$. Then, $\boldsymbol{E} = \begin{bmatrix} \boldsymbol{C} \\ \boldsymbol{D} \end{bmatrix}$. From Theorem 4.20, the $\boldsymbol{x}$ that minimizes $||\boldsymbol{Ax} - \boldsymbol{b}||^2$ subject to $\boldsymbol{Ex} = \boldsymbol{0}$ is obtained by

$$\boldsymbol{x} = (\boldsymbol{A}'\boldsymbol{A} + \boldsymbol{E}'\boldsymbol{E})^{-1}\boldsymbol{A}'\boldsymbol{b} = (\boldsymbol{A}'\boldsymbol{A} + \boldsymbol{C}'\boldsymbol{C} + \boldsymbol{D}'\boldsymbol{D})^{-1}\boldsymbol{A}'\boldsymbol{b}.$$

This $\boldsymbol{x}$ can take various values depending on the choice of $\mathrm{Sp}(\boldsymbol{D}')$.
6. Let $\boldsymbol{P}_{A/T^-} = \boldsymbol{A}(\boldsymbol{A}'\boldsymbol{T}^-\boldsymbol{A})^-\boldsymbol{A}'\boldsymbol{T}^-$ be denoted by $\boldsymbol{P}^*$. Since $\boldsymbol{T}$ is symmetric,

$$(\boldsymbol{P}^*)'\boldsymbol{T}^-\boldsymbol{A} = \boldsymbol{T}^-\boldsymbol{A}(\boldsymbol{A}'\boldsymbol{T}^-\boldsymbol{A})^-\boldsymbol{A}'\boldsymbol{T}^-\boldsymbol{A} = \boldsymbol{T}^-\boldsymbol{A}.$$

7. (i) Let $\boldsymbol{y} \in \mathrm{Ker}(\boldsymbol{A}'\boldsymbol{M})$. Then, $\boldsymbol{Ax} + \boldsymbol{y} = \boldsymbol{0} \Rightarrow \boldsymbol{A}'\boldsymbol{MAx} + \boldsymbol{A}'\boldsymbol{My} = \boldsymbol{0} \Rightarrow \boldsymbol{A}'\boldsymbol{MAx} = \boldsymbol{0} \Rightarrow \boldsymbol{A}(\boldsymbol{A}'\boldsymbol{MA})^-\boldsymbol{AMAx} = \boldsymbol{Ax} = \boldsymbol{0} \Rightarrow \boldsymbol{y} = \boldsymbol{0}$. Hence, $\mathrm{Sp}(\boldsymbol{A})$ and $\mathrm{Ker}(\boldsymbol{A}'\boldsymbol{M})$ are disjoint. On the other hand, $\dim(\mathrm{Ker}(\boldsymbol{A}'\boldsymbol{M})) = \mathrm{rank}(\boldsymbol{I}_n - (\boldsymbol{AM})^-\boldsymbol{AM}) = n - m$, showing that $E^n = \mathrm{Sp}(\boldsymbol{A}) \oplus \mathrm{Ker}(\boldsymbol{A}'\boldsymbol{M})$.

(ii) Clear from $\boldsymbol{P}_{A/M}\boldsymbol{A} = \boldsymbol{A}$ and $\boldsymbol{P}_{A/M}(\boldsymbol{I}_n - (\boldsymbol{A}'\boldsymbol{M})^-\boldsymbol{A}'\boldsymbol{M}) = \boldsymbol{O}$.

(iii) Let $\boldsymbol{M} = \boldsymbol{Q}_B$. Then, $\mathrm{Ker}(\boldsymbol{A}'\boldsymbol{Q}_B) = \mathrm{Sp}(\boldsymbol{I}_n - (\boldsymbol{A}'\boldsymbol{Q}_B)^-\boldsymbol{A}'\boldsymbol{Q}_B)$. Since $\boldsymbol{A}(\boldsymbol{A}'\boldsymbol{Q}_B\boldsymbol{A})^- \in \{(\boldsymbol{A}'\boldsymbol{Q}_B)^-\}$, $\mathrm{Ker}(\boldsymbol{A}'\boldsymbol{Q}_B) = \mathrm{Sp}(\boldsymbol{I}_n - \boldsymbol{A}(\boldsymbol{A}'\boldsymbol{Q}_B\boldsymbol{A})^-\boldsymbol{A}'\boldsymbol{Q}_B) = \mathrm{Sp}(\boldsymbol{B} \times (\boldsymbol{B}'\boldsymbol{Q}_A\boldsymbol{B})^-\boldsymbol{B}'\boldsymbol{Q}_A) = \mathrm{Sp}(\boldsymbol{B})$. Thus, $\mathrm{Ker}(\boldsymbol{A}'\boldsymbol{Q}_B) = \mathrm{Sp}(\boldsymbol{B})$ and $\boldsymbol{T}^-\boldsymbol{P}^*\boldsymbol{A} = \boldsymbol{T}^-\boldsymbol{A} \Rightarrow \boldsymbol{TT}^-\boldsymbol{P}^*\boldsymbol{A} = \boldsymbol{TT}^-\boldsymbol{A}$. On the other hand,

$$\mathrm{Sp}(\boldsymbol{T}) = \mathrm{Sp}(\boldsymbol{G}) + \mathrm{Sp}(\boldsymbol{A}) \Rightarrow \mathrm{Sp}(\boldsymbol{T}) \supset \mathrm{Sp}(\boldsymbol{A}) \Rightarrow \boldsymbol{TT}^-\boldsymbol{P}^*\boldsymbol{A} = \boldsymbol{TT}^-\boldsymbol{A},$$

which implies

$$\boldsymbol{P}^*\boldsymbol{A} = \boldsymbol{A}. \tag{7.1}$$

Also, $(\boldsymbol{P}^*)'\boldsymbol{T}^- = \boldsymbol{T}^-\boldsymbol{A}(\boldsymbol{A}'\boldsymbol{T}^-\boldsymbol{A})^-\boldsymbol{A}'\boldsymbol{T}^- = \boldsymbol{T}^-\boldsymbol{P}^* \Rightarrow \boldsymbol{TP}^*\boldsymbol{T}^- = \boldsymbol{TT}^-\boldsymbol{P}^* = \boldsymbol{P}^* \Rightarrow \boldsymbol{TP}^*\boldsymbol{T}^- = \boldsymbol{TZ} = \boldsymbol{P}^*\boldsymbol{TZ} = \boldsymbol{P}^*\boldsymbol{GZ}$ and $\boldsymbol{T}(\boldsymbol{P}^*)'\boldsymbol{T}^-\boldsymbol{TZ} = \boldsymbol{T}(\boldsymbol{P}^*)'\boldsymbol{Z} = \boldsymbol{TT}^-\boldsymbol{A}(\boldsymbol{A}'\boldsymbol{T}^-\boldsymbol{A})^-\boldsymbol{A}'\boldsymbol{Z} = \boldsymbol{O}$, which implies

$$\boldsymbol{P}^*\boldsymbol{TZ} = \boldsymbol{O}. \tag{7.2}$$

Combining (7.1) and (7.2) above and the definition of a projection matrix (Theorem 2.2), we have $\boldsymbol{P}^* = \boldsymbol{P}_{A\cdot TZ}$.

By the symmetry of $\boldsymbol{A}$,

$$\mu_{\max}(\boldsymbol{A}) = (\lambda_{\max}(\boldsymbol{A}'\boldsymbol{A}))^{1/2} = (\lambda_{\max}(\boldsymbol{A}^2))^{1/2} = \lambda_{\max}(\boldsymbol{A}).$$

Similarly, $\mu_{\min}(\boldsymbol{A}) = \lambda_{\min}(\boldsymbol{A})$, $\mu_{\max}(\boldsymbol{A}) = 2.005$, and $\mu_{\min}(\boldsymbol{A}) = 4.9987 \times 10^{-4}$. Thus, we have $\mathrm{cond}(\boldsymbol{A}) = \mu_{\max}/\mu_{\min} = 4002$, indicating that $\boldsymbol{A}$ is nearly singular. (See Question 13 in Chapter 6 for more details on $\mathrm{cond}(\boldsymbol{A})$.)
8. Let $\boldsymbol{y} = \boldsymbol{y}_1 + \boldsymbol{y}_2$, where $\boldsymbol{y} \in E^n$, $\boldsymbol{y}_1 \in \mathrm{Sp}(\boldsymbol{A})$ and $\boldsymbol{y}_2 \in \mathrm{Sp}(\boldsymbol{B})$. Then, $\boldsymbol{AA}^+_{B\cdot C}\boldsymbol{y}_1 = \boldsymbol{y}_1$ and $\boldsymbol{AA}^+_{B\cdot C}\boldsymbol{y}_2 = \boldsymbol{0}$. Hence, $\boldsymbol{A}^+_{\tilde{B}\cdot C}\boldsymbol{AA}^+_{B\cdot C}\boldsymbol{y} = \boldsymbol{A}^+_{\tilde{B}\cdot C}\boldsymbol{y}_1 = \boldsymbol{x}_1$, where $\boldsymbol{x}_1 \in \mathrm{Sp}(\boldsymbol{Q}_{C'})$.

On the other hand, since $\boldsymbol{A}^+_{\tilde{B}\cdot C}\boldsymbol{y} = \boldsymbol{x}_1$, we have $\boldsymbol{A}^+_{\tilde{B}\cdot C}\boldsymbol{AA}^+_{B\cdot C}\boldsymbol{y} = \boldsymbol{A}^+_{\tilde{B}\cdot C}\boldsymbol{y}_1$, leading to the given equation.

(An alternative proof.)

$$\begin{aligned}&A^+_{\tilde{B}\cdot C}AA^+_{B\cdot C}\\&\quad = Q_{C'}A'(AQ_{C'}A')^-A(A'Q_{\tilde{B}}A)^-A'Q_{\tilde{B}}AQ_{C'}A'(AQ_{C'}A')^-\\&\qquad\qquad A(A'Q_BA)^-A'Q_B\\&\quad = Q_{C'}A'(AQ_{C'}A')^-A(A'Q_{\tilde{B}}A)^-A'Q_B = A^+_{\tilde{B}\cdot C}.\end{aligned}$$

9. Let $K^{1/2}$ denote the symmetric square root factor of K (i.e., $K^{1/2}K^{1/2} = K$ and $K^{-1/2}K^{-1/2} = K^{-1}$). Similarly, let S_1 and S_2 be symmetric square root factors of $A'K^{-1}A$ and $B'KB$, respectively. Define $C = [K^{-1/2}AS_1^{-1/2}, K^{1/2}B \times S_2^{-1/2}]$. Then C is square and $C'C = I$, and so $CC' = K^{-1/2}AS^{-1}A'K^{-1/2} + K^{1/2}BS_2^{-1}B'K^{1/2} = I$. Pre- and postmultiplying both sides, we obtain Khatri's lemma.

10. (i) Let $W = \text{Sp}(F')$ and $V = \text{Sp}(H)$. From (a), we have $Gx \in \text{Sp}(H)$, which implies $\text{Sp}(G) \subset \text{Sp}(H)$, so that $G = HX$ for some X. From (c), we have $GAH = H \Rightarrow HXAH = H \Rightarrow AHXAH = AH$, from which it follows that $X = (AH)^-$ and $G = H(AH)^-$. Thus, $AGA = AH(AH)^-A$. On the other hand, from $\text{rank}(A) = \text{rank}(AH)$, we have $A = AHW$ for some W. Hence, $AGA = AH(AH)^-AHW = AHW = A$, which implies that $G = H(AH)^-$ is a g-inverse of A.

(ii) $\text{Sp}(G') \subset \text{Sp}(F') \Rightarrow G' = F'X' \Rightarrow G = XF$. Hence, $(AG)'F' = F' \Rightarrow FAG = F \Rightarrow FAXF = F \Rightarrow FAXFA = FA \Rightarrow X = (FA)^-$. This and (4.126) lead to (4.127), similarly to (i).

(iii) The G that satisfies (a) and (d) should be expressed as $G = HX$. By $(AG)'F' = F' \Rightarrow FAHX = F$,

$$(1)\quad G = H(FAH)^-F + H(I - (FAH)^-FAH)Z_1.$$

The G that satisfies (b) and (c) can be expressed as $G = XF$. By $GAH = H \Rightarrow XFAH = H$,

$$(2)\quad G = H(FAH)^-F + Z_2(I - FAH(FAH)^-)F.$$

(Z_1 and Z_2 are arbitrary square matrices of orders n and m, respectively.) From $\text{rank}(FAH) = \text{rank}(H)$, the second term in (1) is null, and from $\text{rank}(F) = \text{rank}(FAH)$, the second term in (2) is null. In this case, clearly $AH(FAH)^-FA = A$, and G in (4.129) is a g-inverse of A.

(iv) (4.130): Since $I_m - C'(CC')^-C = Q_{C'}$, we have $G = Q_{C'}(AQ_{C'})^-$. In this case, $\text{rank}(AQ_{C'}) = \text{rank}(A)$, so that $AQ_{C'}(AQ_{C'})^-A = A$. Furthermore, $CQ_{C'}(AQ_{C'})^-A = O$. Since A^-A that satisfies (4.73) also satisfies (4.75), $GA = A^-_{m(C)}A$. On the other hand, since $\text{rank}(G) = \text{rank}(A)$, $G = A^-_{mr(C)}$.

(4.131): Let $G = (FA)^-F = (Q_BA)^-Q_B$. Then, $AGA = A$ and $AGB = O$, from which $AG = AA^-_{\ell(B)}$. Furthermore, $\text{rank}(G) = \text{rank}(A)$, which leads to $G = A^-_{\ell r(B)}$.

(4.132): $G = Q_{C'}(Q_B A Q_{C'})^- Q_B$, from which $AGA = AQ_{C'}(Q_B AQ_{C'})^- Q_B \times A$. Let $G^* = A'(AQ_{C'}A')^- A(A'Q_B A)^- A'$. Then, $Q_B AQ_{C'} G^* Q_B AQ_{C'} = Q_B AQ_{C'}$, indicating that $G^* \in \{(Q_B AQ_{C'})^-\}$. Hence, $AQ_{C'} GQ_B A = AQ_{C'} A' (AQ_{C'} A')^- A(A'Q_B A)^- A'Q_B A = A$. Hence, $AGA = A$. The relation $GAG = G$ can be similarly proven.

Next,

$$\begin{aligned} Q_B AG &= Q_B AQ_{C'}(Q_B AQ_{C'})^- Q_B \\ &= Q_B AQ_{C'} A'(AQ_{C'} A')^- A(A'Q_B A)^- A'Q_B \\ &= Q_B A(A'Q_B A)^- A'Q_B \\ &= P_{A[B]}. \end{aligned}$$

Similarly, $GAQ_{C'} = Q_{C'} A'(AQ_{C'} A')^- AQ_{C'} = P_{A'[C']}$. That is, both $Q_B AG$ and $GAQ_{C'}$ are symmetric. Hence, by Definition 4.4, G coincides with the $B-$, C-constrained Moore-Penrose inverse $A^+_{B \cdot C}$.

(v) We use the matrix rank method to show (4.138). (See the answer to Question 7 in Chapter 1 for a brief introduction to the matrix rank method.) Define $M = \begin{bmatrix} FAH & FA \\ AH & A \end{bmatrix}$. Pre- and postmultiplying M by $\begin{bmatrix} I & O \\ -AH(FAH)^{-1} & I \end{bmatrix}$ and $\begin{bmatrix} I & -(FAH)^{-1}FA \\ O & I \end{bmatrix}$, respectively, we obtain $\begin{bmatrix} FAH & O \\ O & A_1 \end{bmatrix}$, where $A_1 = A - AH(FAH)^{-1}FA$, indicating that

$$\text{rank}(M) = \text{rank}(FAH) + \text{rank}(A_1). \tag{7.3}$$

On the other hand, pre- and postmultiplying M by $\begin{bmatrix} I & -F \\ O & I \end{bmatrix}$ and $\begin{bmatrix} I & O \\ -H & I \end{bmatrix}$, respectively, we obtain $\begin{bmatrix} O & O \\ O & A \end{bmatrix}$, indicating that $\text{rank}(M) = \text{rank}(A)$ Combining this result with (7.3), we obtain (4.138). That $\text{rank}(FAH) = \text{rank}(AH(FAH)^{-1} \times FA)$ is trivial.

11. It is straightforward to verify that these Moore-Penrose inverses satisfy the four Penrose conditions in Definition 3.5. The following relations are useful in this process: (1) $P_{A/M}P_A = P_A$ and $P_A P_{A/M} = P_{A/M}$ (or, more generally, $P_{A/M}P_{A/N} = P_{A/N}$, where N is *nnd* and such that $\text{rank}(NA) = \text{rank}(A)$), (2) $Q_{A/M}Q_A = Q_{A/M}$ and $Q_A Q_{A/M} = Q_A$ (or, more generally, $Q_{A/M}Q_{A/N} = Q_{A/M}$, where N is as introduced in (1)), (3) $P_{A/M}P_{MA} = P_{A/M}$ and $P_{MA}P_{A/M} = P_{MA}$, and (4) $Q_{A/M}Q_{MA} = Q_{MA}$ and $Q_{MA}Q_{A/M} = Q_{A/M}$.

12. Differentiating $\phi(B)$ with respect to the elements of B and setting the result to zero, we obtain

$$\frac{1}{2}\frac{\partial \phi(B)}{\partial B} = -X'(Y - X\hat{B}) + \lambda \hat{B} = O,$$

from which the result follows immediately.

13. (i) $\boldsymbol{R}_X(\lambda)\boldsymbol{M}_X(\lambda)\boldsymbol{R}_X(\lambda) = \boldsymbol{X}(\boldsymbol{X}'\boldsymbol{M}_X(\lambda)\boldsymbol{X})^{-1}\boldsymbol{X}'\boldsymbol{M}_X(\lambda)\boldsymbol{X}(\boldsymbol{X}'\boldsymbol{M}_X(\lambda)\boldsymbol{X})^{-1}$ $\boldsymbol{X}' = \boldsymbol{R}_X(\lambda)$.

(ii) The (i) above indicates that $\boldsymbol{M}_X(\lambda)$ is a g-inverse of $\boldsymbol{R}_X(\lambda)$. That $\boldsymbol{M}_X(\lambda)$ satisfies the three other Penrose conditions can be readily verified.

7.5 Chapter 5

1. Since $\boldsymbol{A}'\boldsymbol{A} = \begin{bmatrix} 6 & -3 \\ -3 & 6 \end{bmatrix}$, its eigenvalues are 9 and 3. Consequently, the singular values of $\boldsymbol{A}$ are 3 and $\sqrt{3}$. The normalized eigenvectors corresponding to the eigenvalues 9 and 3 are, respectively, $\boldsymbol{u}_1 = \left(\frac{\sqrt{2}}{2}, -\frac{\sqrt{2}}{2}\right)'$ and $\boldsymbol{u}_2 = \left(\frac{\sqrt{2}}{2}, \frac{\sqrt{2}}{2}\right)'$. Hence,

$$\boldsymbol{v}_1 = \frac{1}{\sqrt{9}}\boldsymbol{A}\boldsymbol{u}_1 = \frac{1}{3}\begin{bmatrix} 1 & -2 \\ -2 & 1 \\ 1 & 1 \end{bmatrix}\begin{pmatrix} \frac{\sqrt{2}}{2} \\ -\frac{\sqrt{2}}{2} \end{pmatrix} = \frac{\sqrt{2}}{2}\begin{pmatrix} 1 \\ -1 \\ 0 \end{pmatrix},$$

and

$$\boldsymbol{v}_2 = \frac{1}{\sqrt{3}}\boldsymbol{A}\boldsymbol{u}_2 = \frac{1}{\sqrt{3}}\begin{bmatrix} 1 & -2 \\ -2 & 1 \\ 1 & 1 \end{bmatrix}\begin{pmatrix} \frac{\sqrt{2}}{2} \\ \frac{\sqrt{2}}{2} \end{pmatrix} = \frac{\sqrt{6}}{6}\begin{pmatrix} -1 \\ -1 \\ 2 \end{pmatrix}.$$

The SVD of $\boldsymbol{A}$ is thus given by

$$\begin{aligned} \boldsymbol{A} &= \begin{bmatrix} 1 & -2 \\ -2 & 1 \\ 1 & 1 \end{bmatrix} \\ &= 3\begin{pmatrix} \frac{\sqrt{2}}{2} \\ -\frac{\sqrt{2}}{2} \\ 0 \end{pmatrix}\left(\frac{\sqrt{2}}{2}, -\frac{\sqrt{2}}{2}\right) + \sqrt{3}\begin{pmatrix} -\frac{\sqrt{6}}{6} \\ -\frac{\sqrt{6}}{6} \\ \frac{\sqrt{6}}{3} \end{pmatrix}\left(\frac{\sqrt{2}}{2}, \frac{\sqrt{2}}{2}\right) \\ &= \begin{bmatrix} \frac{3}{2} & -\frac{3}{2} \\ -\frac{3}{2} & \frac{3}{2} \\ 0 & 0 \end{bmatrix} + \begin{bmatrix} -\frac{1}{2} & -\frac{1}{2} \\ -\frac{1}{2} & -\frac{1}{2} \\ 1 & 1 \end{bmatrix}. \end{aligned}$$

According to (5.52), the Moore-Penrose inverse of $\boldsymbol{A}$ is given by

$$\begin{aligned} \boldsymbol{A}^+ &= \frac{1}{3}\begin{pmatrix} \frac{\sqrt{2}}{2} \\ -\frac{\sqrt{2}}{2} \end{pmatrix}\left(\frac{\sqrt{2}}{2}, -\frac{\sqrt{2}}{2}, 0\right) + \frac{1}{\sqrt{3}}\begin{pmatrix} \frac{\sqrt{2}}{2} \\ \frac{\sqrt{2}}{2} \end{pmatrix}\left(-\frac{\sqrt{6}}{6}, -\frac{\sqrt{6}}{6}, \frac{\sqrt{6}}{3}\right) \\ &= \frac{1}{3}\begin{bmatrix} 0 & -1 & 1 \\ -1 & 0 & 1 \end{bmatrix}. \end{aligned}$$

(An alternative solution) From $\text{rank}(\boldsymbol{A}) = 2$, $\boldsymbol{A}'(\boldsymbol{A}\boldsymbol{A}')^{-}\boldsymbol{A} = \boldsymbol{I}_2$. Using $\boldsymbol{A}^+ = (\boldsymbol{A}'\boldsymbol{A})^{-1}\boldsymbol{A}'$ in (3.98),

$$\boldsymbol{A}^+ = \begin{bmatrix} 6 & -3 \\ -3 & 6 \end{bmatrix}^{-1} \begin{bmatrix} 1 & -2 & 1 \\ -2 & 1 & 1 \end{bmatrix} = \frac{1}{9}\begin{bmatrix} 2 & 1 \\ 1 & 2 \end{bmatrix}\begin{bmatrix} 1 & -2 & 1 \\ -2 & 1 & 1 \end{bmatrix} = \frac{1}{3}\begin{bmatrix} 0 & -1 & 1 \\ -1 & 0 & 1 \end{bmatrix}.$$

2. Differentiating $f(\boldsymbol{x}, \boldsymbol{y}) = (\boldsymbol{x}'\boldsymbol{A}\boldsymbol{y})^2 - \lambda_1(\boldsymbol{x}'\boldsymbol{x} - 1) - \lambda_2(\boldsymbol{y}'\boldsymbol{y} - 1)$ with respect to $\boldsymbol{x}$ and $\boldsymbol{y}$, and setting the results equal to zero, we obtain

$$(\boldsymbol{x}'\boldsymbol{A}\boldsymbol{y})\boldsymbol{A}\boldsymbol{y} = \lambda_1\boldsymbol{x} \tag{7.4}$$

and

$$(\boldsymbol{x}'\boldsymbol{A}\boldsymbol{y})\boldsymbol{A}'\boldsymbol{x} = \lambda_2\boldsymbol{y}. \tag{7.5}$$

Premultiplying (7.4) and (7.5) by $\boldsymbol{x}'$ and $\boldsymbol{y}'$, respectively, we obtain $(\boldsymbol{x}'\boldsymbol{A}\boldsymbol{y})^2 = \lambda_1 = \lambda_2$ since $||\boldsymbol{x}||^2 = ||\boldsymbol{y}||^2 = 1$. Let $\lambda_1 = \lambda_2 = \mu^2$. Then (1) and (2) become $\boldsymbol{A}\boldsymbol{y} = \mu\boldsymbol{x}$ and $\boldsymbol{A}'\boldsymbol{x} = \mu\boldsymbol{y}$, respectively. Since $\mu^2 = (\boldsymbol{x}'\boldsymbol{A}\boldsymbol{y})^2$, the maximum of $(\boldsymbol{x}'\boldsymbol{A}\boldsymbol{y})^2$ is equal to the square of the largest singular value $\mu(\boldsymbol{A})$ of $\boldsymbol{A}$.
3. $(\boldsymbol{A}+\boldsymbol{A}')^2 = (\boldsymbol{A}+\boldsymbol{A}')'(\boldsymbol{A}+\boldsymbol{A}') = (\boldsymbol{A}\boldsymbol{A}'+\boldsymbol{A}'\boldsymbol{A})+\boldsymbol{A}^2+(\boldsymbol{A}')^2$ and $(\boldsymbol{A}-\boldsymbol{A}')'(\boldsymbol{A}-\boldsymbol{A}') = \boldsymbol{A}\boldsymbol{A}' + \boldsymbol{A}'\boldsymbol{A} - \boldsymbol{A}^2 - (\boldsymbol{A}')^2$. Hence,

$$\boldsymbol{A}\boldsymbol{A}' + \boldsymbol{A}'\boldsymbol{A} = \frac{1}{2}\{(\boldsymbol{A} + \boldsymbol{A}')'(\boldsymbol{A} + \boldsymbol{A}') + (\boldsymbol{A} - \boldsymbol{A}')'(\boldsymbol{A} - \boldsymbol{A}')\}.$$

Noting that $\lambda_j(\boldsymbol{A}\boldsymbol{A}') = \lambda_j(\boldsymbol{A}'\boldsymbol{A})$ by Corollary 1 of Theorem 5.9, $\lambda_j(\boldsymbol{A}'\boldsymbol{A}) \geq \frac{1}{4}\lambda_j(\boldsymbol{A} + \boldsymbol{A}')^2 \Rightarrow 4\mu_j^2(\boldsymbol{A}) \geq \lambda_j^2(\boldsymbol{A} + \boldsymbol{A}') \Rightarrow 2\mu_j(\boldsymbol{A}) \geq \lambda_j(\boldsymbol{A} + \boldsymbol{A}')$.
4. $\tilde{\boldsymbol{A}}'\tilde{\boldsymbol{A}} = \boldsymbol{T}'\boldsymbol{A}'\boldsymbol{S}'\boldsymbol{S}\boldsymbol{A}\boldsymbol{T} = \boldsymbol{T}'\boldsymbol{A}'\boldsymbol{A}\boldsymbol{T}$. Since $\lambda_j(\boldsymbol{T}'\boldsymbol{A}'\boldsymbol{A}\boldsymbol{T}) = \lambda_j(\boldsymbol{A}'\boldsymbol{A})$ from the corollary to Lemma 5.7, $\mu_j(\tilde{\boldsymbol{A}}) = \mu_j(\boldsymbol{A})$. Hence, by substituting $\boldsymbol{A} = \boldsymbol{U}\boldsymbol{\Delta}\boldsymbol{V}'$ into $\tilde{\boldsymbol{A}} = \boldsymbol{S}\boldsymbol{A}\boldsymbol{T}$, we obtain $\tilde{\boldsymbol{A}} = \boldsymbol{S}\boldsymbol{U}\boldsymbol{\Delta}(\boldsymbol{T}'\boldsymbol{V})'$, where $(\boldsymbol{S}\boldsymbol{U})'(\boldsymbol{S}\boldsymbol{U}) = \boldsymbol{U}'\boldsymbol{S}'\boldsymbol{S}\boldsymbol{U} = \boldsymbol{U}'\boldsymbol{U} = \boldsymbol{I}_n$ and $(\boldsymbol{T}'\boldsymbol{V})'(\boldsymbol{T}'\boldsymbol{V}) = \boldsymbol{V}'\boldsymbol{T}\boldsymbol{T}'\boldsymbol{V} = \boldsymbol{V}'\boldsymbol{V} = \boldsymbol{I}_m$. Setting $\tilde{\boldsymbol{U}} = \boldsymbol{S}\boldsymbol{V}$ and $\tilde{\boldsymbol{V}} = \boldsymbol{T}'\boldsymbol{V}$, we have $\tilde{\boldsymbol{A}} = \tilde{\boldsymbol{U}}\boldsymbol{\Delta}\tilde{\boldsymbol{V}}'$.
5. Let k be an integer. Then,

$$\boldsymbol{A}^k = \lambda_1^k\boldsymbol{P}_1^k + \lambda_2^k\boldsymbol{P}_2^k + \cdots + \lambda_n^k\boldsymbol{P}_n^k = \lambda_1^k\boldsymbol{P}_1 + \lambda_2^k\boldsymbol{P}_2 + \cdots + \lambda_n^k\boldsymbol{P}_n.$$

Since $\boldsymbol{I} = \boldsymbol{P}_1 + \boldsymbol{P}_2 + \cdots + \boldsymbol{P}_n$,

$$\begin{aligned} e^A &= \boldsymbol{I} + \boldsymbol{A} + \frac{1}{2}\boldsymbol{A}^2 + \frac{1}{6}\boldsymbol{A}^3 + \cdots \\ &= \sum_{j=1}^n \left\{\left(1 + \lambda_j + \frac{1}{2}\lambda_j^2 + \frac{1}{6}\lambda_j^3 + \cdots\right)\boldsymbol{P}_j\right\} = \sum_{j=1}^n e^{\lambda_j}\boldsymbol{P}_j. \end{aligned}$$

6. (Necessity) Let $\boldsymbol{A}' \in \{\boldsymbol{A}^-\}$. Then $\boldsymbol{A}\boldsymbol{A}'$ is a projector whose eigenvalues are either 1 or 0. That is, nonzero eigenvalues of $\boldsymbol{A}$ are 1.

(Sufficiency) Let $\boldsymbol{A} = \boldsymbol{U}\boldsymbol{\Delta}_r\boldsymbol{V}'$ denote the SVD of $\boldsymbol{A}$, where $\boldsymbol{\Delta}_r$ is a diagonal matrix of order r (where $r = \text{rank}(\boldsymbol{A})$) with unit diagonal elements (i.e., $\boldsymbol{\Delta}_r = \boldsymbol{I}_r$). Hence, $\boldsymbol{A}\boldsymbol{A}'\boldsymbol{A} = \boldsymbol{U}\boldsymbol{\Delta}_r\boldsymbol{V}'\boldsymbol{V}\boldsymbol{\Delta}_r\boldsymbol{U}'\boldsymbol{U}\boldsymbol{\Delta}_r\boldsymbol{V}' = \boldsymbol{U}\boldsymbol{\Delta}_r^3\boldsymbol{V}' = \boldsymbol{U}\boldsymbol{\Delta}_r\boldsymbol{V}' = \boldsymbol{A}$.

7. (i) Use Theorem 5.9 and the fact that $(\boldsymbol{I}_n - \boldsymbol{P}_B)(\boldsymbol{A} - \boldsymbol{B}\boldsymbol{X}) = (\boldsymbol{A} - \boldsymbol{B}\boldsymbol{X}) - \boldsymbol{P}_B\boldsymbol{A} + \boldsymbol{B}\boldsymbol{X} = (\boldsymbol{I}_n - \boldsymbol{P}_B)\boldsymbol{A}$.

(ii) Use Theorem 5.9 and the fact that $(\boldsymbol{I}_p - \boldsymbol{P}_{C'})\boldsymbol{A}'\boldsymbol{C}'\boldsymbol{Y}' = (\boldsymbol{I}_p - \boldsymbol{P}_{C'})\boldsymbol{A}'$, that $\mu_j(\boldsymbol{A}(\boldsymbol{I}_p - \boldsymbol{P}_{C'})) = \mu_j((\boldsymbol{I}_p - \boldsymbol{P}_{C'})\boldsymbol{A}')$, and that $\mu_j(\boldsymbol{A} - \boldsymbol{Y}\boldsymbol{C}) = \mu_j(\boldsymbol{C}'\boldsymbol{Y}' - \boldsymbol{A}')$.

(iii) $\mu_j(\boldsymbol{A} - \boldsymbol{B}\boldsymbol{X} - \boldsymbol{Y}\boldsymbol{C}) \geq \mu_j\{(\boldsymbol{I} - \boldsymbol{P}_B)(\boldsymbol{A} - \boldsymbol{Y}\boldsymbol{C})\} \geq \mu_j\{(\boldsymbol{I} - \boldsymbol{P}_B)(\boldsymbol{A} - \boldsymbol{Y}\boldsymbol{C})(\boldsymbol{I} - \boldsymbol{P}_{C'})\}$.

8. Use $\text{tr}(\boldsymbol{A}\boldsymbol{B}) \leq \text{tr}(\boldsymbol{A})$ on the right-hand side and Theorem 5.9 on the left-hand side.

9. Let $\boldsymbol{A} = \boldsymbol{U}\boldsymbol{\Delta}\boldsymbol{V}'$ denote the SVD of an n by m ($n \geq m$) matrix $\boldsymbol{A}$. Then,

$$\begin{aligned} ||\boldsymbol{y} - \boldsymbol{A}\boldsymbol{x}||^2 &= ||\boldsymbol{U}'\boldsymbol{y} - \boldsymbol{U}'\boldsymbol{U}\boldsymbol{\Delta}\boldsymbol{V}'\boldsymbol{x}||^2 \\ &= ||\boldsymbol{U}'\boldsymbol{y} - \boldsymbol{\Delta}(\boldsymbol{V}'\boldsymbol{x})||^2 = ||\tilde{\boldsymbol{y}} - \boldsymbol{\Delta}\tilde{\boldsymbol{x}}||^2 = \sum_{j=1}^{m}(\tilde{y}_j - \lambda_j\tilde{x}_j)^2 + \sum_{j=m+1}^{n}\tilde{y}_j^2, \end{aligned}$$

where we used the fact that $\boldsymbol{\Delta} = \begin{bmatrix} \lambda_1 & 0 & \cdots & 0 \\ 0 & \lambda_2 & \cdots & 0 \\ \vdots & \vdots & \ddots & \vdots \\ 0 & 0 & \cdots & \lambda_m \\ 0 & 0 & \cdots & 0 \\ \vdots & \vdots & \ddots & \vdots \\ 0 & 0 & \cdots & 0 \end{bmatrix}$. Hence, if $\text{rank}(\boldsymbol{A}) = m$, the equation above takes a minimum $Q = \sum_{j=m+1}^{n}\tilde{y}_j^2$ when $\tilde{x}_j = \frac{\tilde{y}_j}{\lambda_j}$ $(1 \leq j \leq m)$. If, on the other hand, $\text{rank}(\boldsymbol{A}) = r < m$, it takes the minimum value Q when $\tilde{x}_j = \frac{\tilde{y}_j}{\lambda_j}$ $(1 \leq j \leq r)$ and $\tilde{x}_j = z_j$ $(r+1 \leq j \leq m)$, where z_j is an arbitrary constant. Since $\tilde{\boldsymbol{x}} = \boldsymbol{V}'\boldsymbol{x}$ and $\boldsymbol{x} = \boldsymbol{V}\tilde{\boldsymbol{x}}$, so that $||\boldsymbol{x}||^2 = \tilde{\boldsymbol{x}}'\boldsymbol{V}'\boldsymbol{V}\tilde{\boldsymbol{x}} = ||\tilde{\boldsymbol{x}}||^2$, $||\boldsymbol{x}||^2$ takes a minimum value when $z_j = 0$ $(r+1 \leq j \leq m)$. The $\boldsymbol{x}$ obtained this way coincides with $\boldsymbol{x} = \boldsymbol{A}^+\boldsymbol{y}$, where $\boldsymbol{A}^+$ is the Moore-Penrose inverse of $\boldsymbol{A}$.

10. We follow Eckart and Young's (1936) original proof, which is quite intriguing. However, it requires somewhat advanced knowledge in linear algebra:

(1) For a full orthogonal matrix $\boldsymbol{U}$, an infinitesimal change in $\boldsymbol{U}$ can be represented as $\boldsymbol{K}\boldsymbol{U}$ for some skew-symmetric matrix $\boldsymbol{K}$.

(2) Let $\boldsymbol{K}$ be a skew-symmetric matrix. Then, $\text{tr}(\boldsymbol{S}\boldsymbol{K}) = 0 \Longleftrightarrow \boldsymbol{S} = \boldsymbol{S}'$.

(3) In this problem, both $\boldsymbol{B}\boldsymbol{A}'$ and $\boldsymbol{A}'\boldsymbol{B}$ are symmetric.

(4) Both $\boldsymbol{B}\boldsymbol{A}'$ and $\boldsymbol{A}'\boldsymbol{B}$ are symmetric if and only if both $\boldsymbol{A}$ and $\boldsymbol{B}$ are diagonalizable by the same pair of orthogonals, i.e., $\boldsymbol{A} = \boldsymbol{U}\boldsymbol{\Delta}_A\boldsymbol{V}'$ and $\boldsymbol{B} = \boldsymbol{U}\boldsymbol{\Delta}_B\boldsymbol{V}'$.

(5) $\phi(\boldsymbol{B}) = ||\boldsymbol{\Delta}_A - \boldsymbol{\Delta}_B||^2$, where $\boldsymbol{\Delta}_B$ is a diagonal matrix of rank k.

Let us now elaborate on the above:

(1) Since $\boldsymbol{U}$ is fully orthogonal, we have $\boldsymbol{U}\boldsymbol{U}' = \boldsymbol{I}$. Let an infinitesimal change in $\boldsymbol{U}$ be denoted as $d\boldsymbol{U}$. Then, $d\boldsymbol{U}\boldsymbol{U}' + \boldsymbol{U}d\boldsymbol{U}' = \boldsymbol{O}$, which implies $d\boldsymbol{U}\boldsymbol{U}' = \boldsymbol{K}$, where $\boldsymbol{K}$ is skew-symmetric. Postmultiplying both sides by $\boldsymbol{U}$, we obtain $d\boldsymbol{U} = \boldsymbol{K}\boldsymbol{U}$.

(2) Let $\boldsymbol{S}$ be a symmetric matrix. Then, $\text{tr}(\boldsymbol{SK}) = -\text{tr}(\boldsymbol{SK})$, which implies $\text{tr}(\boldsymbol{SK}) = 0$. Conversely, if $\text{tr}(\boldsymbol{SK}) = 0$, then $\text{tr}((\boldsymbol{S} - \boldsymbol{S}')\boldsymbol{K}) = 0$. Since $\boldsymbol{S} - \boldsymbol{S}'$ is skew-symmetric as well as $\boldsymbol{K}$, the only way this can hold is for $\boldsymbol{S} - \boldsymbol{S}' = \boldsymbol{O}$.

(3) $\phi(\boldsymbol{B})$ can be expanded as $\phi(\boldsymbol{B}) = ||\boldsymbol{A}||^2 - 2\text{tr}(\boldsymbol{A}'\boldsymbol{B}) + ||\boldsymbol{B}||^2$. Let $\boldsymbol{B} = \boldsymbol{U}\boldsymbol{\Delta}_B\boldsymbol{V}'$ be the SVD of $\boldsymbol{B}$. Then, $\phi(\boldsymbol{B}) = ||\boldsymbol{A}||^2 - 2\text{tr}(\boldsymbol{A}'\boldsymbol{U}\boldsymbol{\Delta}_B\boldsymbol{V}') + ||\boldsymbol{\Delta}_B||^2$. The change in $\phi(\boldsymbol{B})$ as a result of an infinitesimal change in $\boldsymbol{U}$ has to be 0 at a minimum of ϕ. This implies that $\text{tr}(\boldsymbol{A}'d\boldsymbol{U}\boldsymbol{\Delta}\boldsymbol{V}') = \text{tr}(\boldsymbol{A}'\boldsymbol{K}\boldsymbol{U}\boldsymbol{\Delta}_B\boldsymbol{V}') = \text{tr}(\boldsymbol{U}\boldsymbol{\Delta}_B\boldsymbol{V}'\boldsymbol{A}'\boldsymbol{K}) = \text{tr}(\boldsymbol{B}\boldsymbol{A}'\boldsymbol{K}) = 0$, i.e., $\boldsymbol{B}\boldsymbol{A}'$ must be symmetric. By a similar line of argument for $\boldsymbol{V}$, $\boldsymbol{A}'\boldsymbol{B}$ must also be symmetric.

(4) If $\boldsymbol{A}$ and $\boldsymbol{B}$ are diagonalizable by the same pair of orthonormals (i.e., if $\boldsymbol{A} = \boldsymbol{U}\boldsymbol{\Delta}_A\boldsymbol{V}'$ and $\boldsymbol{B} = \boldsymbol{U}\boldsymbol{\Delta}_B\boldsymbol{V}'$), then we have $\boldsymbol{B}\boldsymbol{A}' = \boldsymbol{U}\boldsymbol{\Delta}_B\boldsymbol{V}'\boldsymbol{V}\boldsymbol{\Delta}_A\boldsymbol{U} = \boldsymbol{U}\boldsymbol{D}\boldsymbol{U}'$ (symmetric) and $\boldsymbol{A}'\boldsymbol{B} = \boldsymbol{V}\boldsymbol{\Delta}_A\boldsymbol{U}'\boldsymbol{U}\boldsymbol{\Delta}_B\boldsymbol{V}' = \boldsymbol{V}\boldsymbol{D}\boldsymbol{V}'$ (symmetric). Conversely, let both $\boldsymbol{B}\boldsymbol{A}'$ and $\boldsymbol{A}'\boldsymbol{B}$ be symmetric. Then, $\boldsymbol{B}\boldsymbol{A}' = \boldsymbol{U}\boldsymbol{D}_1\boldsymbol{U}'$, and $\boldsymbol{A}'\boldsymbol{B} = \boldsymbol{V}\boldsymbol{D}_1\boldsymbol{V}'$ for some orthogonal matrices $\boldsymbol{U}$ and $\boldsymbol{V}$ and diagonal matrices $\boldsymbol{D}_1$ and $\boldsymbol{D}_2$. We have $\boldsymbol{U}\boldsymbol{D}_1^2\boldsymbol{U}' = (\boldsymbol{B}\boldsymbol{A}')^2 = \boldsymbol{B}(\boldsymbol{A}'\boldsymbol{B})\boldsymbol{A}' = \boldsymbol{B}\boldsymbol{V}\boldsymbol{D}_2\boldsymbol{V}'\boldsymbol{A}'$. Pre- and postmultiplying both sides by $\boldsymbol{U}'$ and $\boldsymbol{U}$, respectively, we obtain $\boldsymbol{D}_1^2 = (\boldsymbol{U}'\boldsymbol{B}\boldsymbol{V})\boldsymbol{D}_2(\boldsymbol{V}'\boldsymbol{A}'\boldsymbol{U})$. This implies that both $\boldsymbol{U}'\boldsymbol{B}\boldsymbol{V}$ and $\boldsymbol{V}'\boldsymbol{A}'\boldsymbol{U}$ are diagonal, or $\boldsymbol{A} = \boldsymbol{U}\boldsymbol{\Delta}\boldsymbol{V}'$ and $\boldsymbol{B} = \boldsymbol{U}\boldsymbol{\Delta}_B\boldsymbol{V}'$ for some diagonal matrices $\boldsymbol{\Delta}_A$ and $\boldsymbol{\Delta}_B$.

(5) Let the columns of $\boldsymbol{U}$ or $\boldsymbol{V}$ be permuted and reflected so that the diagonal elements of $\boldsymbol{\Delta}_A$ are all positive and in descending order of magnitude. Then, $\phi(\boldsymbol{B}) = ||\boldsymbol{\Delta}_A - \boldsymbol{\Delta}_B||^2$, where $\boldsymbol{\Delta}_B$ is a diagonal matrix of rank k. Hence, $\phi(\boldsymbol{B})$ is minimized when $\boldsymbol{\Delta}_B$ is a diagonal matrix with the leading k diagonal elements equal to those in $\boldsymbol{\Delta}_A$ and the rest equal to zero. See ten Berge (1993) for an alternative proof.

11. We use the Lagrangean multiplier method to impose the orthogonality constraint on $\boldsymbol{T}$ (i.e., $\boldsymbol{T}'\boldsymbol{T} = \boldsymbol{T}\boldsymbol{T}' = \boldsymbol{I}$). To minimize $\phi(\boldsymbol{T}, \boldsymbol{S}) = ||\boldsymbol{B} - \boldsymbol{A}\boldsymbol{T}||^2 + \text{tr}(\boldsymbol{S}(\boldsymbol{T}'\boldsymbol{T} - \boldsymbol{I}))$, where $\boldsymbol{S}$ is a symmetric matrix of Lagrangean multipliers, we differentiate ϕ with respect to $\boldsymbol{T}$ and set the result to zero. We obtain $\frac{1}{2}\frac{\partial\phi}{\partial\boldsymbol{T}} = -\boldsymbol{A}'(\boldsymbol{B} - \boldsymbol{A}\boldsymbol{T}) + \boldsymbol{T}\boldsymbol{S} = \boldsymbol{O}$. Premultiplying both sides by $\boldsymbol{T}'$, we obtain $\boldsymbol{T}'\boldsymbol{A}'\boldsymbol{A}\boldsymbol{T} + \boldsymbol{S} = \boldsymbol{T}'\boldsymbol{A}'\boldsymbol{B}$. This indicates that $\boldsymbol{T}'\boldsymbol{A}'\boldsymbol{B}$ is symmetric since the left-hand side is obviously symmetric. That is, $\boldsymbol{T}'\boldsymbol{A}'\boldsymbol{B} = \boldsymbol{B}'\boldsymbol{A}\boldsymbol{T}$ or $\boldsymbol{A}'\boldsymbol{B} = \boldsymbol{T}\boldsymbol{B}'\boldsymbol{A}\boldsymbol{T}$. Let the SVD of $\boldsymbol{A}'\boldsymbol{B}$ be denoted as $\boldsymbol{A}'\boldsymbol{B} = \boldsymbol{U}\boldsymbol{\Delta}\boldsymbol{V}'$. Then, $\boldsymbol{U}\boldsymbol{\Delta}\boldsymbol{V}' = \boldsymbol{T}\boldsymbol{V}\boldsymbol{\Delta}\boldsymbol{U}'\boldsymbol{T}$, from which $\boldsymbol{T} = \boldsymbol{U}\boldsymbol{V}'$ follows immediately.

7.6 Chapter 6

1. From $\text{Sp}(\boldsymbol{X}) = \text{Sp}(\tilde{\boldsymbol{X}})$, it follows that $\boldsymbol{P}_X = \boldsymbol{P}_{\tilde{X}}$. Hence, $R^2_{X\cdot y} = \dfrac{\boldsymbol{y}'\boldsymbol{P}_X\boldsymbol{y}}{\boldsymbol{y}'\boldsymbol{y}} = \dfrac{\boldsymbol{y}'\boldsymbol{P}_{\tilde{X}}\boldsymbol{y}}{\boldsymbol{y}'\boldsymbol{y}} = R^2_{\tilde{X}\cdot y}$.

2. We first prove the case in which $\boldsymbol{X} = [\boldsymbol{x}_1, \boldsymbol{x}_2]$. We have

$$1 - R^2_{X\cdot y} = \frac{\boldsymbol{y}'\boldsymbol{y} - \boldsymbol{y}'\boldsymbol{P}_X\boldsymbol{y}}{\boldsymbol{y}'\boldsymbol{y}} = \left(\frac{\boldsymbol{y}'\boldsymbol{y} - \boldsymbol{y}'\boldsymbol{P}_{x_1}\boldsymbol{y}}{\boldsymbol{y}'\boldsymbol{y}}\right)\left(\frac{\boldsymbol{y}'\boldsymbol{y} - \boldsymbol{y}'\boldsymbol{P}_{x_1x_2}\boldsymbol{y}}{\boldsymbol{y}'\boldsymbol{y} - \boldsymbol{y}'\boldsymbol{P}_{x_1}\boldsymbol{y}}\right).$$

The first factor on the right-hand side is equal to $1 - r^2_{x_1 y}$, and the second factor is equal to

$$1 - \frac{\boldsymbol{y}'\boldsymbol{Q}_{x_1}\boldsymbol{x}_2(\boldsymbol{x}_2'\boldsymbol{Q}_{x_1}\boldsymbol{x}_2)^{-1}\boldsymbol{x}_2'\boldsymbol{Q}_{x_1}\boldsymbol{y}}{\boldsymbol{y}'\boldsymbol{Q}_{x_1}\boldsymbol{y}} = 1 - \frac{||\boldsymbol{Q}_{x_1}\boldsymbol{x}_2||^2}{||\boldsymbol{Q}_{x_1}\boldsymbol{y}||^2||\boldsymbol{Q}_{x_1}\boldsymbol{x}_2||^2} = 1 - r^2_{x_2 y|x_1}$$

since $\boldsymbol{P}_{x_1x_2} = \boldsymbol{P}_{x_1} + \boldsymbol{Q}_{x_1}\boldsymbol{x}_2(\boldsymbol{x}_2'\boldsymbol{Q}_{x_1}\boldsymbol{x}_2)^{-1}\boldsymbol{x}_2'\boldsymbol{Q}_{x_1}$.

Let

$$\boldsymbol{X}_{j+1} = [\boldsymbol{x}_1, \boldsymbol{x}_2, \cdots, \boldsymbol{x}_j, \boldsymbol{x}_{j+1}] = [\boldsymbol{X}_j, \boldsymbol{x}_{j+1}].$$

Then, $\boldsymbol{P}_{X_{j+1}} = \boldsymbol{P}_{X_j} + \boldsymbol{Q}_{X_j}\boldsymbol{x}_{j+1}(\boldsymbol{x}_{j+1}'\boldsymbol{Q}_{X_j}\boldsymbol{x}_{j+1})^{-1}\boldsymbol{x}_{j+1}'\boldsymbol{Q}_{X_j}$, and so

$$\begin{aligned} 1 - R^2_{X_{j+1}\cdot y} &= (1 - R^2_{X_j\cdot y})\left(1 - \frac{(\boldsymbol{Q}_{X_j}\boldsymbol{x}_{j+1}, \boldsymbol{Q}_{X_j}\boldsymbol{y})}{||\boldsymbol{Q}_{X_j}\boldsymbol{x}_{j+1}||\,||\boldsymbol{Q}_{X_j}\boldsymbol{y}||}\right) \\ &= (1 - R^2_{X_j\cdot y})(1 - r^2_{x_{j+1}y|x_1x_2\cdots x_j}), \end{aligned}$$

leading to the given equation.

3. ($\Rightarrow$) Let $\boldsymbol{K}'\boldsymbol{y}$ denote an unbiased estimator of $\mathrm{E}(\boldsymbol{L}'y) = \boldsymbol{L}'X\boldsymbol{\beta}$. Then, $\mathrm{E}(\boldsymbol{K}'\boldsymbol{y}) = \boldsymbol{K}'\boldsymbol{X}\boldsymbol{\beta} = \boldsymbol{L}'\boldsymbol{X}\boldsymbol{\beta}$ for $\forall\boldsymbol{\beta} \in E^p$. Hence, $(\boldsymbol{K} - \boldsymbol{L})'\boldsymbol{X} = \boldsymbol{O}$, and $(\boldsymbol{K} - \boldsymbol{L})' = \boldsymbol{P}'(\boldsymbol{I} - \boldsymbol{X}\boldsymbol{X}^-) \Rightarrow \boldsymbol{K}' = \boldsymbol{L}' + \boldsymbol{P}'(\boldsymbol{I} - \boldsymbol{X}\boldsymbol{X}^-)$, where $\boldsymbol{P}$ is arbitrary. $\mathrm{V}(\boldsymbol{K}'\boldsymbol{y}) = \sigma^2\boldsymbol{K}'\boldsymbol{G}\boldsymbol{K} = \sigma^2||\boldsymbol{L} + (\boldsymbol{I} - \boldsymbol{X}\boldsymbol{X}^-)'\boldsymbol{P}||^2_G$. Since $\mathrm{V}(\boldsymbol{L}'\boldsymbol{y}) \le \mathrm{V}(\boldsymbol{K}'\boldsymbol{y})$ holds for arbitrary $\boldsymbol{P}$, we have $(\boldsymbol{I} - \boldsymbol{X}\boldsymbol{X}^-)\boldsymbol{G}\boldsymbol{L} = \boldsymbol{O}$, which implies $\boldsymbol{G}\boldsymbol{L} \in \mathrm{Sp}(\boldsymbol{X})$.

($\Leftarrow$) It suffices to show the reverse of the above. Let $\boldsymbol{K}'\boldsymbol{y}$ denote an unbiased estimator of $\mathrm{E}(\boldsymbol{L}'\boldsymbol{y})$. Then, $\frac{1}{\sigma^2}\mathrm{V}(\boldsymbol{K}'\boldsymbol{y}) = ||\boldsymbol{L}+(\boldsymbol{I}-\boldsymbol{X}\boldsymbol{X}^-)'\boldsymbol{P}||^2_G = \mathrm{tr}(\boldsymbol{L}'\boldsymbol{G}\boldsymbol{L}+\boldsymbol{P}(\boldsymbol{I}-\boldsymbol{X}\boldsymbol{X}^-)'\boldsymbol{G}(\boldsymbol{I}-\boldsymbol{X}\boldsymbol{X}^-)'\boldsymbol{P}+2\boldsymbol{P}'(\boldsymbol{I}-\boldsymbol{X}\boldsymbol{X}^-)\boldsymbol{G}\boldsymbol{L})$. When $\boldsymbol{G}\boldsymbol{L} \in \mathrm{Sp}(\boldsymbol{X})$, the third term in the trace is a zero matrix and the second term is *nnd*. Hence, $\mathrm{V}(\boldsymbol{L}'\boldsymbol{y}) \le \mathrm{V}(\boldsymbol{K}'\boldsymbol{y})$.

4. Let $\boldsymbol{\ell}'\boldsymbol{y}$ denote the BLUE of an estimable function $\boldsymbol{e}'\boldsymbol{\beta}$. Then, $\mathrm{E}(\boldsymbol{\ell}'\boldsymbol{y}) = \boldsymbol{\ell}'\boldsymbol{X}\boldsymbol{\beta} = \boldsymbol{e}'\boldsymbol{\beta}$ for $\forall\boldsymbol{\beta} \in E^p$, which implies that $\boldsymbol{X}'\boldsymbol{\ell} = \boldsymbol{e}$, and $\mathrm{V}(\boldsymbol{\ell}'\boldsymbol{y}) = \sigma^2\boldsymbol{\ell}'\boldsymbol{G}\boldsymbol{\ell} = \sigma^2||\boldsymbol{\ell}||^2_G$ is a minimum. Hence, $\boldsymbol{\ell} = (\boldsymbol{X}')^-_{m(G)}\boldsymbol{e}$. Let $\boldsymbol{Y}' = (\boldsymbol{X}')^-_{m(G)}$. Then,

$$\left\{\begin{array}{l} \boldsymbol{X}'\boldsymbol{Y}'\boldsymbol{X}' = \boldsymbol{X}' \\ \boldsymbol{G}\boldsymbol{Y}'\boldsymbol{X}' = (\boldsymbol{X}\boldsymbol{Y})\boldsymbol{G} \end{array}\right. \Longleftrightarrow \left\{\begin{array}{l} \boldsymbol{X}\boldsymbol{Y}\boldsymbol{X} = \boldsymbol{X} \\ \boldsymbol{X}\boldsymbol{Y}\boldsymbol{G} = \boldsymbol{G}(\boldsymbol{X}\boldsymbol{Y})' \end{array}\right.,$$

where $\boldsymbol{G}(\boldsymbol{X}\boldsymbol{Y})' = \boldsymbol{P}_X\boldsymbol{G}(\boldsymbol{X}\boldsymbol{Y})'$ and $\boldsymbol{P}_X$ is the orthogonal projector onto $\mathrm{Sp}(\boldsymbol{X})$. Transposing both sides, we obtain $\boldsymbol{X}\boldsymbol{Y}\boldsymbol{G} = \boldsymbol{X}\boldsymbol{Y}\boldsymbol{G}\boldsymbol{P}_X \Rightarrow \boldsymbol{X}\boldsymbol{Y}\boldsymbol{G}\boldsymbol{Q}_X = \boldsymbol{O}$. Hence, $\boldsymbol{Z} = \boldsymbol{Q}_X\boldsymbol{Z}$ for $\boldsymbol{Z}$ such that $\mathrm{Sp}(\boldsymbol{Z}) = \mathrm{Sp}(\boldsymbol{X})^\perp$, and so

$$\boldsymbol{X}\boldsymbol{Y}\boldsymbol{G}\boldsymbol{Z} = \boldsymbol{O}.$$

The above shows that $\boldsymbol{Y}$ is a GZ-constrained g-inverse of $\boldsymbol{X}$, denoted as $\boldsymbol{X}^-_{\ell(GZ)}$. That is, $\boldsymbol{\ell}'\boldsymbol{y} = \boldsymbol{e}'\boldsymbol{Y}\boldsymbol{y} = \boldsymbol{e}'\boldsymbol{X}^-_{\ell(GZ)}\boldsymbol{y}$.

5. Choose $\boldsymbol{Z} = \boldsymbol{Q}_X = \boldsymbol{I}_n - \boldsymbol{P}_X$, which is symmetric. Then,

(i) $\mathrm{E}(\boldsymbol{y}'\boldsymbol{Z}'(\boldsymbol{Z}\boldsymbol{G}\boldsymbol{Z})^-\boldsymbol{Z}\boldsymbol{y}) = \mathrm{E}\{\mathrm{tr}(\boldsymbol{Z}(\boldsymbol{Z}\boldsymbol{G}\boldsymbol{Z})^-\boldsymbol{Z}\boldsymbol{y}\boldsymbol{y}')\}$
$= \mathrm{tr}\{\boldsymbol{Z}(\boldsymbol{Z}\boldsymbol{G}\boldsymbol{Z})^-\boldsymbol{Z}\mathrm{E}(\boldsymbol{y}\boldsymbol{y}')\}$
$= \mathrm{tr}\{\boldsymbol{Z}(\boldsymbol{Z}\boldsymbol{G}\boldsymbol{Z})^-\boldsymbol{Z}(\boldsymbol{X}\boldsymbol{\beta}\boldsymbol{\beta}'\boldsymbol{X}' + \sigma^2\boldsymbol{G})\}$

$$= \sigma^2 \mathrm{tr}(\boldsymbol{Z}(\boldsymbol{ZGZ})^- \boldsymbol{ZG}) \qquad (\text{since } \boldsymbol{ZX} = \boldsymbol{O})$$
$$= \sigma^2 \mathrm{tr}\{(\boldsymbol{ZG})(\boldsymbol{ZG})^-\}$$
$$= \sigma^2 \mathrm{tr}(\boldsymbol{P}_{GZ}).$$

On the other hand, $\mathrm{tr}(\boldsymbol{P}_{GZ}) = \mathrm{rank}([\boldsymbol{X}, \boldsymbol{G}]) - \mathrm{rank}(\boldsymbol{X}) = f$ since $\mathrm{Sp}(\boldsymbol{X}) \oplus \mathrm{Sp}(\boldsymbol{G}) = \mathrm{Sp}(\boldsymbol{X}) \oplus \mathrm{Sp}(\boldsymbol{GZ})$, establishing the proposition.

(ii) From $\boldsymbol{y} \in \mathrm{Sp}([\boldsymbol{X}, \boldsymbol{G}])$, it suffices to show the equivalence between $\boldsymbol{TZ}(\boldsymbol{ZG} \times \boldsymbol{Z})^- \boldsymbol{ZT}$ and $\boldsymbol{TT}^-(\boldsymbol{I} - \boldsymbol{P}_{X/T^-})\boldsymbol{T}$. Let $\boldsymbol{T} = \boldsymbol{XW}_1 + (\boldsymbol{GZ})\boldsymbol{W}_2$. Then,

$$\begin{aligned} \boldsymbol{TZ}(\boldsymbol{ZGZ})^- \boldsymbol{ZT} &= \boldsymbol{TZ}(\boldsymbol{ZGZ})^- \boldsymbol{Z}(\boldsymbol{XW}_1 + \boldsymbol{GZW}_2) \\ &= \boldsymbol{TZ}(\boldsymbol{ZGZ})^- \boldsymbol{ZGZW}_2 \\ &= \boldsymbol{GZ}(\boldsymbol{ZGZ})^- \boldsymbol{ZGZW}_2 = \boldsymbol{GZW}_2, \end{aligned}$$

where we used $\boldsymbol{T} = \boldsymbol{G} + \boldsymbol{XUX}'$ to derive the second-to-last equality.

Furthermore, from the result of Exercise 6 in Chapter 4, $\boldsymbol{TT}^-(\boldsymbol{I} - \boldsymbol{P}_{X/T^-})\boldsymbol{T} = \boldsymbol{TT}^- \boldsymbol{P}_{GZ \cdot X} \boldsymbol{T}$, and the last equality follows from $\boldsymbol{T} = \boldsymbol{XW}_1 + (\boldsymbol{GZ})\boldsymbol{W}_2$.

6. (i) Let $\boldsymbol{G}^* = [\boldsymbol{G}, \boldsymbol{1}_n]$. Since $\mathrm{Sp}(\boldsymbol{1}_n) \subset \mathrm{Sp}(\boldsymbol{G})$,

$$\boldsymbol{P}_{G^*} = \boldsymbol{P}_G = \boldsymbol{P}_M + \boldsymbol{Q}_M \boldsymbol{G}(\boldsymbol{G}'\boldsymbol{Q}_M \boldsymbol{G})^- \boldsymbol{G}'\boldsymbol{Q}_M. \tag{7.6}$$

On the other hand, let $\tilde{\boldsymbol{G}} = [\boldsymbol{g}_1, \boldsymbol{g}_2, \cdots, \boldsymbol{g}_{m-1}]$. Then, $\mathrm{Sp}([\tilde{\boldsymbol{G}}, \boldsymbol{1}_n]) = \mathrm{Sp}(\boldsymbol{G})$. Therefore, $\boldsymbol{P}_G = \boldsymbol{P}_{\tilde{G} \cup 1} = \boldsymbol{P}_M + \boldsymbol{Q}_M \tilde{\boldsymbol{G}}(\tilde{\boldsymbol{G}}'\boldsymbol{Q}_M \tilde{\boldsymbol{G}})^- \tilde{\boldsymbol{G}}\boldsymbol{Q}_M$.

(ii) $\min_\alpha ||\boldsymbol{y} - \boldsymbol{G}^*\boldsymbol{\alpha}||^2 = ||\boldsymbol{y} - \boldsymbol{P}_{G^*}\boldsymbol{y}||^2$, and $\boldsymbol{P}_{G^*} = \boldsymbol{P}_G$. Let $\boldsymbol{y}_R$ be a vector of raw scores. Then, $\boldsymbol{y} = \boldsymbol{Q}_M \boldsymbol{y}$, so using (7.6) we obtain

$$\begin{aligned} ||\boldsymbol{y} - \boldsymbol{P}_{G^*}\boldsymbol{y}||^2 &= ||\boldsymbol{y} - \boldsymbol{P}_G \boldsymbol{y}||^2 \\ &= ||\boldsymbol{y} - \boldsymbol{P}_M \boldsymbol{y} - \boldsymbol{Q}_M \tilde{\boldsymbol{G}}(\tilde{\boldsymbol{G}}'\boldsymbol{Q}_M \tilde{\boldsymbol{G}})^{-1} \tilde{\boldsymbol{G}}'\boldsymbol{Q}_M \boldsymbol{y}||^2 \\ &= \boldsymbol{y}'(\boldsymbol{I} - \tilde{\boldsymbol{G}}(\tilde{\boldsymbol{G}}\boldsymbol{Q}_M \tilde{\boldsymbol{G}})^{-1} \tilde{\boldsymbol{G}}')\boldsymbol{y}. \end{aligned}$$

Note that $\boldsymbol{P}_M \boldsymbol{y} = \boldsymbol{0}$ and $\boldsymbol{Q}_M \boldsymbol{y} = \boldsymbol{y}$, since $\boldsymbol{y}$ is a vector of deviation scores from the means.

7. (i) Clear from $\mathrm{Sp}(\boldsymbol{Q}_G \boldsymbol{D}_x) \supset \mathrm{Sp}(\boldsymbol{Q}_G \boldsymbol{x})$.

(ii) $\boldsymbol{P}_x \boldsymbol{P}_{D_x[G]} = \boldsymbol{x}(\boldsymbol{x}'\boldsymbol{x})^{-1}\boldsymbol{x}'\boldsymbol{Q}_G \boldsymbol{D}_x(\boldsymbol{D}_x'\boldsymbol{Q}_G \boldsymbol{D}_x)^{-1}\boldsymbol{D}_x'\boldsymbol{Q}_G$
$= \boldsymbol{x}(\boldsymbol{x}'\boldsymbol{x})^{-1}\boldsymbol{1}_n'\boldsymbol{D}_x'\boldsymbol{Q}_G \boldsymbol{D}_x(\boldsymbol{D}_x'\boldsymbol{Q}_G \boldsymbol{D}_x)^{-1}\boldsymbol{D}_x'\boldsymbol{Q}_G$
$= \boldsymbol{x}(\boldsymbol{x}'\boldsymbol{x})^{-1}\boldsymbol{1}_n'\boldsymbol{D}_x'\boldsymbol{Q}_G = \boldsymbol{P}_x \boldsymbol{Q}_G$.

Noting that $\boldsymbol{P}_x \boldsymbol{P}_{x[G]} = \boldsymbol{x}(\boldsymbol{x}'\boldsymbol{x})^{-1}\boldsymbol{x}'\boldsymbol{Q}_G \boldsymbol{x}(\boldsymbol{x}'\boldsymbol{Q}_G \boldsymbol{x})^{-1}\boldsymbol{x}'\boldsymbol{Q}_G = \boldsymbol{P}_x \boldsymbol{Q}_G$ leads to the given equation.

(iii) and (iv) Use (4.47b) in the corollary to Theorem 4.8.

(v) Let a_i and b_i denote the estimates of parameters α_i and β_i in the model $y_{ij} = \alpha_i + \beta_i x_{ij} + \epsilon_{ij}$. Let

$$f(a_i, b_i) = \sum_{i=1}^{m} \sum_{j=1}^{n_i} (y_{ij} - a_i - b_i x_{ij})^2.$$

To minimize f defined above, we differentiate f with respect to a_i and set the result equal to zero. We obtain $a_i = \bar{y}_i - b_i\bar{x}_i$. Using the result in (iv), we obtain

$$f(\boldsymbol{b}) = \sum_{i=1}^{m}\sum_{j=1}^{n_i}\{(y_{ij} - \bar{y}_i) - b_i(x_{ij} - \bar{x}_i)\}^2 = ||\boldsymbol{y} - \boldsymbol{D}_x\boldsymbol{b}||^2_{Q_G} \geq ||\boldsymbol{y} - \boldsymbol{P}_{D_x[G]}\boldsymbol{y}||^2_{Q_G}.$$

Let b denote the estimate of β_i under the restriction that $\beta_i = \beta$ $(i = 1, \cdots, m)$. Then,

$$f(b) = \sum_{i=1}^{m}\sum_{j=1}^{n_i}\{(y_{ij} - \bar{y}_i) - b(x_{ij} - \bar{x}_i)\}^2 = ||\boldsymbol{y} - b\boldsymbol{x}||^2_{Q_G} \geq ||\boldsymbol{y} - \boldsymbol{P}_{x[G]}\boldsymbol{y}||^2_{Q_G},$$

leading to the given equation.

8. From

$$\begin{aligned} \boldsymbol{S}\boldsymbol{S}' &= \boldsymbol{\Delta}_X^{-1}\boldsymbol{U}_X\boldsymbol{C}_{XY}\boldsymbol{U}_Y'\boldsymbol{\Delta}_Y^{-2}\boldsymbol{U}_Y\boldsymbol{C}_{YX}\boldsymbol{U}_X'\boldsymbol{\Delta}_X^{-1} \\ &= \boldsymbol{\Delta}_X^{-1}\boldsymbol{U}_X\boldsymbol{C}_{XY}\boldsymbol{C}_{YY}^{-1}\boldsymbol{C}_{YX}\boldsymbol{U}_X'\boldsymbol{\Delta}_X^{-1}, \end{aligned}$$

we have $(\boldsymbol{S}\boldsymbol{S}')\boldsymbol{a} = (\boldsymbol{\Delta}_X^{-1}\boldsymbol{U}_X\boldsymbol{C}_{XY}\boldsymbol{C}_{YY}^{-1}\boldsymbol{C}_{YX}\boldsymbol{U}_X'\boldsymbol{\Delta}_X^{-1})\boldsymbol{\Delta}_X\boldsymbol{U}_X\tilde{\boldsymbol{a}} = \lambda\boldsymbol{\Delta}_X\boldsymbol{U}_X\tilde{\boldsymbol{a}}$, where $\tilde{\boldsymbol{a}} = \boldsymbol{U}_X'\boldsymbol{\Delta}_X^{-1}\boldsymbol{a}$. Premultiplying both sides by $\boldsymbol{U}_X'\boldsymbol{\Delta}_X$, we obtain $\boldsymbol{C}_{XY}\boldsymbol{C}_{YY}^{-1}\boldsymbol{C}_{YX}\tilde{\boldsymbol{a}}$ $= \lambda\boldsymbol{C}_{XX}\tilde{\boldsymbol{a}}$. The λ is an eigenvalue of $\boldsymbol{S}\boldsymbol{S}'$, and the equation above is the eigenequation for canonical correlation analysis, so that the singular values of $\boldsymbol{S}$ correspond to the canonical correlation coefficients between $\boldsymbol{X}$ and $\boldsymbol{Y}$.

9. Let $\boldsymbol{X}\boldsymbol{A}$ and $\boldsymbol{Y}\boldsymbol{B}$ denote the matrices of canonical variates corresponding to $\boldsymbol{X}$ and $\boldsymbol{Y}$, respectively. Furthermore, let $\rho_1, \rho_2, \cdots, \rho_r$ represent r canonical correlations when $\text{rank}(\boldsymbol{X}\boldsymbol{A}) = \text{rank}(\boldsymbol{Y}\boldsymbol{B}) = r$. In this case, if $\dim(\text{Sp}(\boldsymbol{Z})) = m$ $(m \leq r)$, m canonical correlations are 1. Let $\boldsymbol{X}\boldsymbol{A}_1$ and $\boldsymbol{Y}\boldsymbol{B}_1$ denote the canonical variates corresponding to the unit canonical correlations, and let $\boldsymbol{X}\boldsymbol{A}_2$ and $\boldsymbol{Y}\boldsymbol{B}_2$ be the canonical variates corresponding to the canonical correlations less than 1. Then, by Theorem 6.11, we have

$$\boldsymbol{P}_X\boldsymbol{P}_Y = \boldsymbol{P}_{XA}\boldsymbol{P}_{YB} = \boldsymbol{P}_{XA_1}\boldsymbol{P}_{YB_1} + \boldsymbol{P}_{XA_2}\boldsymbol{P}_{YB_2}.$$

From $\text{Sp}(\boldsymbol{X}\boldsymbol{A}_1) = \text{Sp}(\boldsymbol{Y}\boldsymbol{B}_1)$, we have

$$\boldsymbol{P}_{XA_1} = \boldsymbol{P}_{YB_2} = \boldsymbol{P}_Z,$$

where $\boldsymbol{Z}$ is such that $\text{Sp}(\boldsymbol{Z}) = \text{Sp}(\boldsymbol{X}) \cap \text{Sp}(\boldsymbol{Y})$. Hence, $\boldsymbol{P}_X\boldsymbol{P}_Y = \boldsymbol{P}_Z + \boldsymbol{P}_{XA_2}\boldsymbol{P}_{YB_2}$. Since $\boldsymbol{A}_2'\boldsymbol{X}'\boldsymbol{X}\boldsymbol{A}_2 = \boldsymbol{B}_2'\boldsymbol{Y}'\boldsymbol{Y}\boldsymbol{B}_2 = \boldsymbol{I}_{r-m}$, we also have $\boldsymbol{P}_{XA_2}\boldsymbol{P}_{YB_2} = \boldsymbol{X}\boldsymbol{A}_2(\boldsymbol{A}_2'\boldsymbol{X}'$ $\times \boldsymbol{Y}\boldsymbol{B}_2)\boldsymbol{B}_2'\boldsymbol{Y}' \Rightarrow (\boldsymbol{P}_{XA_2}\boldsymbol{P}_{YB_2})^k = \boldsymbol{X}\boldsymbol{A}_2(\boldsymbol{A}_2'\boldsymbol{X}'\boldsymbol{Y}\boldsymbol{B}_2)^k\boldsymbol{B}_2'\boldsymbol{Y}'$. Since

$$\boldsymbol{A}_2'\boldsymbol{X}\boldsymbol{Y}\boldsymbol{B}_2 = \begin{bmatrix} \rho_{m+1} & 0 & \cdots & 0 \\ 0 & \rho_{m+2} & \cdots & 0 \\ \vdots & \vdots & \ddots & \vdots \\ 0 & 0 & \cdots & \rho_r \end{bmatrix},$$

where $0 < \rho_j < 1$ $(j = m+1, \cdots, r)$, we obtain $\lim_{k\to\infty}(\boldsymbol{P}_{XA_2}\boldsymbol{P}_{YB_2})^k = \boldsymbol{O}$, leading to the given equation.
10. (i) From

$$\begin{bmatrix} \boldsymbol{X}'\boldsymbol{X} & \boldsymbol{X}'\boldsymbol{Y} \\ \boldsymbol{Y}'\boldsymbol{X} & \boldsymbol{Y}'\boldsymbol{Y} \end{bmatrix} = \begin{bmatrix} \boldsymbol{X}' \\ \boldsymbol{Y}' \end{bmatrix} [\ \boldsymbol{X} \quad \boldsymbol{Y}\ ] = \begin{bmatrix} \boldsymbol{X}' \\ \boldsymbol{Y}' \end{bmatrix} \begin{bmatrix} \boldsymbol{X}' \\ \boldsymbol{Y}' \end{bmatrix}',$$

$\boldsymbol{R}\boldsymbol{R}^- = \begin{bmatrix} \boldsymbol{X}' \\ \boldsymbol{Y}' \end{bmatrix} \begin{bmatrix} \boldsymbol{X}' \\ \boldsymbol{Y}' \end{bmatrix}^-$. From (3.12), $\{(\boldsymbol{R}\boldsymbol{R}^-)'\} = \{[\boldsymbol{X}, \boldsymbol{Y}]^-[\boldsymbol{X}, \boldsymbol{Y}]\}$, and so

$$\mathrm{Sp}\{(\boldsymbol{I}_{p+q} - \boldsymbol{R}\boldsymbol{R}^-)'\} = \mathrm{Sp}\{(\boldsymbol{I}_{p+q} - [\boldsymbol{X}, \boldsymbol{Y}]^-[\boldsymbol{X}, \boldsymbol{Y}])\}.$$

(ii) From $\begin{bmatrix} \boldsymbol{X}' \\ \boldsymbol{Y}' \end{bmatrix} \begin{bmatrix} \boldsymbol{X}' \\ \boldsymbol{Y}' \end{bmatrix}^- \begin{bmatrix} \boldsymbol{X}' \\ \boldsymbol{Y}' \end{bmatrix} = \begin{bmatrix} \boldsymbol{X}' \\ \boldsymbol{Y}' \end{bmatrix}$, $\boldsymbol{R}\boldsymbol{R}^- \begin{bmatrix} \boldsymbol{X}' \\ \boldsymbol{Y}' \end{bmatrix} = \begin{bmatrix} \boldsymbol{X}' \\ \boldsymbol{Y}' \end{bmatrix}$. It follows that $\boldsymbol{S}_{11}\boldsymbol{X}' + \boldsymbol{S}_{12}\boldsymbol{Y}' = \boldsymbol{X}' \Rightarrow \boldsymbol{S}_{12}\boldsymbol{Y}' = (\boldsymbol{I}_p - \boldsymbol{S}_{11})\boldsymbol{X}'$. Premultiply both sides by $\boldsymbol{Q}_Y$.

(iii) From (ii), $(\boldsymbol{I}_p - \boldsymbol{S}_{11})\boldsymbol{X}' = \boldsymbol{S}_{12}\boldsymbol{Y}' \Rightarrow \boldsymbol{X}(\boldsymbol{I}_p - \boldsymbol{S}_{11})' = \boldsymbol{Y}\boldsymbol{S}_{12}'$. Similarly, $(\boldsymbol{I}_p - \boldsymbol{S}_{22})\boldsymbol{Y}' = \boldsymbol{S}_{21}\boldsymbol{X}' \Rightarrow \boldsymbol{Y}(\boldsymbol{I}_q - \boldsymbol{S}_{22}) = \boldsymbol{X}\boldsymbol{S}_{21}'$. Use Theorem 1.4.
11. (i) Define the factor analysis model as

$$\boldsymbol{z}_j = a_{j1}\boldsymbol{f}_1 + a_{j2}\boldsymbol{f}_2 + \cdots + a_{jr}\boldsymbol{f}_r + u_j\boldsymbol{v}_j \quad (j = 1, \cdots, p),$$

where $\boldsymbol{z}_j$ is a vector of standardized scores, $\boldsymbol{f}_i$ is a vector of common factor scores, a_{ji} is the factor loading of the jth variable on the ith common factor, $\boldsymbol{v}_j$ is the vector of unique factors, and u_j is the unique factor loading for variable j. The model above can be rewritten as

$$\boldsymbol{Z} = \boldsymbol{F}\boldsymbol{A}' + \boldsymbol{V}\boldsymbol{U}$$

using matrix notation. Hence,

$$\begin{aligned} \frac{1}{n}||\boldsymbol{P}_F\boldsymbol{z}_j||^2 &= \frac{1}{n}\boldsymbol{z}_j'\boldsymbol{F}\left(\frac{1}{n}F'F\right)^{-1}\left(\frac{1}{n}\boldsymbol{F}'\boldsymbol{z}_j\right) \\ &= \frac{1}{n}(\boldsymbol{F}'\boldsymbol{z}_j)'(\boldsymbol{F}'\boldsymbol{z}_j) = \boldsymbol{a}_j'\boldsymbol{a}_j = \sum_{i=1}^{r} a_{ji}^2 = h_j^2. \end{aligned}$$

(ii) $\mathrm{tr}(\boldsymbol{P}_F\boldsymbol{P}_Z) \le \min(\mathrm{rank}(\boldsymbol{F}), \mathrm{rank}(\boldsymbol{Z})) = \mathrm{rank}(\boldsymbol{F}) = r$.

(iii) $\boldsymbol{H}_j = [\boldsymbol{F}, \boldsymbol{Z}_{(j)}] \Rightarrow R^2_{H_j\cdot z_j} = \frac{1}{n}||\boldsymbol{P}_{H_j}\boldsymbol{z}_j||^2 = \frac{1}{n}||(\boldsymbol{P}_F + \boldsymbol{P}_{Z_{(j)}[F]}\boldsymbol{z}_j||^2$. On the other hand, from $\frac{1}{n}\boldsymbol{Z}_{(j)}'\boldsymbol{Q}_F\boldsymbol{z}_j = \frac{1}{n}(\boldsymbol{Z}_{(j)}'\boldsymbol{z}_j - \boldsymbol{Z}_{(j)}'\boldsymbol{P}_F\boldsymbol{z}_j) = \boldsymbol{r}_j - \boldsymbol{A}'\boldsymbol{a}_j = \boldsymbol{0}$, $R^2_{H_j\cdot z_j} = h_j^2$. From $\boldsymbol{P}_{H_j} = \boldsymbol{P}_{Z_{(j)}} + \boldsymbol{P}_{F[Z_{(j)}]}$, $R^2_{H_j\cdot z_j} = R^2_{Z_{(j)}\cdot z_j} + \boldsymbol{S}$, where $\boldsymbol{S} \ge \boldsymbol{O}$. Hence, $R^2_{Z_{(j)}\cdot z_j} \le h_j$. (See Takeuchi, Yanai, and Mukherjee (1982, p. 288) for more details.)
12. (i) Use the fact that $\mathrm{Sp}(\boldsymbol{P}_{X\cdot Z}\boldsymbol{P}_{Y\cdot Z}) = \mathrm{Sp}(\boldsymbol{X}\boldsymbol{A})$ from $(\boldsymbol{P}_{X\cdot Z}\boldsymbol{P}_{Y\cdot Z})\boldsymbol{X}\boldsymbol{A} = \boldsymbol{X}\boldsymbol{A}\boldsymbol{\Delta}$.

(ii) Use the fact that $\mathrm{Sp}(\boldsymbol{P}_{Y\cdot Z}\boldsymbol{P}_{X\cdot Z}) = \mathrm{Sp}(\boldsymbol{YB})$ from $(\boldsymbol{P}_{Y\cdot Z}\boldsymbol{P}_{X\cdot Z})\boldsymbol{YB} = \boldsymbol{YB\Delta}$.

(iii) $\boldsymbol{P}_{XA\cdot Z}\boldsymbol{P}_{X\cdot Z} = \boldsymbol{XA}(\boldsymbol{A}'\boldsymbol{X}'\boldsymbol{Q}_Z\boldsymbol{XA})^-\boldsymbol{A}'\boldsymbol{X}'\boldsymbol{Q}_Z\boldsymbol{X}(\boldsymbol{X}'\boldsymbol{Q}_Z\boldsymbol{X})^-\boldsymbol{X}\boldsymbol{Q}_Z$
$= \boldsymbol{XA}(\boldsymbol{A}'\boldsymbol{X}'\boldsymbol{Q}_Z\boldsymbol{XA})^-\boldsymbol{A}'\boldsymbol{X}'\boldsymbol{Q}_Z = \boldsymbol{P}_{XA\cdot Z}$.

Hence, $\boldsymbol{P}_{XA\cdot Z}\boldsymbol{P}_{Y\cdot Z} = \boldsymbol{P}_{XA\cdot Z}\boldsymbol{P}_{X\cdot Z}\boldsymbol{P}_{Y\cdot Z} = \boldsymbol{P}_{X\cdot Z}\boldsymbol{P}_{Y\cdot Z}$.

We next show that $\boldsymbol{P}_{X\cdot Z}\boldsymbol{P}_{YB\cdot Z} = \boldsymbol{P}_{X\cdot Z}\boldsymbol{P}_{Y\cdot Z}$. Similar to the proof of $\boldsymbol{P}_{XA\cdot Z}$ $\boldsymbol{P}_{Y\cdot Z} = \boldsymbol{P}_{X\cdot Z}\boldsymbol{P}_{Y\cdot Z}$ above, we have $\boldsymbol{P}_{YB\cdot Z}\boldsymbol{P}_{X\cdot Z} = \boldsymbol{P}_{Y\cdot Z}\boldsymbol{P}_{X\cdot Z}$. Premultiplying both sides by $\boldsymbol{Q}_Z$, we get

$$\boldsymbol{P}_{YB[Z]}\boldsymbol{P}_{X[Z]} = \boldsymbol{P}_{Y[Z]}\boldsymbol{P}_{X[Z]},$$

and, by transposition, we obtain

$$\boldsymbol{P}_{X[Z]}\boldsymbol{P}_{Y[Z]} = \boldsymbol{P}_{Y[Z]}\boldsymbol{P}_{X[Z]}.$$

Premultiplying both sides by $\boldsymbol{X}(\boldsymbol{X}'\boldsymbol{Q}_Z\boldsymbol{X})^-\boldsymbol{X}'$, we obtain $\boldsymbol{P}_{X\cdot Z}\boldsymbol{P}_{Y\cdot Z} = \boldsymbol{P}_{X\cdot Z} \times \boldsymbol{P}_{YB\cdot Z}$, from which it follows that

$$\begin{aligned} \boldsymbol{P}_{XA\cdot Z}\boldsymbol{P}_{YB\cdot Z} &= \boldsymbol{P}_{XA\cdot Z}\boldsymbol{P}_{X\cdot Z}\boldsymbol{P}_{YB\cdot Z} = \boldsymbol{P}_{XA\cdot Z}\boldsymbol{P}_{X\cdot Z}\boldsymbol{P}_{Y\cdot Z} \\ &= \boldsymbol{P}_{XA\cdot Z}\boldsymbol{P}_{Y\cdot Z} = \boldsymbol{P}_{X\cdot Z}\boldsymbol{P}_{Y\cdot Z}. \end{aligned}$$

13.

$$\boldsymbol{Ax} = \boldsymbol{b} \Rightarrow ||\boldsymbol{A}||||\boldsymbol{x}|| \geq ||\boldsymbol{b}||. \tag{7.7}$$

From $\boldsymbol{A}(\boldsymbol{x} + \Delta\boldsymbol{x}) = \boldsymbol{b} + \Delta\boldsymbol{b}$,

$$\boldsymbol{A}\Delta\boldsymbol{x} = \Delta\boldsymbol{b} \rightarrow \Delta\boldsymbol{x} = \boldsymbol{A}^{-1}\Delta\boldsymbol{b} \Rightarrow ||\Delta\boldsymbol{x}|| \leq ||\boldsymbol{A}^{-1}||||\Delta\boldsymbol{b}||. \tag{7.8}$$

From (7.7) and (7.8),

$$\frac{||\Delta\boldsymbol{x}||}{||\boldsymbol{x}||} \leq \frac{||\boldsymbol{A}||||\boldsymbol{A}^{-1}||||\Delta\boldsymbol{b}||}{||\boldsymbol{b}||}.$$

Let $||\boldsymbol{A}||$ and $||\boldsymbol{A}^{-1}||$ be represented by the largest singular values of $\boldsymbol{A}$ and $\boldsymbol{A}^{-1}$, respectively, that is, $||\boldsymbol{A}|| = \mu_{\max}(\boldsymbol{A})$ and $||\boldsymbol{A}^{-1}|| = (\mu_{\min}(\boldsymbol{A}))^{-1}$, from which the assertion follows immediately.

Note Let

$$\boldsymbol{A} = \begin{bmatrix} 1 & 1 \\ 1 & 1.001 \end{bmatrix} \text{ and } \boldsymbol{b} = \begin{pmatrix} 4 \\ 4.002 \end{pmatrix}.$$

The solution to $\boldsymbol{Ax} = \boldsymbol{b}$ is $\boldsymbol{x} = (2, 2)'$. Let $\Delta\boldsymbol{b} = (0, 0.001)'$. Then the solution to $\boldsymbol{A}(\boldsymbol{x} + \Delta\boldsymbol{x}) = \boldsymbol{b} + \Delta\boldsymbol{b}$ is $\boldsymbol{x} + \Delta\boldsymbol{x} = (1, 3)'$. Notably, $\Delta\boldsymbol{x}$ is much larger than $\Delta\boldsymbol{b}$.

Chapter 8

References

Baksalary, J. K. (1987). Algebraic characterizations and statistical implications of the commutativity of orthogonal projectors. In T. Pukkila and S. Puntanen (eds.), *Proceedings of the Second International Tampere Conference in Statistics*, (pp. 113–142). Tampere: University of Tampere.

Baksalary, J. K., and Styan, G. P. H. (1990). Around a formula for the rank of a matrix product with some statistical applications. In R. S. Rees (ed.), *Graphs, Matrices and Designs*, (pp. 1–18). New York: Marcel Dekker.

Ben-Israel, A., and Greville, T. N. E. (1974). *Generalized Inverses: Theory and Applications.* New York: Wiley.

Brown, A. L., and Page, A. (1970). *Elements of Functional Analysis.* New York: Van Nostrand.

Eckart, C., and Young, G. (1936). The approximation of one matrix by another of lower rank. *Psychometrika*, **1**, 211–218.

Groß, J., and Trenkler, G. (1998). On the product of oblique projectors. *Linear and Multilinear Algebra*, **44**, 247–259.

Guttman, L. (1944). General theory and methods of matric factoring. *Psychometrika*, **9**, 1–16.

Guttman, L. (1952). Multiple group methods for common-factor analysis: Their basis, computation and interpretation. *Psychometrika*, **17**, 209–222.

Guttman, L. (1957). A necessary and sufficient formula for matric factoring. *Psychometrika*, **22**, 79–81.

Hayashi, C. (1952). On the prediction of phenomena from qualitative data and the quantification of qualitative data from the mathematico-statistical point of view. *Annals of the Institute of Statistical Mathematics*, **3**, 69–98.

Hoerl, A. F., and Kennard, R. W. (1970). Ridge regression: Biased estimation for nonorthogonal problems. *Technometrics*, **12**, 55–67.

Kalman, R. E. (1976). Algebraic aspects of the generalized inverse of a rectangular matrix. In M. Z. Nashed (ed.), *Generalized Inverse and Applications*, (pp. 267–280). New York: Academic Press.

Khatri, C. G. (1961). A simplified approach to the derivation of the theorems on the rank of a matrix. *Journal of the Maharaja Sayajirao University of Baroda*, **10**, 1–5.

Khatri, C. G. (1966). Note on a MANOVA model applied to problems in growth curve. *Annals of the Institute of Statistical Mathematics*, **18**, 75–86.

Khatri, C. G. (1968). Some results for the singular multivariate regression models. *Sankhyā A*, **30**, 267–280.

Khatri, C. G. (1990). Some properties of BLUE in a linear model and canonical correlations associated with linear transformations. *Journal of Multivariate Analysis*, **34**, 211–226.

Magnus, J. R., and Neudecker, H. (1988). *Matrix Differential Calculus.* Chichester: Wiley.

Marsaglia, G., and Styan, G. P. H. (1974). Equalities and inequalities for ranks of matrices. *Linear and Multilinear Algebra*, **2**, 269–292.

Mitra, S. K. (1968). A new class of g-inverse of square matrices. *Sankhyā A*, **30**, 323–330.

Mitra, S. K. (1975). Optimal inverse of a matrix. *Sankhyā A*, **37**, 550–563.

Moore, E. H. (1920). On the reciprocals of the general algebraic matrix. *Bulletin of the American Mathematical Society*, **26**, 394–395.

Nishisato, S. (1980). *Analysis of Categorical Data: Dual Scaling and Its Applications.* Toronto: University of Toronto Press.

Penrose, R. (1955). A generalized inverse for matrices. *Proceedings of the Cambridge Philosophical Society*, **51**, 406–413.

Rao, C. R. (1962). A note on a generalized inverse of a matrix with applications to problems in mathematical statistics. *Journal of the Royal Statistical Society B*, **24**, 152–158.

Rao, C. R. (1964). The use and interpretation of principal component analysis in applied research. *Sankhyā A*, **26**, 329–358.

Rao, C. R. (1973). Representation of best linear unbiased estimators in the Gauss-Markoff model with singular covariance matrices. *Journal of Multivariate Analysis*, **3**, 276–292.

Rao, C. R. (1974). Projectors, generalized inverses and the BLUEs. *Journal of the Royal Statistical Society B*, **36**, 442–448.

Rao, C. R. (1979). Separation theorems for singular values of matrices and their applications in multivariate analysis. *Journal of Multivariate Analysis*, **9**, 362–377.

Rao, C. R. (1980). Matrix approximations and reduction of dimensionality in multivariate statistical analysis. In P. R. Krishnaiah (ed.), *Multivariate Analysis V* (pp. 3–34). Amsterdam: Elsevier-North-Holland.

Rao, C. R., and Mitra, S. K. (1971). *Generalized Inverse of Matrices and Its Applications*. New York: Wiley.

Rao, C. R., and Rao, M. B. (1998). *Matrix Algebra and Its Applications to Statistics and Econometrics*. Singapore: World Scientific.

Rao, C. R., and Yanai, H. (1979). General definition and decomposition of projectors and some applications to statistical problems. *Journal of Statistical Planning and Inference*, **3**, 1–17.

Rao, C. R., and Yanai, H. (1985). Generalized inverse of linear transformations: A geometric approach. *Linear Algebra and Its Applications*, **70**, 105–113.

Schönemann, P. H. (1966). A general solution of the orthogonal Procrustes problems. *Psychometrika*, **31**, 1–10.

Takane, Y., and Hunter, M. A. (2001). Constrained principal component analysis: A comprehensive theory. *Applicable Algebra in Engineering, Communication, and Computing*, **12**, 391–419.

Takane, Y., and Shibayama, T. (1991). Principal component analysis with external information on both subjects and variables. *Psychometrika*, **56**, 97–120.

Takane, Y., and Yanai, H. (1999). On oblique projectors. *Linear Algebra and Its Applications*, **289**, 297–310.

Takane, Y., and Yanai, H. (2005). On the Wedderburn-Guttman theorem. *Linear Algebra and Its Applications*, **410**, 267–278.

Takane, Y., and Yanai, H. (2008). On ridge operators. *Linear Algebra and Its Applications*, **428**, 1778–1790.

Takeuchi, K., Yanai, H., and Mukherjee, B. N. (1982). *The Foundations of Multivariate Analysis*. New Delhi: Wiley Eastern.

ten Berge, J. M. F. (1993). *Least Squares Optimization in Multivariate Analysis*. Leiden: DSWO Press.

Tian, Y. (1998). The Moore-Penrose inverses of $m \times n$ block matrices and their applications. *Linear Algebra and Its Applications*, **283**, 35–60.

Tian, Y. (2002). Upper and lower bounds for ranks of matrix expressions using generalized inverses. *Linear Algebra and Its Applications*, **355**, 187–214.

Tian, Y. and Styan, G. P. H. (2009). On some matrix equalities for generalized inverses with applications. *Linear Algebra and Its Applications*, **430**, 2716–2733.

Tikhonov, A. N., and Arsenin, V. Y. (1977). *Solutions of Ill-Posed Problems.* Washington, DC: Holt, Rinehart and Winston.

Torgerson, W. S. (1958). *Theory and Methods of Scaling.* New York: Wiley.

Van den Wollenberg, A. L. (1977). Redundancy analysis: An alternative for canonical correlation analysis. *Psychometrika*, **42**, 207–219.

Werner, H. J. (1992). G-inverses of matrix products. In S. Schach and G. Trenkler (eds.), *Data Analysis and Statistical Inference* (pp. 531–546). Bergish-Gladbach: Eul-Verlag.

Yanai, H. (1980). A proposition of generalized method for forward selection of variables. *Behaviormetrika*, **7**, 95–107.

Yanai, H. (1981). Explicit expression of projectors on canonical variables and distances between centroids of groups. *Journal of the Japanese Statistical Society*, **11**, 43–53.

Yanai, H. (1990). Some generalized forms of least squares g-inverse, minimum norm g-inverses and Moore-Penrose inverse matrix. *Computational Statistics and Data Analysis*, **10**, 251–260.

Yoshida, K. (1981). *Functional Analysis* (sixth edition). New York: Springer.

Index